GENERAL MEDICINE
RADIOLOGY:
Clinical Cases

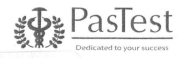

D0413671

GENERAL MEDICINE RADIOLOGY:
Clinical Cases

PRABHAKAR RAJIAH MBBS MD FRCR
Diagnostic Radiologist
Cleveland Clinic
USA

BISWARANJAN BANERJEE MBBS FRCS DMRD FRCR
Consultant Diagnostic Radiologist
Tameside General Hospital
UK

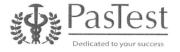
PasTest
Dedicated to your success

© 2008 PASTEST LTD
Egerton Court
Parkgate Estate
Knutsford
Cheshire
WA16 8DX
Telephone: 01565 752000

First Published 2008

Reprinted 2010

ISBN: 1905 635 32X
978 1905 635 320

A catalogue record for this book is available from the British Library.
The information contained within this book was obtained by the author from
reliable sources. However, while every effort has been made to ensure its accu-
racy, no responsibility for loss, damage or injury occasioned to any person acting or refraining from action as a result of information contained herein can be
accepted by the publishers or author.

PasTest Revision Books and Intensive Courses
PasTest has been established in the field of postgraduate medical education since
1972, providing revision books and intensive study courses for doctors preparing for
their professional examinations.
Books and courses are available for the following specialties:

**MRCGP, MRCP Parts 1 and 2, MRCPCH Parts 1 and 2, MRCS,
MRCOG Parts 1 and 2, DRCOG, DCH, FRCA, Dentistry.**

For further details contact:
PasTest, Freepost, Knutsford, Cheshire WA16 7BR
Tel: 01565 752000 Fax: 01565 650264
www.pastest.co.uk enquiries@pastest.co.uk

Cover image: MRI scans BSIP, LAURENT/SCIENCE PHOTO LIBRARY
Text prepared by Carnegie Book Production, Lancaster
Printed and bound in the UK by CPI Antony Rowe, Chippenham, Wiltshire

CONTENTS

Introduction   vii

1 Cardiovascular radiology
    QUESTIONS   1
    ANSWERS   23

2 Chest radiology
    QUESTIONS   49
    ANSWERS   101

3 Gastrointestinal and hepatobiliary radiology
    QUESTIONS   155
    ANSWERS   201

4 Genitourinary radiology
    QUESTIONS   253
    ANSWERS   273

5 Endocrinology and haematology
    QUESTIONS   295
    ANSWERS   315

6 Neuroradiology
    QUESTIONS   335
    ANSWERS   367

7 Musculoskeletal radiology
    QUESTIONS   399
    ANSWERS   427

Colour Images   455

Index   461

INTRODUCTION

Radiology is a rapidly evolving field with new technological developments every year. It has become an integral component of the diagnostic and therapeutic dimension of every speciality and plays a vital role in management of patients. Although the role of plain X-rays in diagnosis is progressively decreasing, they still have their place in the initial stages of patient management. Ultrasound and CT have become the commonly used modalities in diagnosis. MRI is very useful in assessment of musculoskeletal, central nervous and cardiovascular systems.

Radiological pictures are also increasingly used in many postgraduate examinations. Hence it is essential for clinicians and radiologists alike to be well informed in the appropriate investigation for any clinical case and be aware of the radiological findings in each clinical scenario.

General Medicine Radiology: Clinical Cases consists of 205 cases and approximately 350 images. The book is divided into seven sections – Cardiovascular radiology, Chest radiology, Gastrointestinal and hepatobiliary radiology, Genitourinary radiology, Endocrinology and haematology, Neuroradiology and Musculoskeletal radiology. Each case is presented with pertinent history, followed by radiological pictures and several questions. The second part of each chapter contains the case diagnosis, clinical features, and radiological findings, imaging techniques, diagnostic algorithm, differential diagnosis and management.

The book covers almost the entire gamut of radiological findings in common general medical conditions. The cases include pictures from multiple modalities such as X-rays, ultrasound, Doppler, CT scan, MRI and nuclear medicine, reflecting the current practice. The cases range from the very common to unusual and challenging.

The format of the book, images and discussion would be ideal not only for medicine and radiology trainees preparing for postgraduate exams, but also for medical students intending to specialise in either of these fields. Physicians and radiologists who wish to update their knowledge on the radiological aspects of common and uncommon medical conditions will also find this book useful.

Dr Prabhakar Rajiah
Dr Biswaranjan Banerjee

1

CARDIOVASCULAR
RADIOLOGY
QUESTIONS

Case 1.1

A 63-year-old man presented with sudden onset of severe, tearing, left-sided chest pain. On examination, he had a systolic murmur. His blood pressure was 160/84 mmHg on the right arm and 190/110 mmHg on the left arm.

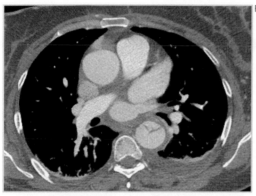

Fig 1.1a

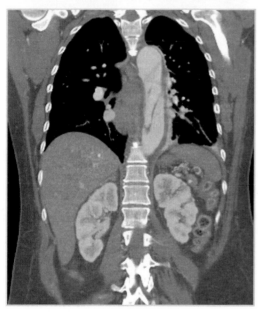

Fig 1.1b

1. What do you find on the computed tomography (CT) scan?
2. What is the diagnosis?
3. What are the causes and the locations?
4. What are the types and the radiological features?
5. What are the complications and management?

Answers *on pages 23–47*

Case 1.2

A 57-year-old man presents with chest pain on exertion, radiating to the neck and left arm. He also complains of dyspnoea. Clinical examination showed no cardiac murmurs.

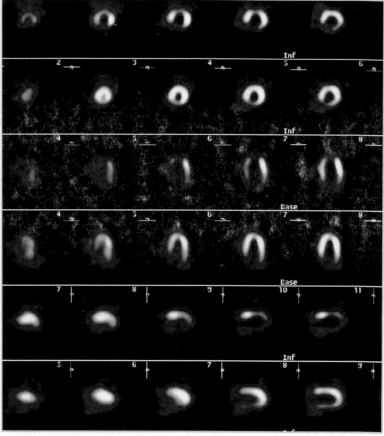

For colour version, see *Colour Images* section from page 455.

Fig 1.2

1. What is this investigation and what are the findings?
2. How is this procedure done?
3. What is the diagnosis?
4. What are the different types of abnormalities detected on this scan? What are the indications?
5. What are the false-positive and -negative signs?

Answers *on pages 23–47*

Case 1.3

A 51-year-old presents with intermittent episodes of severe chest pain, which is predominantly on the left side of the chest. He also complains of sweating and dyspnoea.

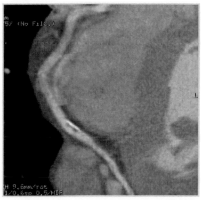

Fig 1.3a

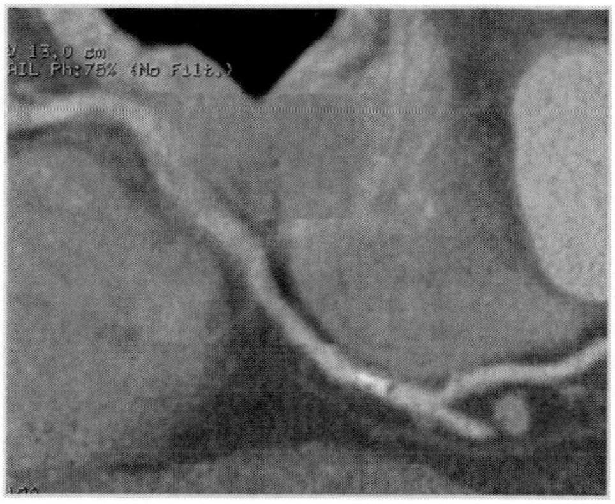

Fig 1.3b

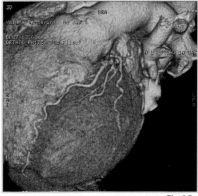

Fig 1.3c

For colour version, see *Colour Images* section from page 455.

1. What is this investigation?
2. What are the findings and what is the diagnosis?
3. What are the indications for these investigations?
4. What are the limitations and contraindications of this technique?
5. What further course of management is indicated in such a patient?

Answers *on pages 23–47*

Case 1.4

A 64-year-old woman presents with severe headache, facial swelling and frequent episodes of loss of consciousness. Clinical examination reveals oedematous face and neck with prominent veins.

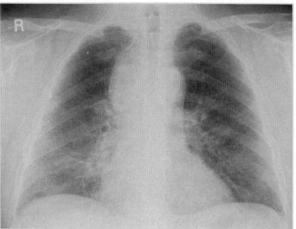
Fig 1.4a

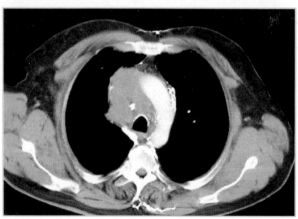
Fig 1.4b

1. What can you find on the X-ray and CT scan of the chest?
2. What is the cause of the patient's symptoms?
3. What are the underlying conditions that lead to this disease?
4. What are natural methods of compensating for this condition?
5. What are the radiological features and what is the treatment?

Answers on pages 23–47

Case 1.5

A 64-year-old man with a history of medically controlled hypertension presents with severe chest pain.

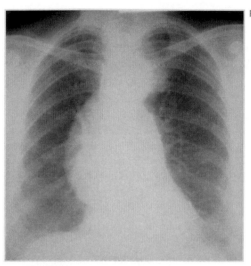

Fig 1.5a

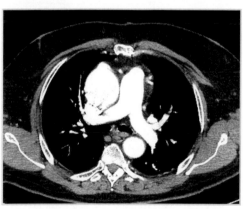

Fig 1.5b

1. What can you find on the X-ray and CT scan?
2. What is the diagnosis?
3. What are the causes, associations and types of this disease?
4. What are the radiological features?
5. What is the management?

Answers *on pages 23–47*

Case 1.6

A 8-year-old boy presented with chest pain, headache and dyspnoea on exertion. Clinical examination revealed a systolic murmur in the cardiac apex. Blood pressure in the upper extremities was 150/110 mmHg and 140/78 mmHg in the lower extremities.

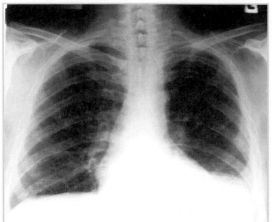

Fig 1.6a

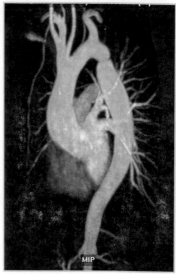

Fig 1.6b

1. What do you see on the plain film?

2. What does MRI show? What is the diagnosis?

3. What are the clinical features and associations?

4. What are the radiological findings?

5. What is the management?

Answers on pages 23–47

Case 1.7

A 1-year-old girl presents with cyanosis, respiratory distress and failure to thrive. On clinical examination, the baby is cyanotic and tachypnoeic, and has features of cardiac failure.

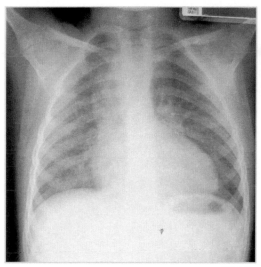
Fig 1.7a

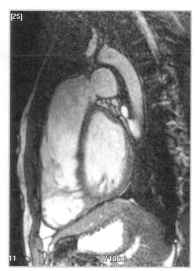
Fig 1.7b

1. What do you observe on the plain X-ray of the chest in this kid?
2. What is the diagnosis?
3. What is the second investigation and how does it help?
4. What are the physiology and clinical features of this condition?
5. What are the radiological features?
6. What are the associations and treatment?

Answers *on pages 23–47*

Case 1.8

A 57-year-old woman presents with chest pain and difficulty in breathing. On examination, the patient is tachypnoeic and the heart sounds are muffled.

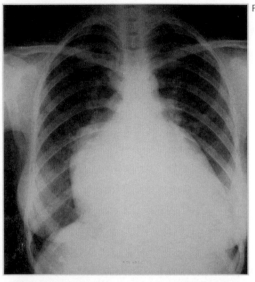

Fig 1.8a

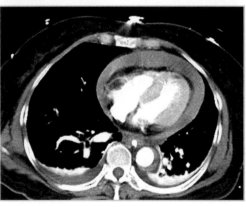

Fig 1.8b

1. What do you see on the plain X-ray?
2. What do you see on the CT scan and what is the diagnosis?
3. What are the causes?
4. What are the radiological findings?
5. What are the complications and treatment?

Answers on pages 23–47

Case 1.9

A 33-year-old woman presents with sudden onset of right-sided chest pain and dyspnoea. On clinical examination, she is tachypnoeic. No abnormal breath sounds are heard. An ECG shows right heart strain and her oxygen saturation is low.

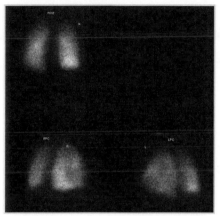

Fig 1.9a

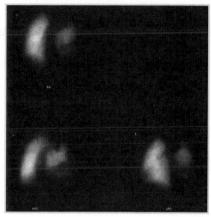

Fig 1.9b

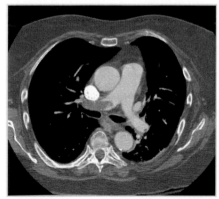

Fig 1.9c

1. What is the investigation shown in Figs 1.9a and 1.9b? What are the findings?
2. What is the investigation shown in Fig 1.9c? What does it show?
3. What is the diagnosis? What is the imaging protocol for this condition?
4. What are the predisposing factors and clinical features?
5. What is the differential diagnosis?
6. How is this condition managed and what are the complications?

Answers *on pages 23–47*

Case 1.10

A 56-year-old presents with chest pain, dypsnoea and difficulty in breathing at night. On examination, she has generalised oedema and crackles in the lungs.

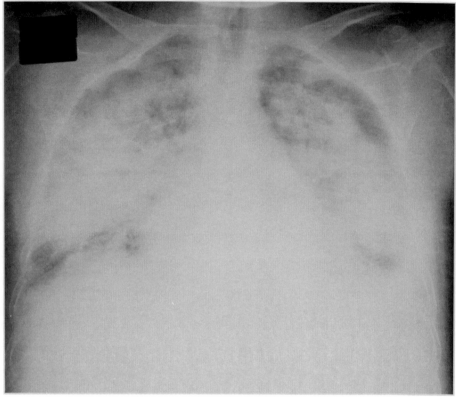

Fig 1.10

1. What can you see on the chest X-ray?
2. What is the diagnosis?
3. What are the causes?
4. What are the radiological findings and what is the reason for this appearance?
5. What is the differential diagnosis?

Answers on pages 23–47

Case 1.11

A 10-year-old presents with chest pain, difficulty in breathing, haemoptysis and palpitations. On examination he had a palpable thrill and a loud S1. There were bilateral crackles in his lungs.

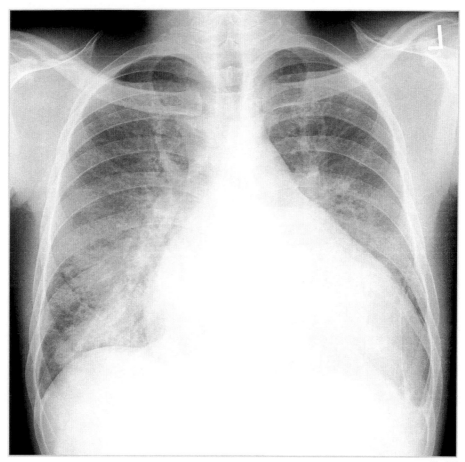

Fig 1.11

1. What do you observe on the chest X-ray?
2. What is the diagnosis?
3. What are the causes and haemodynamics of this condition?
4. What are the radiological features?
5. What are the clinical features and treatment?

Answers *on pages 23–47*

Case 1.12

A 59-year-old man with a recent MI (myocardial infarction) presents with chest pain, dyspnoea and fatigue. On clinical examination, there is a prominent apical impulse. ECG shows ST-segment elevation.

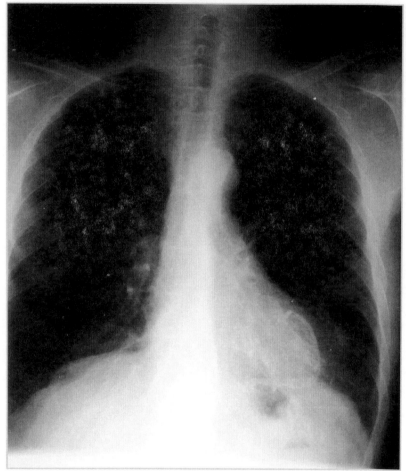

Fig 1.12

1. What do you observe on the chest X-ray?
2. What is the diagnosis?
3. What are the causes and types?
4. What further investigations are required?
5. How will you manage this condition?

Answers on pages 23–47

Case 1.13

A 57-year-old male patient presents with chest pain, dyspnoea and fatigue. On examination there is generalised oedema, muffled heart sounds and prominent venous pulsations.

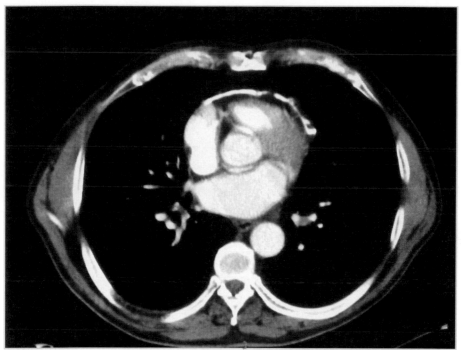

Fig 1.13

1. What do you observe on the CT scan?
2. What is the cause of the patient's symptoms?
3. What is the pathology of this condition? What are the causes?
4. What are the clinical features? What further investigations are required?
5. What is the differential diagnosis? How will you manage this condition?

Answers *on pages 23–47*

Case 1.14

A 36-year-old woman, who has recovered from a recent haemorrhagic stroke, presents with chest pain worse on breathing and bilateral leg pain. Clinical examination showed bilateral, swollen, oedematous legs. The patient was tachypnoeic and afebrile.

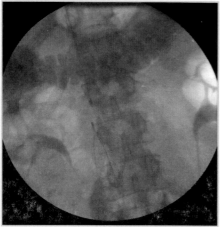

Fig 1.14a

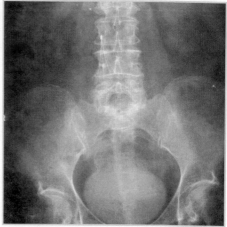

Fig 1.14b

1. What procedure is being done in the first film? What do you note in the second film?
2. What are the indications for this?
3. What are the types and where are they placed?
4. What are the precautions?
5. What are the contraindications for this procedure?

Answers on pages 23–47

Case 1.15

A 31-year-old woman presents with hypertension, malaise and loss of weight. Clinical examination revealed abnormal pulses in the upper and lower extremities.

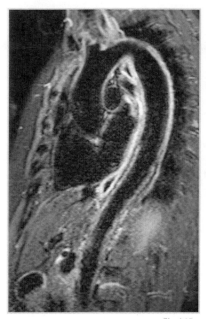

Fig 1.15a

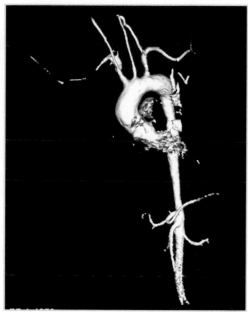

Fig 1.15b

1. What are the findings in this MRI and MR angiography (3D reconstruction)?
2. What is the diagnosis?
3. What is the pathology and what are the clinical features?
4. What are the different types of the disease?
5. What are the radiological features and what is the differential diagnosis?

Answers on pages 23–47

Case 1.16

A 12-year-old girl presents with difficulty in breathing and cyanosis on exertion, palpitations and frequent respiratory infections. Clinical examination showed a heaving impulse in the parasternal region and a pansystolic murmur in the tricuspid area. The ECG showed a right bundle-branch block (RBBB) pattern.

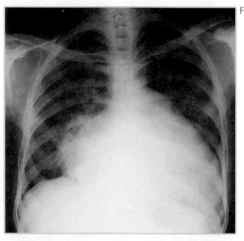
Fig 1.16a

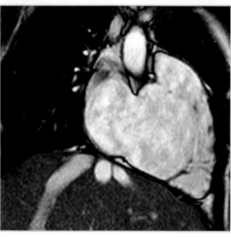
Fig 1.16b

1. What do you see on the plain X-ray of the chest?
2. What is the diagnosis? What do you see on the MR scan?
3. What are the pathophysiology and the development of this condition?
4. What are the radiological features and differential diagnosis?
5. What are the clinical features, complications and treatment of this condition?

Answers on pages 23–47

Case 1.17

A 33-year-old woman presents with chest pain, dyspnoea on exertion, palpitations and frequent syncope. Clinical examination reveals an enlarged heart with displaced apex and forceful apical impulse. A systolic murmur is also heard.

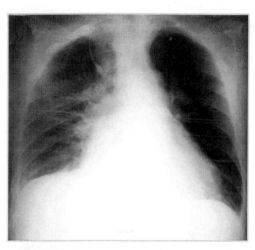

Fig 1.17a

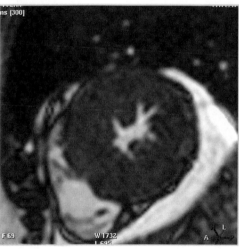

Fig 1.17b

1. What do you observe on the chest X-ray and MRI?
2. What is the diagnosis?
3. What are the types and variations of this disease?
4. What are the clinical features and what is the treatment?
5. What are the radiological features?

Answers on pages 23–47

Case 1.18

A 21-year-old man presents with fever, lumps and chest pain. On clinical examination, he is febrile and tachypnoeic, with multiple, enlarged lymph nodes in the groin and axilla. A systolic murmur was heard in the apical region.

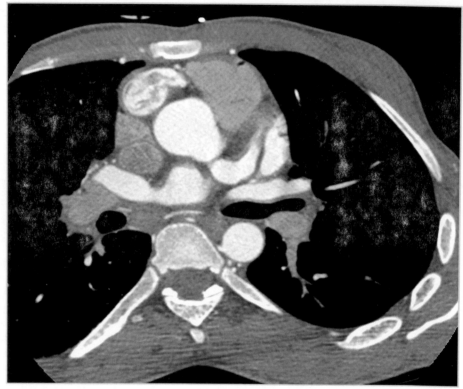

Fig 1.18

1. What do you observe on this CT angiography?
2. What are the diagnosis and differential diagnosis?
3. What are the clinical features of this disease?
4. What are the radiological features?
5. What is the treatment?

Answers on pages 23–47

Case 1.19

A 45-year-old man presents with difficult in breathing and chest pain on exertion. Clinical examination revealed a split in the S2, with a faint murmur. The lungs were normal with no abnormal breath sounds.

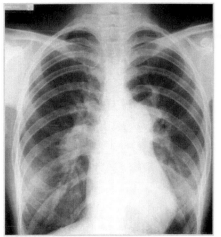

Fig 1.19a

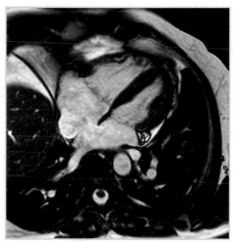

Fig 1.19b

1. What do you observe on the plain X-ray?
2. What are the findings on MRI?
3. What is the diagnosis?
4. What are the types of this disease?
5. What is the pathophysiology and what are the radiological features?
6. What is the treatment?

Answers on pages 23–47

Case 1.20

A 35-year-old woman presents with severe pain in her left thigh and leg. On examination, her left leg is swollen, tender and oedematous. The pulses are normal.

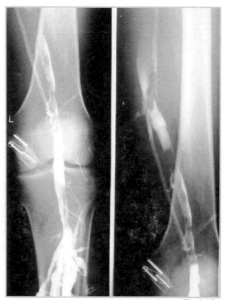

Fig 1.20a

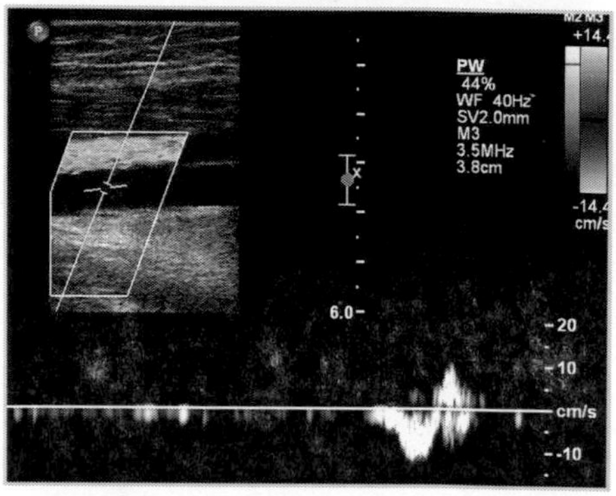

Fig 1.20b

For colour version, see *Colour Images* section from page 455.

1. What are the findings on the venogram and Doppler ultrasonography?
2. What is the diagnosis?
3. What are the causes of this disease?
4. What are the common locations?
5. What are the imaging features?
6. What are the complications and management?

Answers *on pages 23–47*

Case 1.1: Answers

1. The CT scan shows a normal appearance of the ascending aorta. In the descending aorta, a flap is seen anteriorly. This is better seen in the coronal view, where the flap is seen to extend for most of the length of the descending thoracic aorta.

2. Aortic dissection, affecting the descending aorta, type B.

3. Dissection is separation of aortic intima and adventitia by blood accessing the media of aorta, splitting it into two. It is caused by a combination of medial degeneration, which decreases the cohesiveness within the aortic wall, and hydrodynamic forces of systemic hypertension. No intimal tear is seen in 5%. Common causes of dissection are hypertension, Marfan syndrome, Ehler–Danlos syndrome, coarctation of aorta, bicuspid aortic valve, prosthetic valve, trauma, aortic stenosis, relapsing polychondritis, Turner syndrome, pregnancy, systemic lupus erythematosus (SLE) and cocaine usage. Syphilis does not cause dissection. The most common site is the anterior and right lateral wall of the ascending aorta just distal to the valve. Other sites are the superior and posterior walls of the transverse aortic arch, and the posterior left lateral wall of the upper descending aorta distal to the left subclavian artery.

4. There are two classification systems:

    (a) Stanford: type A – affects ascending aorta; type B – ascending aorta not involved.

    (b) DeBakey: I – entire aorta; II – ascending aorta only; III – descending aorta.

    The chest X-ray may show displacement of calcification in a patient with known disease, by 4–10 mm from the outer aortic contour. The contour of the aorta is irregular. The superior mediastinum is widened (> 8 cm). Left pleural effusion and left basal atelectasis may be present. CT with contrast is the investigation of choice. Non-contrast CT may show high-density clot within a false lumen. Contrast scan shows intimal flap separating the true and false lumina. Calcification is displaced internally by the flap. Magnetic resonance imaging (MRI) shows similar appearances and may also show cobwebs, marking the false lumen. The differential diagnosis is penetrating ulcer of the thoracic aorta. Imaging with CT or MRI is useful in confirming the diagnosis, assessing the extent of dissection and evaluating the complications, which are useful in planning treatment.

5. Complications are aortic insufficiency, coronary artery occlusion causing myocardial ischaemia, pericardial and pleural effusions and rupture into the right ventricle/left atrium/superior vena cava (SVC)/pulmonary artery, producing a left to right shunt. Occlusion of branch vessels can occur as a result of flap entering the branch vessel origin or covering it like a curtain. Occlusion of carotid/vertebral arteries can result in stroke. Compromise of spinal arteries arising from the descending aorta may cause paraplegia. The dissection can extend distally to the abdominal aorta. Aneurysm can originate from the false or true lumen. Type A dissections require immediate surgical graft reinforcement of the aortic wall to prevent rupture and aortic insufficiency. There is 10–35% mortality from surgery. Type B dissections are treated with antihypertensive drugs.

Case 1.2: Answers

1. This is a thallium stress test (myocardial perfusion imaging). The images are acquired in stress and rest. The first two rows are images in the short axis of the heart, the next two rows in the horizontal long axis and the last two rows in vertical long axis. In each set, the first row is the stress image and the second row the rest image. In the other images there is normal uptake in all regions of heart in the rest images, but, in stress images, defects (areas without uptake) are in the inferior wall, apical region and part of the septal wall.

2. Thallium-201 chloride is the isotope used in stress test. Thallium uptake depends on Na^+/K^+ ATPase; it is similar to normal K^+, but less readily released than K^+. The distribution is proportionate to regional blood flow and uptake in the myocardium depends on the perfusion, mass and cellular integrity. Thallium is injected and images are acquired at rest. After exercise blood flow increases through coronary artery dilatation, heart rate increases and unveils coronary artery disease, and can separate viable and non-viable myocardium. It can detect very severe ischaemia with stenosis > 95%, but cannot detect most coronary artery disease (CAD), with narrowing < 90%. Stress is induced by exercise according to the Bruce treadmill protocol or by pharmacological agents such as adenosine, dipyridamole, dobutamine or arbutamine . Initially, exercise images are performed, redistribution images are obtained at 2–6 hours and delayed images at 24 hours. Other agents that could be used are technetium-99m-labelled (99mTc) radiopharmaceuticals such as sestamibi, tetrofosmin and teboroxime , for single-photon imaging (single photon emission CT or SPECT) and rubidium-82 (82Rb) for positron emission tomography (PET).

3. This patent has ischaemic heart disease resulting from coronary artery disease.

4. A defect in rest images indicates infarct. A defect in stress, but a normal rest scan, indicate ischaemia. The indications for scan are:

(a) Known or suspected CAD:

– diagnosis of physiologically significant CAD (presence and severity)

– determine prognosis (risk stratification based on perfusion defects, left ventricular [LV] function)

– differentiating coronary and non-coronary causes of acute chest pain.

(b) Follow-up of patients with known CAD to evaluate the immediate and long-term effects of:

– revascularisation procedures (bypass, angioplasty, stents, growth factors)

– drugs for ischaemia or hypercholesterolaemia.

(c) Known or suspected congestive heart failure:

– differentiate ischaemic from idiopathic cardiomyopathy

– determine presence of viable myocardium after infarct for revascularisation.

5. A false-positive thallium test is seen in sarcoidosis, amyloidosis, cardiomyopathy, valvular aortic stenosis, mitral valve prolapse, cardiac contusion, myocardial fibrosis, coronary artery spasm, apical myocardial thinning, attenuation caused by diaphragm/breast/pacemakers. False-negative tests are seen in β blockers, poor technique, balanced ischaemia with symmetrical three-vessel disease, insignificant obstruction, inadequate stress and overestimation of stenosis in angiography.

Case 1.3: Answers

1. This is a cardiac CT coronary angiography. The first two pictures are curved oblique reformats of the right coronary artery (RCA). The third picture is a three-dimensional volume-rendered image.

2. The coronary angiography shows areas of calcification and plaque, narrowing the coronary artery, which is narrowing the lumen.

3. The indications of cardiac CT are:

   − exclusion of CAD in the low- to intermediate-risk patient with symptoms (detects early disease, can image structures outside the lumen and in the wall, can diagnose and quantify stenosis, identify type of plaque and determine who needs coronary angiography/surgery)

   − evaluation of bypass grafts and stents

   − triple rule-out study in patients presenting with chest pain (for pulmonary embolism, aortic dissection and coronary disease)

   − evaluation of wall motion and valve function

   − evaluation of cardiac/pericardial masses/thrombus

   − evaluation of the pulmonary veins before ablation for atrial fibrillation

   − calcium scoring (the overall calcium burden in the coronary arteries can be calculated without any contrast and this is an independent marker for coronary atherosclerosis)

   − congenital cardiac diseases

   − anomalous coronary arteries

   − new-onset heart failure

   − equivocal stress test

   − coronary artery mapping before repeat sternotomy

   − coronary vein mapping before pacemaker insertion.

The advantages of CT angiography are: non-invasive, fast, easy, can identify plaques (calcified and soft), can assess extraluminal structures, capable of multiplanar reconstruction and assessment of function.

4. Cardiac CT is a non-invasive, effective test in evaluation of chest problems. Images of the heart and coronary arteries are acquired at a high speed. Modern multislice CT scanners have 64 detectors and can perform 3 rotations in a second, so the entire heart can be scanned in 4−5 heart beats at specific phases of the cardiac cycle, which is obtained by ECG gating. Metoprolol 100 mg is given before the scan, to reduce the heart rate to less than 60/min. The images are reconstructed by the computer in multiple planes. The limitations are: radiation (less than coronary angiography and stress testing); difficult in patients with fast and irregular heart beats; requires premedication; quantification of stenosis might be difficult with severe calcification; visualisation difficult in stents and grafts; overestimation of stenosis; retrograde filling and occlusion cannot be differentiated. Contraindications are: inability to breathhold, contraindications for intravenous contrast use due to renal failure and allergy, marked arrhythmia, classic cardiac chest pain, very young patients.

5. In patients with significant stenosis or occlusion, revascularisation with balloon angioplasty or bypass surgery is performed, after assessing the viability of the myocardium with a stress test.

Case 1.4: Answers

1. The X-ray of the chest shows a large soft tissue mass in the right paratracheal region, which is seen as a bulge. Contrast enhanced scans of the chest show a large non-enhancing soft tissue mass in the anterior mediastinum, which is encasing and grossly compressing the SVC (the contrast-filled structure in the middle).

2. SVC syndrome caused by lymphoma.

3. SVC syndrome is caused by obstruction of the SVC with development of collaterals. Malignant tumours such as bronchial carcinoma and lymphoma account for 80–90% of the causes. Other uncommon causes are large retrosternal goitre, granulomatous mediastinitis (tuberculosis [TB], histoplasmosis, sarcoidosis), ascending aortic aneurysm, constrictive pericarditis and complications related to placement of central venous catheters and pacer wires.

4. SVC obstruction may be bypassed by the development of a collateral circulation. Blood may be diverted by downhill oesophageal varices, through aygos/hemiazygous, accessory hemiazygos/superior intercostal, lateral thoracic and vertebral veins. Symptoms are head and neck oedema, headache, syncope, prominent collaterals, proptosis, dyspnoea, cyanosis, chest pain and haematemesis.

5. Palliative treatment consists of placing a stent in the SVC. Radiation of a bronchogenic tumour or lymphoma also alleviates the symptoms. Chemotherapy may be indicated in some cases.

Case 1.5: Answers

1. The X-ray shows a smooth and dilated structure in the mediastinum, to the right side of the heart, which is continuous with the aortic arch, indicating that this is a dilated aorta. A contrast-enhanced axial CT scan of the chest shows a massively enlarged ascending aorta. There is no evidence of dissection. The descending aorta is normal and there is no mediastinal haematoma.

2. Ascending aortic aneurysm.

3. Causes of ascending aortic aneurysm: atherosclerosis, dissection, Marfan syndrome, Ehler–Danlos syndrome, infection (syphilitic, mycotic), dissection, trauma, arteritis (Takayasu's, giant cell, rheumatic, ankylosing spondylitis). The true aetiology of aortic aneurysms is probably multifactorial, and the condition occurs in individuals with multiple risk factors, which include smoking, hypertension, atherosclerosis, bicuspid or unicuspid aortic valves, and genetic disorders. It is common in men, especially those aged over 60 years. The aneurysm can be **true** (all layers of wall present) or **false** (focal perforation with all layers disrupted, contained by adventitia). Based on shape it can be fusiform or saccular. Most patients are hypertensive but remain relatively asymptomatic until the aneurysm expands, when they present with pain. Patients with acute dissection develop complications such as rupture, tamponade, acute aortic insufficiency, myocardial infarction (MI) or end-organ ischaemia. Normal growth rates average 0.07 cm/year in the ascending aorta and 0.19 cm/year in the descending aorta. Crawford classification:

   – type I involves the descending thoracic aorta from the left subclavian artery down to the abdominal aorta above the renal arteries

   – type II extends from the left subclavian artery to the renal arteries and may continue distally to the aortic bifurcation

   – type III begins at the mid-to-distal descending thoracic aorta and involves most of the abdominal aorta as far distal as the aortic bifurcation

   – type IV extends from the upper abdominal aorta and all or none of the infrarenal aorta.

4. In chest X-rays, an aneurysm causes widening of the mediastinum, with enlargement of the aortic knob and displacement of the trachea when the aneurysm is big. Ascending aortic aneurysms are often discovered incidentally on CT or MRI. In contrast-enhanced CT the aorta is enlarged, with eccentric thrombus and a small, but patent, lumen. Ascending aorta > 3 cm is ectactic and > 4 cm is aneurysmal. When the aneurysm ruptures, it is seen as soft-tissue opacity on the plain X-ray with mediastinal widening. A crescent sign indicates a high-density crescent in the aneurysm, in turn indicating impending rupture. When there is frank rupture, CT shows a large mediastinal haematoma in the non-contrast scan. Contrast extravasation is seen in post-contrast scans. MRI and MR angiography (MRA) are also very useful in diagnosis and follow-up of patients with aortic aneurysm.

5. In patients without familial disorders such as Marfan syndrome, elective repair is performed when the ascending aneurysm measures 5.5 cm and the descending aneurysm reaches 5 cm. In patients with familial disorders, elective repair is performed when the ascending aorta reaches 5 cm and descending aorta 6 cm. A growth rate of 1 cm/year or faster is an indication for elective surgical repair. Emergency repair is indicated for acute dissection involving ascending aorta. Aortic valve replacement is indicated when the root measures > 4.5 cm, with aortic insufficiency or stenosis.

Case 1.6: Answers

1. The plain X-ray shows bilateral, severe, inferior rib notching. The aorta has an abnormal configuration. The '3' sign is present with a central notch and protrusions on either side of it.

2. This is an MR angiography, which shows a notch in the isthmus of the aorta, just distal to the left subclavian artery origin. The findings reflect the plain film findings and confirm coarctation of the aorta.

3. Coarctation of the aorta is part of spectrum of abnormalities ranging from discrete narrowing at one end to an interrupted aortic arch at the other. Discrete coarctation is the most common type, seen in older children. It is usually juxtaductal and postductal, depending on the relationship of the narrowing to the insertion of ductus or ligamentum arteriosum. They are most commonly seen distal to the left subclavian artery and at (juxta) or

just beyond (post) the ligamentum arteriosum. Very rarely, they are seen proximal to the left subclavian artery. Usually they are asymptomatic and discovered as a result of an incidental finding of hypertension. Complications of hypertension ensue if they are left untreated. Associated cardiovascular conditions include ventricular septal defect, mitral valve abnormalities, bicuspid aortic valve, right-sided and double aortic arch. Coarctation is also associated with an increased incidence of berry aneurysm. Associated berry aneurysms can rupture and cause subarachnoid haemorrhage. An associated bicuspid aortic valve can predispose to endocarditis.

4. On the chest X-ray, the heart is usually normal in size. The aortic arch is prominent if there is an associated bicuspid aortic valve. Classically, a notch is seen between the pre-stenotic dilatation of the distal transverse arch and the post-stenotic dilatation of the descending thoracic aorta. (Figure of '3' sign – midportion of '3' representing notch at site of narrowing.) The reverse '3' sign is the corresponding finding in barium swallow. Rib notching results from pressure erosion from collateral vessels on the adjacent ribs. It is rarely seen before age 7–8 years. They are classically seen posteriorly from rib 4 to rib 8. Dilated internal mammary arteries cause retrosternal notching. An echocardiogram is more useful in neonates. MRI gives qualitative and quantitative information. The site and extent of stenosis, and the relationship to subclavian arteries and collateral vessels, are all demonstrated. Information can also be obtained on peak pressure gradient and LV function. It is very useful in postoperative cases in assessment of re-coarctation.

5. Coarctation is treated by balloon angioplasty, stenting or surgical repair, depending on the severity and complexity of the lesion. Postoperative complications include re-stenosis and aneurysm formation. Balloon angioplasty is the preferred method for re-stenosis.

Case 1.7: Answers

1. The X-ray shows a boot-shaped heart with prominent right sided aortic arch and a narrowed cardiac waist.

2. Tetralogy of Fallot with right-sided aortic arch.

3. This is an MR scan done after surgery. MRI shows a wide right ventricular (RV) outflow tract, secondary to surgery. This patient has pulmonary regurgitation, which is a common complication after RV surgery.

4. Tetralogy of Fallot consists of infundibular pulmonary stenosis, ventral septal defect (VSD), overriding of the aortic arch and RV hypertrophy (RVH). If there is an associated atrial septal defect (ASD) as well, it is called pentalogy of Fallot. It accounts for 10% of congenital heart diseases and the most common cause of cyanosis after age 1 year. The affected children usually present with cyanosis by 3–4 months of age (patent ductus arteriosus [PDA] conceals cyanosis at birth). The other features are dyspnoea, cyanosis, clubbing, episodic spells of unconsciousness, squatting position when fatigued, polycythaemia, lowered Po_2 and systolic murmur in the pulmonary area.

5. The radiological features of tetralogy of Fallot are a boot-shaped heart caused by uplifting of the cardiac apex secondary to RVH and absence of the normal main pulmonary artery segment, which results in a concavity in the region of the pulmonary artery. Heart size is normal as a result of lack of pulmonary blood flow or congestive heart failure. Decreased numbers and calibre of pulmonary vessels are seen. Pulmonary oligaemia is seen, which is noted as increased lucency in the lungs. Reticular opacities in horizontal distribution are seen in the periphery as a result of prominent bronchopulmonary collaterals. A right-sided aortic arch is seen in 20–25% of these patients, which indents the leftward-positioned tracheobronchial shadow. The X-ray can be normal in acyanotic tetralogy of Fallot and there may be findings of small- to moderate-sized VSD with mild RVH, right atrial enlargement and increased pulmonary vascular markings.

6. The associations are bicuspid pulmonic valve, pulmonary artery stenosis, right aortic arch, tracheo-oesophageal fistula, Down syndrome, forked ribs, scoliosis, coronary artery anomalies (single right coronary artery [RCA] or lateral anterior ascending [LAD] from RCA). Treatments include palliative shunts such as the Blalock–Taussig shunt where the subclavian and pulmonary arteries are anastomosed on the side opposite to the aortic arch. Corrective cardiac surgery includes closure of the VSD and reconstruction of the RV outflow tract by excision of obstructing tissue. MRI is very useful in the follow-up of these patients. Complications such as pulmonary regurgitation are very well demonstrated and quantified by MRI.

Case 1.8: Answers

1. The X-ray shows an enlarged heart, which is globular. The pulmonary vasculature appears normal.

2. The CT scan shows a thick layer of fluid collection around the heart and within the pericardium, consistent with pericardial effusion. Small pleural effusions and atelectasis are also noted at both lung bases.

3. A normal pericardium contains 50 ml fluid. Pericardial effusion can be serous, exudative, lymphatic or haemorrhagic. Serous effusion is seen in cardiac failure, hypoalbuminaemia and radiation. Exudate is seen in infections (TB, pyogenic, viral), uraemia, collagen vascular diseases and hypersensitivity. Lymph accumulates in tumours, trauma and after surgery. Haemopericardium is seen after trauma, surgery, anticoagulants, aortic aneurysm rupture, acute myocardial infarction (MI) and tumours.

4. The X-ray shows a water-bottle configuration of the heart, which is enlarged and globular, with narrowing of the vascular pedicle. As a result of diminished cardiac pulsations, a clear interface can be seen between the heart and the lungs. In the lateral view, there is separation of the retrosternal from the epicardial line by > 2 mm with loss of retrosternal clear space. The X-ray is normal if the fluid is < 250 ml or there is acute pericarditis. Echocardiography shows the fluid collection between the pericardial and epicardial layers. If the accumulations are seen only in the posterior part, it indicates a collection of less than 300 ml; if the separation occurs throughout the cardiac cycle, it indicates 300–500 ml and, if there is separation anteriorly, it indicates a collection of 1000 ml or more. The CT scan is not used for diagnosis, but pericardial effusion can be an incidental finding. It shows pericardial effusion as a low-density fluid collection around the heart. The fluid is clear in transudate and may show high density when it is exudative or haemorrhagic.

5. Cardiac tamponade occurs when the effusion is large. A combination of a fall in systolic pressure, rising jugular venous pressure and suppressed heart sounds is called Beck's triad and is typical of cardiac tamponade. Pericardiocentesis is carried out to drain pericardial fluid.

Case 1.9: Answers

1. The first test is a ventilation-perfusion lung scintigraphy (V/Q scan). The first picture (Fig 1.9a) is the ventilation scan, which is normal in this patient. The second picture (Fig 1.9b) is the perfusion scan, which shows defects in the right upper lobe and to a lesser extent in the right lower lobe.

2. This is CT pulmonary angiography; 150 ml of iodinated contrast is injected at the rate of 4–5 ml/s into the antecubital vein, and images are acquired throughout the chest during peak enhancement in the pulmonary arteries. There is a hypodense filling defect within the right pulmonary artery. The left pulmonary artery is normal.

3. This patient has pulmonary embolism (PE). The imaging protocol varies from centre to centre. In a patient with chest pain and suspected PE, a chest X-ray should be performed. If the chest X-ray is normal, a ventilation perfusion lung scintigraphy may be considered as the next step. Ventilation scan is done by inhalation of radioactive tracer gas such as Krypton or Xenon. Areas of lung that do not receive enough air are seen as cold spots. In perfusion scan, technetium (Tc^{99m}) labeled microspheres or albumin macroaggregates are injected into a vein, which travels through the blood stream into the lungs. Areas of the lungs that are not receiving enough blood will be seen as filling defects. In pulmonary embolism, the ventilation scans will be normal and perfusion scans show cold areas, giving the characteristic mismatched ventilation and perfusion defects. If chest X-ray is abnormal or the ventilation perfusion scan is indeterminate, a CT pulmonary angiography is performed. With the modern 64 slice CT scanners, embolus can be detected even in tiny peripheral pulmonary arterial branches. In some centres, a CT pulmonary angiography is undertaken in all patients with suspected PE, since it is fast, accurate and efficient way of diagnosing pulmonary embolism.

4. Hypercoagulable states, deep venous thrombosis (DVT), recent surgery, pregnancy, immobilisation and underlying malignancy are predisposing features. Chest pain, back pain, shoulder pain, dyspnoea, haemoptysis, wheeze, syncope and cardiac arrhythmia are clinical features. Low Po_2, and raised D-dimer and white blood cell (WBC) counts are useful laboratory findings.

5. MI, angina, pneumonia and oesophageal reflux are differential diagnoses.

6. Oxygen, fluids, anticoagulants and fibrinolytics are used for treating a PE. An inferior vena cava (IVC) filter is deployed into the IVC, in those patients with a contraindication to anticoagulation. Sudden death, cardiac arrest, pulmonary hypertension and cor pulmonale are the complications.

Case 1.10: Answers

1. The heart is enlarged and there are prominent pulmonary vessels; there are also bilateral, peihilar, fluffy, airspace opacities and small lines in the lung bases, with small pleural effusion.

2. Congestive cardiac failure.

3. Causes of cardiac failure:

(a) underlying cause: structural abnormalities that affect coronary, peripheral arterial circulation, myocardium, pericardium, valves

(b) fundamental causes: biochemical or physiological mechanisms that increase haemodynamic burden

(c) precipitating cause: arrhythmia, infection, PE, exertion, drugs, high-output states.

4. X-rays show enlarged heart (heart is not usually enlarged in acute heart failure). The radiological changes depend on the pulmonary capillary wedge pressure. When the pressure > 10 mmHg, the fluid leaks into the interstitium and compresses the lower lobes first; this recruits the resting upper lobe vessels to carry more blood, resulting in prominent upper lobe vessels (cephalisation).

Other features are peribronchial cuffing (interstitial fluid around the bronchi), loss of definition of vessels, thickened fissures and pleural effusions. Laminar effusions are seen beneath the visceral pleura in the loose connective tissue between the pleura and lung. Pseudotumours caused by loculated collections in fissures can be seen. Kerley B lines may be seen which are distended interlobular septa, 1–2 cm long at bases, horizontal, perpendicular to pleural surface. (Kerley A – connective tissue near bronchoarterial bundle, near hilum, oblique, longer; Kerley C lines represent a reticular network of lines.)

There is a 12-hour radiographic lag from onset of symptoms. Radiological findings persist for several days despite clinical recovery. Batwing/butterfly shape shadowing in lung fields is a result of increased accumulation of oedematous fluid in the parahilar region. Various theories exist for this appearance. The autoregulation is poorer in the central than in the peripheral region; lymphatics are not efficient in the central region, probably secondary to reduced ventilation in the centre. The lower lung zones are more affected than the upper. Usually it clears in 2–3 days from the periphery to the centre.

5. Cardiac failure results in clinical symptoms such as dyspnoea, orthopnoea, paroxysmal nocturnal dyspnoea (PND), fatigue, weakness, nocturia and syncope. The differential diagnoses for alveolar opacities include infection, haemorrhage, aspiration, lymphoma and pulmonary alveolar proteinosis. Causes of pulmonary oedema can be cardiac, renal or acute respiratory distress syndrome (ARDS). In **cardiac** causes, the distribution is even in 90%; in renal, central distribution in 70%; in **ARDS**, peripheral in 45% and even in 35%. Air bronchograms are more common in ARDS, and pleural effusions are more common in cardiac than renal failure.

Case 1.11: Answers

1. The X-ray shows cardiomegaly, straightening of the left heart border and a shadow within the shadow on the right side of the cardiac contour. There are also prominent vessels in the upper lobe, indicating pulmonary venous hypertension.

2. Mitral stenosis.

3. Rheumatic fever is the most common cause of mitral stenosis. Other causes include infective endocarditis, carcinoid, eosinophilic endocarditis, rheumatoid arthritis, SLE, mucopolysaccharidosis, left atrial myxoma, thrombus, congenital, Fabry's disease, Whipple's disease and methysergide therapy. Lutimbachir syndrome is a combination of mitral stenosis and ASD. Shone's complex is a combination of mitral stenosis, aortic stenosis and coarctation of the aorta. Mitral stenosis leads to elevated left atrial pressure, which sequentially results in increased pulmonary vascular pressure, dilatation of the left atrium, pulmonary venous hypertension, post-capillary pulmonary arterial hypertension, RVH, tricuspid regurgitation, RV dilatation and right heart failure.

4. X-ray shows features of left atrial enlargement – dilated left atrial appendage resulting in straight left cardiac border; **shadow within shadow** – double density of left atrium within the right cardiac shadow (normal left atrium is not visualized in X-rays); splaying of the carina; displacement of the oesophagus posterior and to the right; bulge of posterior superior cardiac border below the carina; Calcification of valve leaflets is seen in 60%. Aorta can be small due to low cardiac output. The increased vascular resistance results in the following stages – Pressures of **16–19 mm Hg** results in pulmonary venous hypertension, which causes upper lobar diversion of blood; Pressure of **20–25 mm Hg** results in interstitial pulmonary oedema, which is seen as septal lines, reticular opacities and pleural effusion; Pressure of **26–30 mm Hg** results in frank alveolar oedema, which is seen as patchy alveolar opacities. Pulmonary arterial hypertension manifests as enlarged pulmonary arteries and peripheral arterial pruning with subsequent hypertrophy of RV and secondary tricuspid insufficiency. **Pulmonary hemosiderosis** is seen as 1–3 mm ill-defined nodules in middle and lower lobes. **Pulmonary ossification** is seen as calcified 1–3 mm nodules in middle and lower lungs. Echocardiography is useful for assessing morphology of mitral valve, measuring orifice, mobility, thickness and calcification. Doppler is useful for quantifying haemodynamic severity.

5. Patients are asymptomatic or present with chest pain, dyspnoea, orthopnoea, PND, haemoptysis (rupture of anastomosis between bronchial veins) and Ortner syndrome (hoarseness of voice as a result of impingement on left recurrent laryngeal nerve). Complications include atrial fibrillation, systemic embolism and infective endocarditis. Clinical examination reveals a palpable diastolic thrill, a loud S1 followed by S2 and opening snap, and a characteristic low-pitched, mid-diastolic, rumbling murmur with presystolic accentuation, which is augmented by expiration, coughing, exercise, squatting and nitrites. Features of cardiac failure may also be seen. Definitive treatment is commissurotomy if the valves are pliable and valve replacement if they are not.

Case 1.12: Answers

1. The X-ray shows a curvilinear calcification in the wall of the heart, conforming to the shape of the LV wall. The heart is not enlarged and the lungs are normal.

2. LV aneurysm.

3. LV aneurysms can be true or false: a **true aneurysm** contains myocardial wall; a **false aneurysm** is myocardial rupture limited by pericardial adhesions; a **functional aneurysm** protrudes during systole, but not in diastole. Aneurysms interfere with ventricular performance, because they do not have contractile function. True aneurysms usually result after an acute MI; 90% of them involve the LAD territory and are seen in 10% of patients with LAD occlusion. Intraventricular tension stretches infarcted heart muscle, expanding the infarct and fibrous tissue, which bulges with each cardiac contraction. The wall becomes fibrotic and bulges with systole, reducing the effectiveness of contraction. Impaired motion can result in the formation of thrombus, which can embolise. The rest of the ventricle becomes hyperkinetic. In large aneurysms, stroke volume decreases or is maintained at the expense of increased end-diastolic volume, increasing the wall tension and myocardial oxygen demand Other causes of aneurysm are blunt chest injury, resulting in contusion and vascular damage causing necrosis.

4. X-ray, echocardiography, CT and MRI are useful in diagnosis. LV aneurysms are usually 1–8 cm, and are common in the apex and anterior wall (90%). They occur in 10% of those with an occluded LAD, and poor collateral supply. The X-ray shows characteristic bulge of the silhouette of the left ventricle with calcification in the apical and anterolateral aspects. The calcification is curvilinear and seen in the periphery of the aneurysm's infarct. False aneuryms are usually seen in the posterolateral wall of the left ventricle. A true aneurysm protrudes in systole and diastole, with the mouth wide or wider than its maximal diameter, and the wall formed by the left ventricle with fibrous tissue and myocardium; it never ruptures and may contain thrombus. A false aneurysm protrudes in both systole and diastole, with a mouth smaller than the maximal diameter of the aneurysm and the wall made up of parietal pericardium; it always contains thrombus and prone to rupture. A functional aneurysm protrudes during systole, but not in diastole. Multidetector CT scans are very fast and reliable in diagnosing aneurysms. MRI is useful for assessing the anatomy of the aneurysm and function of the heart. Delayed enhancement is seen in the infarcted and scarred myocardium. In echocardiography, the true and false aneuryms can be differentiated and abnormal flow is demonstrated within the aneurysm. Thrombus can also be detected using echocardiography, CT and MRI.

5. True LV aneurysms have a low risk of rupture, because the density of the fibrous tissue increases with time. Clinical features are angina, heart failure and arrhythmias. Surgical excision is done only to improve function Aggressive management of MI diminishes the incidence of LV aneurysms. Aneurysmectomy or a Dor procedure (LV reconstructive surgery) is done only when the remaining heart is not too small for normal cardiac output.

Case 1.13: Answers

1. The CT scan shows a curvilinear, thin sheet of calcification in the pericardium, surrounding the heart.

2. Constrictive calcific pericarditis.

3. Constrictive pericarditis occurs when a thickened fibrotic pericardium, of whatever cause, impedes normal diastolic filling. This usually involves the parietal pericardium, although it can involve the visceral pericardium. Pericarditis may deposit fibrin, which results in pericardial effusion. This often leads to pericardial organisation, chronic fibrotic scarring, calcification and restricted cardiac filling. Half the patients with constrictive pericarditis have some degree of pericardial calcification. Causes are idiopathic, infectious (TB [common in developing countries], streptococci and others), radiation, post-surgical, uraemia, neoplasms, connective tissue disorders, drug induced (procainamide, hydralazine, methysergide), trauma and MI. Occasionally the clues to the aetiology can be seen, such as apical fibrosis and calcification in lung TB. Constrictive pericarditis usually develops insidiously and may be secondary to any cause of acute pericarditis. It is more common when the pericardial fluid is purulent or haemorrhagic, eg TB or malignancy.

4. The clinical picture is that of right heart failure with severe ascites and hepatosplenomegaly. Constrictive pericarditis restricts diastolic filling as a result of confining the pericardium. Dyspnoea, oedema, abdominal swelling, fatigue, orthopnoea, chest pain, nausea, vomiting and right upper quadrant pain are seen. Other signs are elevated jugular venous pressure, which rises on inspiration (Kussmaul's sign), pulsus paradoxus and loud third heart sound (pericardial knock). The X-ray can show severe pericardial calcification. The cardiac contour is normal in the absence of pericardial effusion. The SVC may be prominent along with the azygos. Pleural effusions can be seen. Pulmonary oedema is rare. An echocardiogram is required for further assessment and to differentiate constrictive pericarditis and restrictive cardiomyopathy. Constriction limits ventricular filling and enhances ventricular interaction, but restriction generally limits ventricular distensibility and the myocardium is abnormal. In both, there is early diastolic filling with early ventricular pressure equilibration. CT and MRI show the pericardial thickening and calcification. MRI is also useful in assessing the function.

5. Differential diagnosis includes: restrictive cardiomyopathy (sarcoidosis, amyloidosis, haemochromatosis), cardiac fibrosis, congestive cardiac failure, cardiac tamponade, right-sided valvular abnormalities and right atrial tumours. Subacute constrictive pericarditis may respond to steroids. Diuretics are used to relieve congestion. Pericardectomy (surgical resection of the pericardium) is the treatment of choice.

Case 1.14: Answers

1. The first picture shows a catheter in the IVC. A metallic device is being deployed in the distal aspect of the catheter. The second film shows an IVC filter in position and the catheter has been removed.

2. Indications for IVC filter are:

(a) DVT or PE in a patient with a contraindication to anticoagulation

(b) DVT/PE in a patient with a complication from anticoagulation

(c) failure of anticoagulation therapy.

(d) free floating iliofemoral or caval thrombosis

(e) prophylaxis to prevent PE in high-risk patients (surgery, chronic pulmonary hypertension, trauma).

3. There are many different types of IVC filter, including the Mobin–Uddin umbrella filter, titanium Greenfield filter, etc. Characteristics of a good filter are: should trap most of the thrombi, should be non-thrombogenic, biocompatible and structurally strong; should not migrate or cause perforation; should be non-ferromagnetic; and should be retrievable when required. Filters are placed under fluoroscopic guidance. Most are placed in the infrarenal IVC. Indications for a suprarenal filter are: renal vein thrombosis, IVC thrombosis extending above the level of the renal veins, thrombus in the infrarenal IVC, recurrent PE despite an infrarenal filter, PE after ovarian vein thrombosis and pregnancy. One of the femoral veins is punctured. A guidewire is passed into the femoral vein and the filter system is passed over the guidewire. The filter is then deployed at the infrarenal portion of IVC.

4. Before the procedure, DVT/PE is confirmed. The coagulation profile is tested and, if the patient is already on anticoagulants, it is discontinued before the procedure. The IVC should be assessed for size, configuration, anatomical variation and thrombosis. This can be done by Doppler, cavography, CT or MRI.

5. Contraindications are thrombus between the venous access and deployment sites and therapeutic anticoagulation.

Case 1.15: Answers

1. MRI of the aorta without contrast shows abnormal thickening and high signal in the wall of the aortic arch and descending thoracic aorta consistent with an active inflammatory disease. Volume rendered 3D MR angiogram (Fig 1.15b) shows narrowing of the descending thoracic aorta, proximal left subclavian artery and brachiocephalic artery.

2. Takayasu's arteritis.

3. Takayasu's arteritis is granulomatous vasculitis of unknown aetiology that causes fibroproliferation of the aorta, great vessels, pulmonary arteries and renal arteries, and causes segmental stenosis, occlusion, dilatation and aneurysms. It is more common in women, seen in the third and fourth decades, and common in Asians. Clinical features are fever, tachycardia, pain, bruits, hypertension, diminished or absent pulses, and ischaemic symptoms

4. **Type I**: involvement of arch and its branches; **type II**: entire aorta; **type III**: arch and its branches, thoracic and abdominal aorta distal to arch; **type IV**: dilated type. Type II is the most common and the left subclavian artery is most commonly involved, followed by the left common carotid artery. Pulmonary arteries are involved in 50%. Treatment is with steroids. Short segment stenosis can be managed with angioplasty, which is contraindicated in the acute phase.

5. Diagnosis is made with conventional angiography, CT angiography or MRA. The classic appearance is involvement of the larger arteries with thickened walls and narrowing of the lumen and focal areas of dilatation and aneurysms. Smooth, symmetrical, focal narrowing is the most

common appearance. The differential diagnosis is **atherosclerosis** (> 40, men, origin of vessels and bifurcations), **fibromuscular dysplasia** (beaded appearance, does not affect aorta, rare in subclavian artery), **temporal arteritis** (only temporal arteries, no involvement of carotid or aorta), **syphilitic aortitis** (calcification in ascending aorta), **neurofibromatosis I, Williams syndrome, rubella** and **radiation.**

Case 1.16: Answers

1. The X-ray shows an enlarged, box-shaped heart and gross right atrial enlargement. There is decreased vascularity in both the lungs.

2. Ebstein's anomaly. In the MRI, the right atrium is enlarged. The septal leaflet of tricuspid valve is not where it should be, but situated far inferiorly into the right ventricle.

3. Ebstein's anomaly is a congenital malformation, in which the septal and posterior tricuspid leaflets of the tricuspid valve are displaced apically, leading to atrialisation of the right ventricle. Tricuspid regurgitation is caused by leaflet anomaly. The regurgitation may be mild or severe depending on the extent of the leaflet displacement. Although the atrialised portion of the right ventricle is anatomically part of the right atrium, it contracts and relaxes with the right ventricle. This discordant contraction leads to stagnation of blood in the right atrium. During ventricular systole, the atrialised portion of the right ventricle contracts with the right ventricle, causing backward flow of blood into the right atrium, which makes the tricuspid regurgitation worse. Maternal lithium, benzodiazepine, varnishing substance and previous fetal loss are associated.

4. In normal infants, the heart can occupy up to 60% of the chest. Presence of pulmonary vasculature in the peripheral third of the lungs indicates plethora. Absence of vasculature in the central portions indicates oligaemia and peripheral pruning indicates pulmonary arterial hypertension. In Ebstein's anomaly, the heart is enlarged with a huge right atrium. The classic appearance is a squared-/boxed-off heart. There is decreased pulmonary vasculature (right-to-left shunt at atrial level) with small aortic root and main pulmonary artery. On the lateral chest X-ray, distortion of the RV outflow or displacement by the atrialised segment of the right ventricle may cause abnormal filling of the retrosternal space.

This finding is of use in older children and adults. The differential diagnosis for an enormously enlarged heart is: pericardial effusion, valvular heart disease, cardiomyopathy, cardiac failure and giant right atrial aneurysm. Echocardiography or MRI can diagnose the condition. There is apical displacement of the septal leaflet of tricuspid valve, > 20 mm or 8 mm/m^2. The right ventricle is dilated with decreased contractility.

5. Clinical features are: cyanosis, heart failure, fatigue, exertional dyspnoea and palpitations. Auscultation may reveal a triple or quadruple gallop rhythm and a split S2. A pansystolic murmur of tricuspid regurgitation or an ejection murmur of pulmonary stenosis may be heard. The ECG shows an RBBB pattern, giant P waves and sometimes first-degree atrioventricular (AV) block or Wolff–Parkinson–White (WPW) syndrome (delta wave). Brain abscesses caused by a right-to-left shunt, bacterial endocarditis and paradoxical embolism are other complications. Ebstein's anomaly should be suspected in patients with WPW syndrome, cyanotic congenital heart disease, ASD, severe right heart failure, severe tricuspid regurgitation and left transposition of the great arteries. Antibiotic prophylaxis for endocarditis and treatment of heart failure and arrhythmia are given. Radiofrequency ablation is used for treating supraventricular tachycardia. Surgical care includes correction of the underlying tricuspid valve and RV abnormalities and correction of any associated intracardiac defects. Indications for surgery are: severe heart failure, paradoxical embolism, refractory arrhythmias and significant cyanosis.

Case 1.17: Answers

1. The X-ray shows an enlarged heart with LV configuration. On MRI, the heart is enlarged. There is massive concentric thickening of the myocardium.

2. Hypertrophic cardiomyopathy.

3. Hypertrophic cardiomyopathy is an autosomal dominant disorder, resulting in abnormal, often asymmetrical hypertrophy of the myocardium; it is caused by myocyte disarray without other discernible causes for hypertrophy. Myocardial disarray results in abnormal myocardial hypertrophy and hypertrophy of endomyocardial coronary arteries. It is usually septal, but can involve any portion of the myocardium or can be concentric (concentric may indicate secondary cause). LV outflow tract (LVOT) dynamic pressure gradient related to septal hypertrophy and elevated LVOT velocities results in a Venturi effect pulling the anterior leaflet of the mitral valve towards the interventricular septum, which causes more obstruction and potentially mitral regurgitation. Endomyocardial arterial hypertrophy can result in ischaemia with normal epicardial coronaries. Diastolic dysfunction results in impaired ventricular filling and increased filling pressures despite small or normal ventricular size. Myocardial disarray can result in arrhythmias such as ventricular tachycardia or fibrillation. Other types of cardiomyopathy are dilated, restrictive and arrhythmogenic RV cardiomyopathy. Amyloidosis, sarcoidosis and haemochromatosis produce specific types of cardiomyopathy.

4. Hypertrophic cadiomyopathy can present with a wide range of clinical symptoms, including sudden cardiac death, dyspnoea, syncope, angina, palpitations, orthopnoea, PND, congestive heart failure and dizziness. Most patients have a benign clinical course, but complications can be catastrophic such as sudden death (caused by ventricular tachyarrhythmias). Heart failure is secondary to valve dysfunction. Endocarditis is seen. Treatment is with LV myomectomy, alcohol septal ablation to scar the hypertrophied myocardium or defibrillator/pacemaker to treat arrhythmia.

5. On the X-ray, the heart is enlarged with an LV pattern. The diagnosis is usually made with echocardiography. The typical feature is a ratio of end-diastolic septal thickness:posterolateral wall > 1.3. In concentric hypertrophy, the wall measures > 1.2 cm in end-diastole and there is no cause for concentric hypertrophy such as hypertension. MRI enables delineation of location and extent of hypertrophic myocardium. The important role of MRI is to identify unusual forms of hypertrophy that are difficult to assess with echocardiography. It can identify areas not well seen on echocardiography, such as the apex and LV free wall. It shows abnormal wall motion in thickened segments, increased myocardial mass, diastolic dysfunction, LVOT narrowing and delayed enhancement (as a result of collagen) in hypertrophied areas. MRI can also be used to monitor response to therapy.

Case 1.18: Answers

1. In the CT scan, there is massive enlargement of the left main coronary artery and LAD artery. (The sternum is the dense structure anteriorly. The dense opacity under the sternum is the SVC. Deep to it the aortic root is seen as a round opacity. The left main coronary artery is arising from the left side of it.)

2. Coronary artery aneurysm. Causes are: atherosclerosis, congenital, Kawasaki's disease, arteritis (Takayasu's, SLE, syphilis, polyarteritis nodosa), mycotic infections, connective tissue disorders (Marfan and Ehler–Danlos syndromes), polycystic kidney disease, cocaine abuse, trauma, metastatic tumours and after angioplasty. This patient has Kawasaki's disease.

3. Coronary artery aneurysms can be asymptomatic or present with ischemic or congestive cardiac failure symptoms (due to aneurysm or coronary artery disease). Myocardial infarction, thromboemboli and sudden cardiac death with acute rupture can occur. Kawasaki disease, also known as mucocutaneous lymph node syndrome is a self-limiting vasculitis of unknown etiology. Prolonged fever, rash, mucocutaneous involvement, cervical adenopathy, conjunctivitis, extremity changes and coronary artery aneurysms are characteristic features of Kawasaki disease.

4. Conventional coronary angiography is the best modality for diagnosing aneurysms. But multidetector CT is equally good and very fast, and images can be reconstructed in multiple planes. Coronary aneurysms can be saccular or fusiform. A diameter more than 1.5 times the normal artery is called an aneurysm. If there is diffuse dilatation involving > 50% of the artery, it is caused ectasia. Kawasaki's disease is the most common cause of aneurysms worldwide. The RCA is the most commonly involved followed by the LAD. A CT scan helps in preoperative planning by demonstrating the size, neck and relationship of the aneurysm to adjacent vessels. MRI and MRA are also good at diagnosing aneurysms. Differential diagnoses are cardiac wall aneurysm, post-traumatic pseudoaneurysm of aorta/ pulmonary artery, tumour of heart/pericardium and thymoma.

5. Prognosis of a coronary artery aneurysm depends on the severity of the CAD. Treatment is with anticoagulants and antiplatelets. Surgery with a bypass graft or stent is indicated if there is significant coronary stenosis/angina in spite of medical treatment. γ-Globulin, aspirin and anticoagulants are used in the treatment of Kawasaki's disease.

Case 1.19: Answers

1. The X-ray shows small aortic knuckle, and prominent main pulmonary arteries with pulmonary plethora. Lung fields are hyperinflated but no focal lung lesion is seen.

2. MRI shows a defect in the middle of the interatrial septum.

3. ASD. In ASD, there is left-to-right shunting of the blood, resulting in an admixture of oxygenated blood and deoxygenated blood in the right atrium, and a volume overload of the right atrium and right ventricle; if untreated this results in pulmonary hypertension and heart failure. When the pressure in the right side increases, the shunt will decrease and eventually there will be a reversal of the shunt to a right-to-left shunt, which is called Eisenmenger syndrome.

4. There are four types of ASD: **ostium secundum, ostium primum, sinus venosus** and **coronary sinus type**. Ostium secundum is the most common type of defect and is located in the region of the fossa ovalis, which is in the middle of the septum. Ostium primum is situated in the lower part of the septum and often a component of the endocardial cushion defect. Sinus venosus is seen in either the upper or the lower part of the septum, bordering the SVC/IVC ostium. This is usually associated with partial anomalous pulmonary venous return. In a coronary sinus defect there is absence of the wall separating the coronary sinus from the left atrium, so the left SVC drains into the left atrium. Ostium secundum defects can present late in life, with dyspnoea on exertion and other signs of cardiac failure or stroke. RV lift is felt along the lower left sternal edge. Fixed, wide splitting of S2 and a pulmonary ejection systolic murmur are heard.

5. X-rays show an enlarged right atrium, right ventricle, main and hilar pulmonary arteries, with small ascending aorta, aortic arch and SVC shadow. There is disparity in the enlargement of central and lobar arteries to the peripheral arteries. Calcification of main or central pulmonary arteries can be seen. A two-to-one shunt should be present before pulmonary plethora is universally present. Pulmonary oedema rarely occurs in a simple atrial defect. The septal defect is identified in echocardiography. Contrast ultrasonography can demonstrate the shunt. Transoesophageal echocardiography is more sensitive in detection. In MRI, the left-to-right shunt is identified and quantified.

6. The ASD can be closed surgically or percutaneously. Closure is successful if performed before the development of pulmonary hypertension. An Amplatzer septal occluder is used if the ASD is ostium secundum and there is a large enough rim of tissue around the defect so that the device does not impinge on the SVC, IVC or valves. Small defects can be directly sutured and closed. Larger defects require a pericardial or Dacron patch.

Case 1.20: Answers

1. Venogram shows multiple, small, filling defects in the popliteal vein, extending to the femoral vein. Doppler ultrasonography shows colour flow within the femoral artery, but no colour flow within the femoral vein, which is distended with intraluminal hypoechoic thrombus.

2. DVT in the left leg.

3. DVT is caused in hypercoagulability states, stasis, intimal injury or platelet aggregation. The predisposing factors are surgery, trauma, prolonged immobilisation, obesity, malignancy, diabetes, pregnancy, oral contraceptive pills, cardiac failure, MI, old age, varicose veins, previous DVT, polycythaemia and smoking.

4. The most common location is the dorsal vein of calf. Other locations are the iliac, femoral and popliteal veins. It is rare in the internal iliac, ovarian and ascending lumbar veins. It is more common in the left side as a result of compression of the left common iliac vein by the left common iliac artery, which leads to chronic endothelial injury. Patients present with

swelling, pain, warmth, tenderness and calf pain, with dorsiflexion of the foot (Homan's sign). The Wells' clinical prediction guide quantifies the pretest probability of DVT. The model enables physicians to stratify their patients reliably into high-, moderate- or low-risk categories. Combining this with objective tests simplifies the diagnosis and management of DVT. The D-dimer level is elevated, but it may be elevated in trauma, recent surgery, haemorrhage, cancer and sepsis. It is used to rule out DVT, but not to confirm the diagnosis of DVT. A negative D-dimer assay rules out DVT in patients with low-to-moderate risk and a Wells' DVT score < 2. All patients with a positive D-dimer assay result and all patients with a moderate-to-high risk of DVT (Wells' DVT score ≥ 2) require a diagnostic study (duplex ultrasonography).

5. Doppler ultrasonography shows expansion of the veins. Thrombus is hypoechoic or isoechoic. Normal veins can be compressed with the ultrasonic probe, but this is not possible with a thrombosed vein. There is no cyclical variation in flow with respiration and there is no augmentation on distal compression. Soft tissue oedema can be seen. Doppler ultrasonography is not very good for below-calf veins and for iliac veins. Doppler ultrasonography also excludes Baker's cyst, abscess, haematoma and other causes of leg swelling. Venography shows filling defect in deep veins, but it does not fill all the calf veins or the common femoral or iliac veins. ^{125}I-labelled fibrinogen localises to the clot. Venous occlusion plethysmography shows delay in venous outflow. CT venography can be done and combined with CT of the chest to diagnose PE. It is very useful for iliofemoral DVT. MRI can also be used for diagnosis.

6. Complications are PE (77% risk from iliac veins, 35–70% for femoropopliteal veins, 0–50% for calf veins), post-phlebitic syndrome and phlegmasia cerulea/alba dolens with gangrene. Tibial/peroneal venous thrombi resolve in 40%. Treatment is with intravenous heparin, systemic anticoagulation with warfarin for > 3 months. An IVC filter is placed in patients with contraindications/complications from DVT, or recurrent DVT.

2
CHEST RADIOLOGY
QUESTIONS

Case 2.1

A 31-year-old man presents with fever, cough and chest pain. On examination he is febrile and tachypnoeic, and there is bronchial breathing in the right lower lobe. His white blood cell (WBC) count is 20000μl.

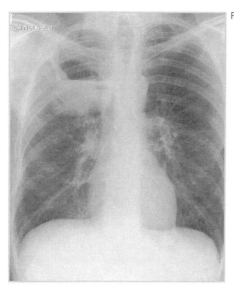

Fig 2.1a

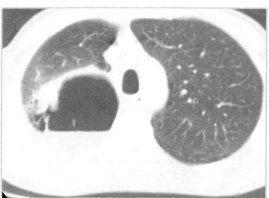

Fig 2.1b

1. What can you find on the X-ray and CT scan?
2. What is the diagnosis?
3. What are the causes and clinical features?
4. What are the radiological features?
5. What are the common differential diagnoses?

Answers on pages 101–153

Case 2.2

A 37-year-old man presents with fever, night sweats, weight loss and haemoptysis. Clinical examination showed dullness on percussion in the right upper zone and crackles.

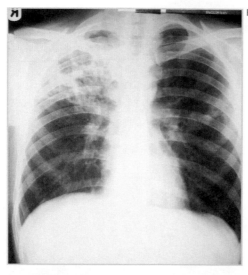
Fig 2.2a

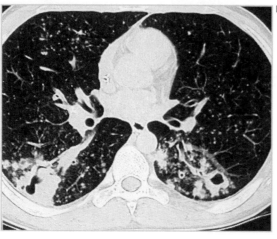
Fig 2.2b

1. What can you see on the chest X-ray and CT scan?
2. What is the diagnosis?
3. What are the pathological types and common locations?
4. What are the radiological features?
5. What is the differential diagnosis?

Answers on pages 101–153

Case 2.3

A 35-year-old man presents with cough, haemoptysis and chest pain. Clinical examination showed tenderness and bronchial breathing in the right upper lobe.

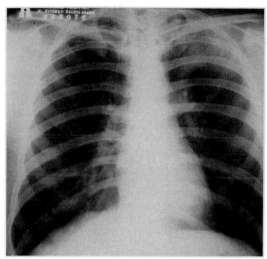

Fig 2.3a

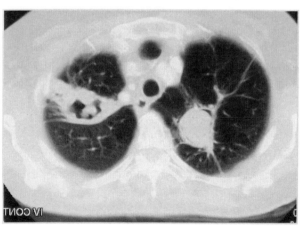

Fig 2.3b

1. What can you find on the X-ray and CT scan?
2. What is the diagnosis?
3. What is the causative agent?
4. What are the predisposing factors?
5. What are the radiological features?
6. What is the differential diagnosis?

Answers *on pages 101–153*

Case 2.4

A 38-year-old man presents with severe dyspnoea and wheezing. On examination, he is severely tachypnoeic and there are bilateral diffuse rhonchi.

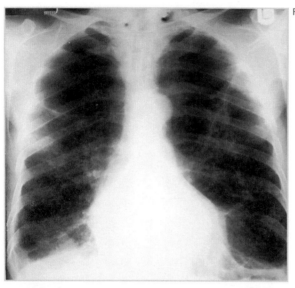

Fig 2.4a

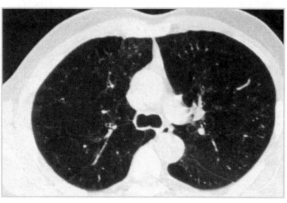

Fig 2.4b

1. What can you find on the X-ray and CT scan?
2. What is the diagnosis?
3. What are the pathology and types of the disease?
4. What are the radiological features?
5. What is the role of the CT scan?
6. What are the complications and associations?

Answers *on pages 101–153*

Case 2.5

A 42-year-old woman presents with sudden onset of chest pain, dyspnoea, fever and night sweats. On examination, she is dyspnoeic, febrile and in respiratory distress. There is no lymphadenopathy. Bronchial breathing is heard on the right side of the chest. Percussion was normal.

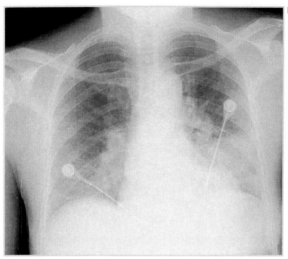

Fig 2.5a

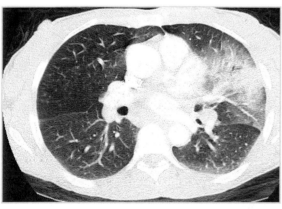

Fig 2.5b

1. What do you observe on the chest X-ray?
2. What is the diagnosis and what are the types?
3. What is the most common causative aetiology?
4. What are the predisposing factors?
5. What are the radiological features and differential diagnosis?
6. What are the complications and treatment?

Answers on pages 101–153

Case 2.6

A 56-year-old woman presents with cough, chest pain, haemoptysis and dyspnoea. Clinical examination revealed decreased breath sounds on the left side.

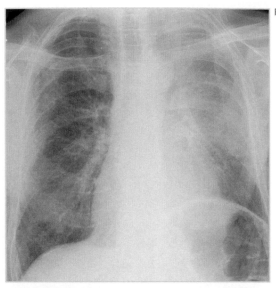

Fig 2.6a

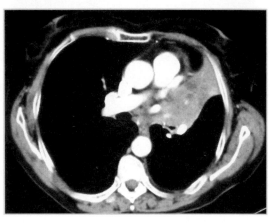

Fig 2.6b

1. What do you find on the chest X-ray?
2. What is the diagnosis?
3. What additional information does the CT scan add?
4. What are the radiological features of this pathological process?
5. What is the management of this patient?

Answers *on pages 101–153*

Case 2.7

A 56-year-old woman presents with cough and difficulty in breathing. On examination, bilateral basal end-inspiratory crackles were heard. Lung function tests showed a restrictive pattern.

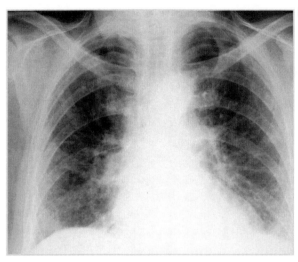
Fig 2.7a

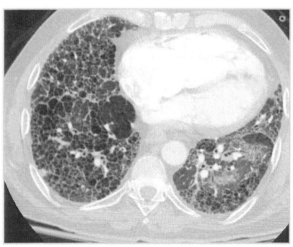
Fig 2.7b

1. What do you find on the X-ray and CT scan?
2. What is the diagnosis?
3. What are the pathology and location of this disease?
4. What are the radiological features?
5. What is the differential diagnosis?

Answers *on pages 101–153*

Case 2.8

A 47-year-old patient with a history of a neoplasm presents with gradual onset of dyspnoea, chest pain and cough. Clinical examination showed reduced breath sounds in the right upper lobe.

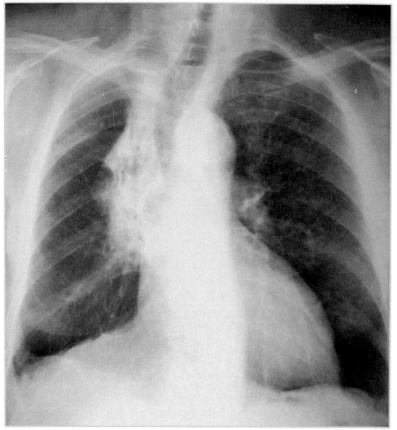

Fig 2.8

1. What do you find on the chest X-ray?
2. What is the diagnosis?
3. What are the types and time of onset of this disease process?
4. What are the critical factors in the development of this disease?
5. What are the radiological features and differential diagnosis?

Answers on pages 101–153

Case 2.9

A 41-year-old man presents with sudden onset of chest pain, dyspnoea, fever and night sweats. On clinical examination, he is febrile and tachypnoeic. The breath sounds are decreased on the right side and there is a stony dull note on percussion.

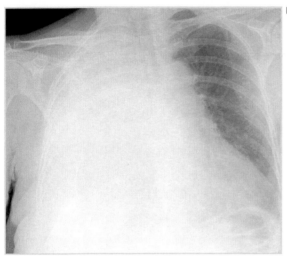
Fig 2.9a

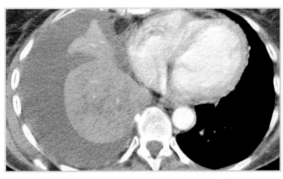
Fig 2.9b

1. What do you observe on the plain film and CT scan of the chest?
2. What is the diagnosis? What is the radiological differential diagnosis?
3. What are the causes?
4. What are the characteristic features of an exudative process that differentiates it from a transudate?
5. What is the most sensitive method in the diagnosis of this condition and what are the radiological features?

Answers *on pages 101–153*

Case 2.10

A 41-year-old man presents with fever, chest pain, muscle and joint pain, sinusitis and haemoptysis. Clinical examination showed tachypnoea and bilateral bronchial breathing and ulcerating lesions in the nasal cavity.

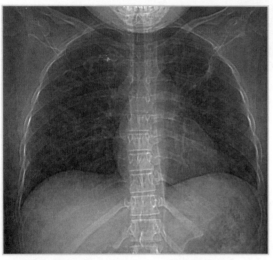

Fig 2.10a

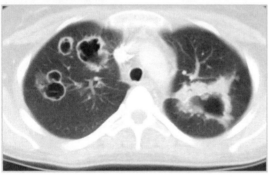

Fig 2.10b

1. What are the findings on the X-ray and HRCT?
2. What is the most likely diagnosis?
3. What is the pathology?
4. What are the radiological features?
5. What is the differential diagnosis?
6. What other systems are affected?

Answers on pages 101–153

Case 2.11

A 35-year-old woman with chronic muscle weakness presents with dyspnoea, chest pain and hoarseness of voice.

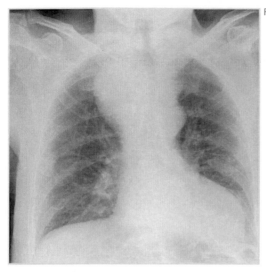

Fig 2.11a

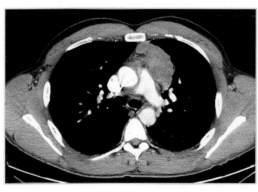

Fig 2.11b

1. What are the findings on the chest X-ray and CT scan?
2. What is the diagnosis?
3. What are the pathology and clinical features?
4. What is the most important association and how strong is it?
5. What are the radiological features and differential diagnosis?

Answers *on pages 101–153*

Case 2.12

A 10-year-old boy presents with head and neck swelling, dyspnoea and hoarseness of voice. On examination there is oedema in the face and neck with prominent veins. There are multiple lymph nodes palpable in the axilla and groin. There are decreased breath sounds in both the lungs.

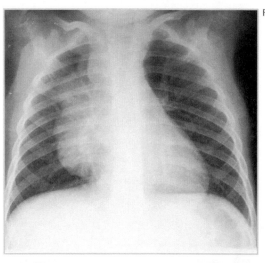

Fig 2.12a

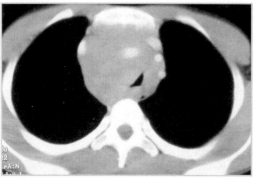

Fig 2.12b

1. What do you find on the X-ray and CT scan?
2. What is the diagnosis?
3. What are the types of disease?
4. What are the common locations?
5. What are the radiological features?
6. What is the differential diagnosis?

Answers on pages 101–153

Case 2.13

A 56-year-old man working in a sheep farm presents with fever, weight loss and dyspnoea. On clinical examination, there are bronchial breath sounds in the right lung.

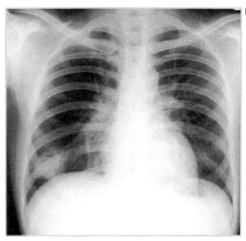

Fig 2.13a

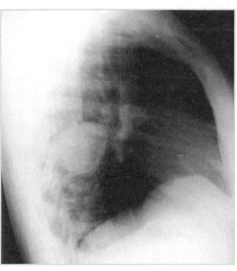

Fig 2.13b

1. What are the findings on X-rays?
2. What is the diagnosis?
3. What are the causative agent and the pathophysiology?
4. What are the different radiological signs?
5. What is the differential diagnosis?

Answers *on pages 101–153*

Case 2.14

A 27-year-old man with a long-standing infectious disease presents with chest pain, cough, weight loss and fever.

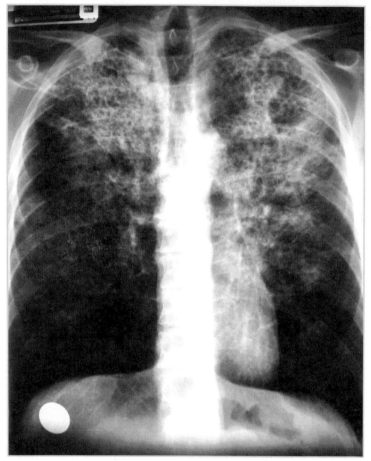

Fig 2.14

1. What are the findings on the chest X-ray?
2. What are the diagnosis and cause of this distribution?
3. What is the underlying disease in this patient?
4. What are the radiological features?
5. What is the differential diagnosis?

Answers on pages 101–153

Case 2.15

A 12-year-old boy presents with frequent episodes of cough and fever. On examination, the patient is febrile and tachypnoeic. Bronchial breathing is heard on the right side.

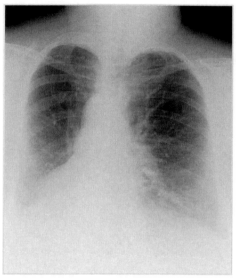

Fig 2.15a

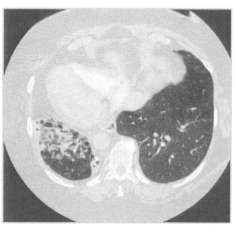

Fig 2.15b

1. What do you find on the chest X-ray?
2. What do you find on the CT scan of the chest?
3. What is the diagnosis?
4. What is the pathophysiology of this disease?
5. What are the radiological features and treatment?

Answers *on pages 101–153*

Case 2.16

A 33-year-old man presents with fever and cough with purulent sputum. Clinical examination showed decreased breath sounds in the right upper lobe.

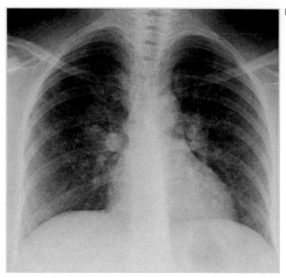

Fig 2.16a

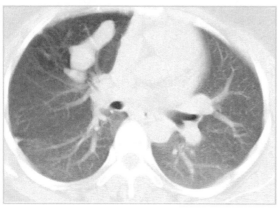

Fig 2.16b

1. What do you observe on the X-ray and CT scan of the chest?
2. What is the diagnosis?
3. What are the development and pathophysiology of this disease?
4. What are the radiological features?
5. What is the differential diagnosis?

Answers *on pages 101–153*

Case 2.17

A 35-year-old woman presents with dyspnoea and red eye. On examination, there are bilateral crepitations in the lungs.

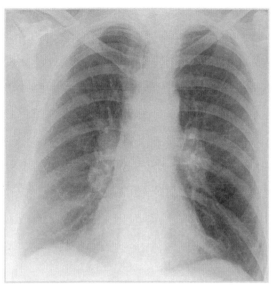

Fig 2.17a

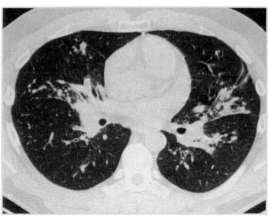

Fig 2.17b

1. What do you find on the X-ray and CT scan?
2. What is the diagnosis?
3. What are the stages and how do you confirm the disease?
4. What are the radiological features?
5. What are the common differential diagnoses?
6. What are the complications?

Answers on pages 101–153

Case 2.18

A 23-year-old woman presents with recurrent bouts of productive cough and fever. On examination, he is febrile and has bronchial breathing and crackles in the bases.

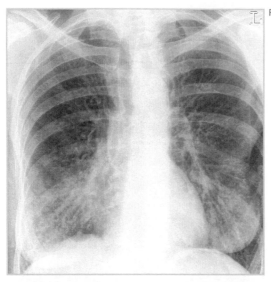

Fig 2.18a

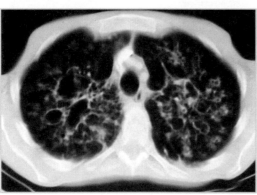

Fig 2.18b

1. What are the findings on the chest X-ray and CT scan?
2. What is the diagnosis?
3. What is the classification of this disease? What are the radiological features?
4. What are the common causes?
5. What is the differential diagnosis?

Answers on pages 101–153

Case 2.19

A 43-year-old woman presents with cough, dyspnoea, chest pain, episodes of cutaneous flushing and diarrhoea.

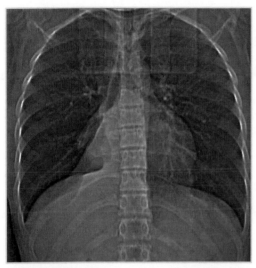
Fig 2.19a

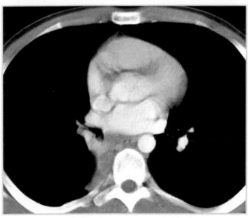
Fig 2.19b

1. What do you see on the chest X-ray and CT scan?
2. What is the diagnosis?
3. What are the cell of origin and locations?
4. What are the radiological features?
5. What is the differential diagnosis?

Answers *on pages 101–153*

Case 2.20

A 57-year-old man presented with cough with sputum and fever. Clinical examination showed reduced breath sounds in the right middle and lower zones.

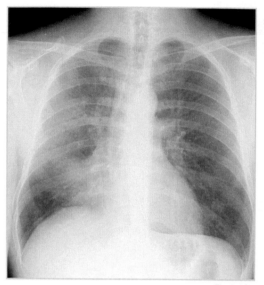

Fig 2.20a

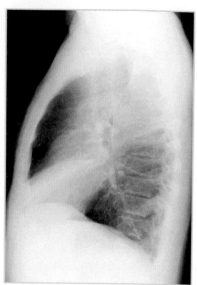

Fig 2.20b

1. What do you observe on the chest X-ray?
2. What is the diagnosis?
3. What are the causes of this appearance?
4. What are the radiological features?
5. What is the differential diagnosis?

Answers on pages 101–153

Case 2.21

A 67-year-old man presented with chest pain and difficult in breathing. He has retired after working for 30 years in a shipyard. Clinically there are reduced breath sounds on the right side with a dull note on percussion.

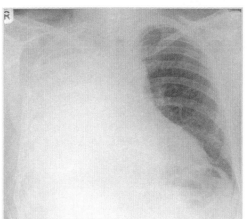
Fig 2.21a

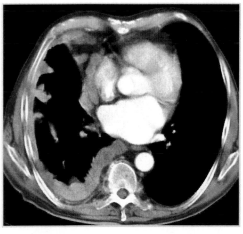
Fig 2.21b

1. What are the findings on the chest X-ray and a CT scan carried out after pleural aspiration?
2. What is the diagnosis?
3. What are the predisposing factors, latency period and histological types?
4. What are the clinical features and pattern of spread?
5. What are the radiological findings?
6. What is the differential diagnosis?

Answers *on pages 101–153*

Case 2.22

A 61-year-old man presents with cough and dyspnoea. He has retired after working for 40 years in a mine. Clinically, he has tachypnoea and bilateral bronchial breath sounds.

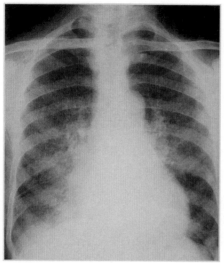
Fig 2.22a

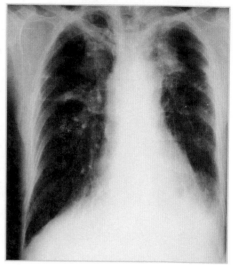
Fig 2.22b

1. What are the findings on the X-rays? The first X-ray was done 2 years earlier.
2. What is the diagnosis? What complication has developed?
3. What is the pathophysiology of this disease?
4. What are the radiological features?
5. What is the differential diagnosis?
6. What are the complications?

Answers on pages 101–153

Case 2.23

A 68-year-old man presents who has long-standing dyspnoea. He has developed new onset of chest pain and haemoptysis. Clinical examination shows decreased breath sounds in the right lung.

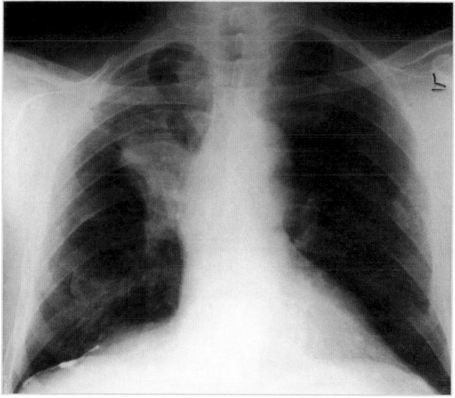

Fig 2.23

1. What are the findings on the chest X-ray?
2. What is the diagnosis? What complication is seen?
3. What are the pathology and causes of this condition?
4. What are the radiological features?
5. What is the time frame for various lesions in this condition?

Answers *on pages 101–153*

Case 2.24

A 45-year-old woman with a chronic joint condition develops cough and dyspnoea. On clinical examination, she has tenderness and stiffness in multiple joints. Chest examination revealed bronchial breathing bilaterally.

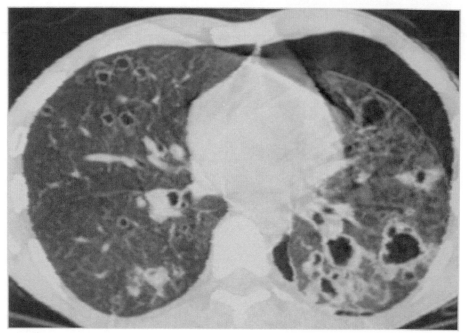

Fig 2.24

1. What are the findings on the chest CT?
2. What is the diagnosis? What complication do you see?
3. What are the various types of presentations of this disease in the lung?
4. What are the radiological features?
5. What is the differential diagnosis?
6. What are the features of Caplan syndrome?

Answers on pages 101–153

Case 2.25

A 46-year-old woman with a chronic connective tissue disorder presents with cough and difficulty in breathing. On examination, bilateral basal crepitations were heard. Joint contractures were also noted. A lung function test showed a restrictive pattern.

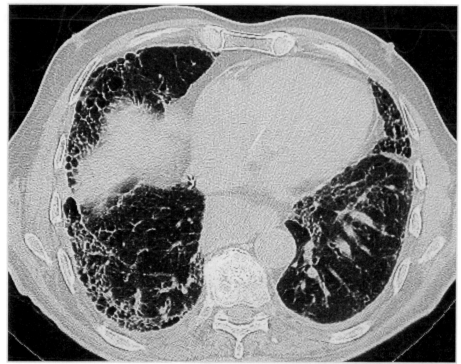

Fig 2.25

1. What do you find on the CT scan?
2. What is the diagnosis?
3. What are the pathology and location of this disease?
4. What are the radiological features?
5. What is the common differential diagnosis?

Answers *on pages 101–153*

Case 2.26

A 20-year-old man presents with chest pain and tachypnoea. Clinical examination showed mild crackles in the right base.

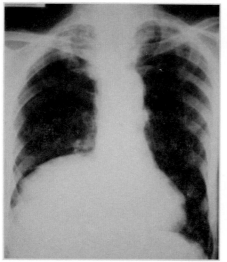

Fig 2.26a

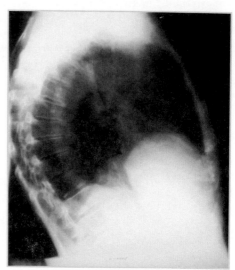

Fig 2.26b

1. What are the findings on the X-ray ?
2. What is the diagnosis?
3. What is the development of this lesion? What are the clinical features?
4. What are the radiological features? What is the differential diagnosis?
5. What is the most common location of a traumatic defect?

Answers on pages 101–153

Case 2.27

A 43-year-old patient involved in major road traffic accident was recovering well from fractures of the pelvis and tibia. He developed sudden onset of hypoxia, not responding to oxygen therapy and dyspnoea.

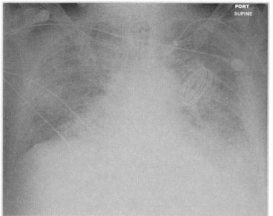

Fig 2.27a

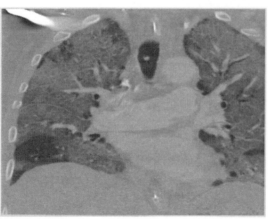

Fig 2.27b

1. What do you find on the chest X-ray and the CT scan?
2. What is the diagnosis?
3. What are the causes of this disease?
4. What are the stages of this disease?
5. What are the radiological features and differential diagnosis?
6. What is the treatment of this disease?

Answers *on pages 101–153*

Case 2.28

A 29-year-old man with renal problems presents with sudden onset of severe haemoptysis and dyspnoea. Clinical examination showed bilateral, diffuse crackles and decreased breath sounds.

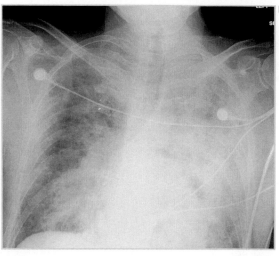

Fig 2.28a

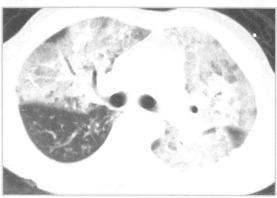

Fig 2.28b

1. What do you see on the plain X-ray and CT scan?
2. What is the diagnosis?
3. What other causes of haemoptysis may mimic this appearance?
4. What are the radiological features?
5. What is the radiological differential diagnosis?

Answers on pages 101–153

Case 2.29

A 27-year-old man presents with intermittent coughing and malaise. Clinical examination is unremarkable, except for faint crackles.

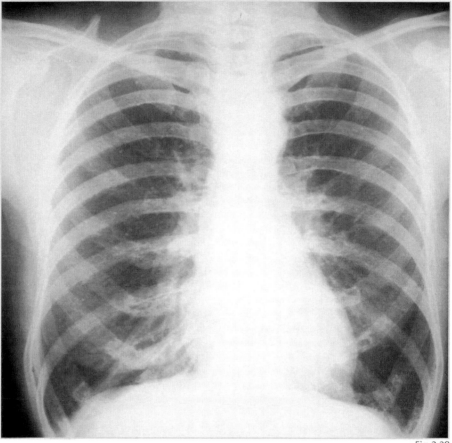

Fig 2.29

1. What do you find on the chest X-ray?
2. What is the diagnosis?
3. What are the clinical features?
4. What are the radiological features?
5. What is the differential diagnosis?

Answers *on pages 101–153*

Case 2.30

A 47-year-old man had a recent operation for a perforated duodenal ulcer. On the third postoperative day, he develops a cough and difficulty breathing. On examination, bronchial breathing is heard in the right side.

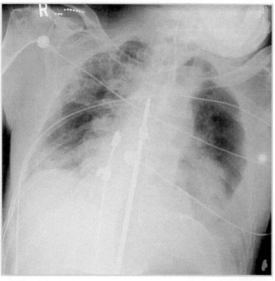

Fig 2.30a

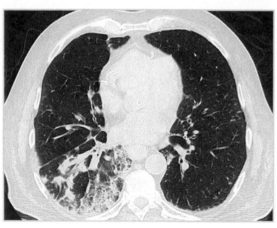

Fig 2.30b

1. What do you see on the plain X-ray and CT scan?
2. What is the diagnosis?
3. What are the predisposing factors and causes?
4. What is the most common location?
5. What are the radiological features and complications?

Answers on pages 101–153

A 30-year-old woman with a past history of spontaneous pneumothorax, presents with cough, dyspnoea and haemoptysis. Clinical examination shows bilateral rhonchi. Pulmonary function tests show an obstructive pattern.

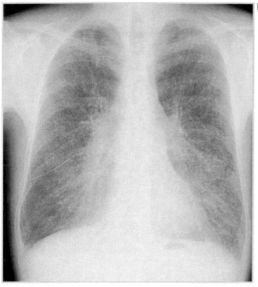
Fig 2.31a

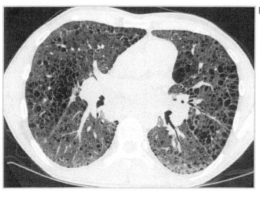
Fig 2.31b

1. What are the findings on the X-ray and CT scan?
2. What is the diagnosis?
3. What is the pathology?
4. What are the other associations of this disease?
5. What are the radiological features?
6. What is the differential diagnosis?

Answers on pages 101–153

Case 2.32

A 58-year-old man presents with a chronic problem of chest pain, difficulty breathing and fever. On examination there are crackles in both lungs. Breath sounds are normal.

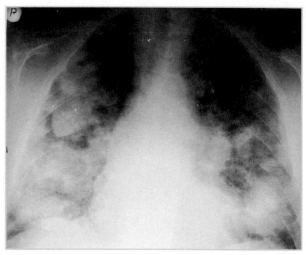
Fig 2.32a

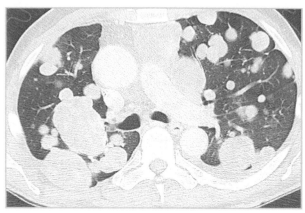
Fig 2.32b

1. What are the findings on the X-ray and CT scan through the upper lobes of the lungs?
2. What is the diagnosis?
3. What are the aetiological factors?
4. What are the radiological features and differential diagnosis?
5. What are the variations in presentation of this disease?

Answers on pages 101–153

Case 2.33

A 43-year-old man presents with fever, non-productive cough, chest pain and dyspnoea. On clinical examination, bilateral bronchial breathing is heard.

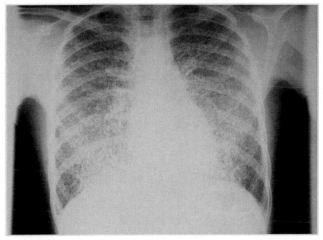
Fig 2.33a

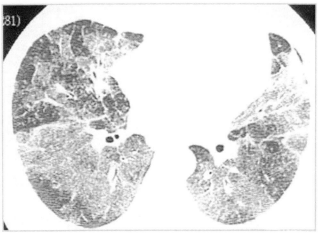
Fig 2.33b

1. What do you find on the chest X-ray and HRCT scan?
2. What is the diagnosis?
3. What are the pathology and pathophysiology of this disease?
4. What are the radiological features?
5. What is the differential diagnosis?

Answers on pages 101–153

Case 2.34

A 53-year-old man presents with right-sided chest pain, fever and dyspnoea. Clinical examination shows decreased breath sounds, stony dullness and tenderness on the left side.

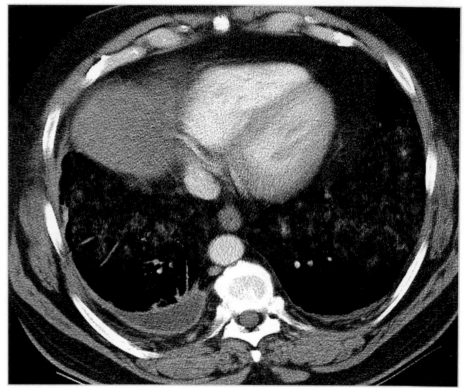

Fig 2.34

1. What do you see on the CT scan?

2. What is the diagnosis?

3. What are the causative agents?

4. What are the pathological stages of this disease process?

5. What are the radiological features?

6. What is the treatment and what is the role of radiology?

Answers on pages 101–153

Case 2.35

A 27-year-old man presents with sudden worsening of his chronic medical problem. On examination he has diffuse, bilateral rhonchi.

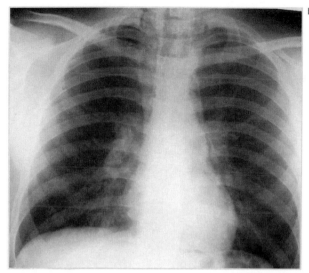

Fig 2.35a

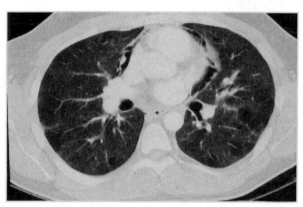

Fig 2.35b

1. What do you see on the plain X-ray and CT scan?
2. What is the diagnosis?
3. What is the cause?
4. What are the common causes?
5. What are the radiological findings?
6. What is the radiological differential diagnosis?

Answers *on pages 101–153*

Case 2.36

A 52-year-old man presents with difficult in breathing and chest pain. The physical examination was unremarkable. An X-ray showed a solitary nodule in the left lower lobe.

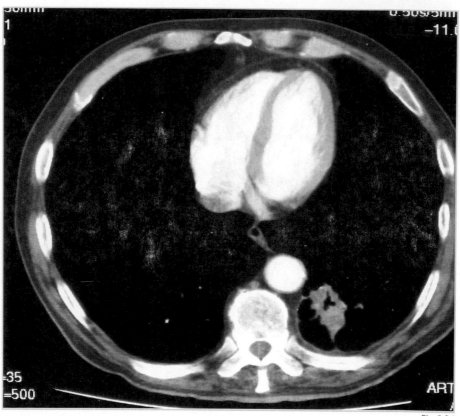

Fig 2.36

1. What do you find on the CT scan?
2. What is the diagnosis?
3. What are the pathology and location of this disease?
4. What are the radiological features?
5. What are the common differential diagnoses?
6. What is Carney's triad?

Answers *on pages 101–153*

Case 2.37

A 37-year-old man presents with long-standing dyspnoea and wheezing.
Clinical examination revealed bronchial breathing and tachypnoea.
Pulmonary function tests revealed an obstructive pattern. The chest X-ray
was unremarkable.

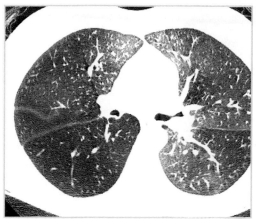

Fig 2.37a

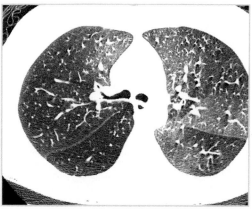

Fig 2.37b

1. What do you find on the CT scan?
2. What is the diagnosis?
3. What is the pathology and what are the types?
4. What are the radiological features?
5. What is the differential diagnosis?

Answers *on pages 101–153*

Case 2.38

A 64-year-old man presents with chest pain, dyspnoea and pain in the right arm. Clinical examination revealed tenderness in the right chest wall, with bronchial breathing in the upper lobe.

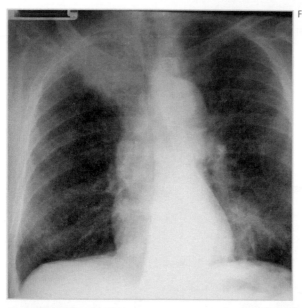

Fig 2.38a

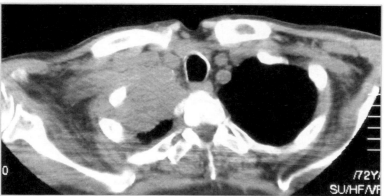

Fig 2.38b

1. What do you observe on the chest X-ray and CT scan?
2. What is the diagnosis?
3. What are the clinical features and treatment?
4. What are the radiological features?
5. What is the differential diagnosis?

Answers on pages 101–153

Case 2.39

A 27-year-old man presents with sudden onset of dyspnoea and chest pain. On examination, the patient is tachycardic, with decreased breath sounds on the right side and a hyperresonant chest on percussion.

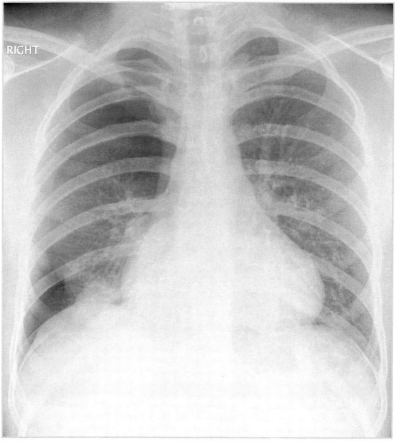

RIGHT

Fig 2.39

1. What are the findings on the chest X-ray?
2. What is the diagnosis?
3. What are the types and causes of this condition?
4. What are the radiological features?
5. What is the indication for treatment?

Answers on pages 101–153

Case 2.40

A 15-year-old girl presents with fever and dyspnoea. On examination the girl is febrile and has tachypnoea. Reduced breath sounds were heard on the right side.

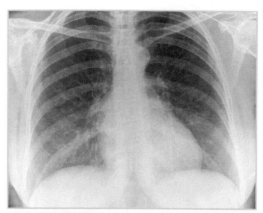

Fig 2.40a

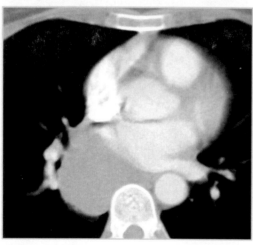

Fig 2.40b

1. What can you see on the chest X-ray?
2. What do you see on the chest CT scan?
3. What are the diagnosis and differential diagnosis?
4. What is the development of this disease?
5. What are the clinical and radiological features of this disease?

Answers on pages 101–153

Case 2.41

A 36-year-old patient with HIV presents with chest pain, dyspnoea and haemoptysis. He gives a past history of skin lesions, which were treated with local resection. Clinically the patient was apyrexial, but bilateral breath sounds were detected on auscultation.

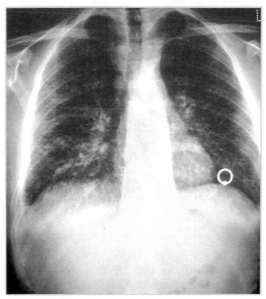
Fig 2.41a

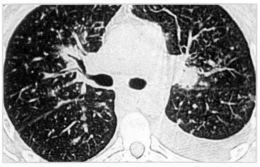
Fig 2.41b

1. What do you find on the chest X-ray and CT scan?
2. What is the diagnosis?
3. What are the clinical features?
4. What are the radiological features?
5. What is the differential diagnosis and how the diagnosis is confirmed?

Answers on pages 101–153

Case 2.42

A 56-year-old miner presents with chronic cough and dyspnoea. Clinical examination was unremarkable.

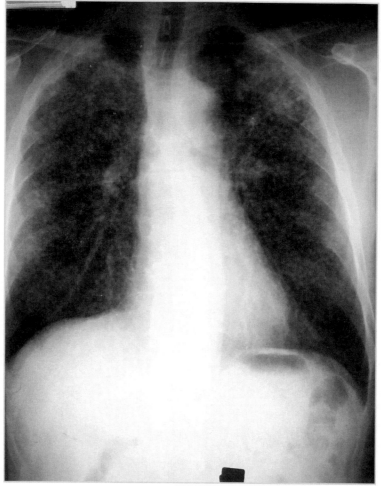

Fig 2.42

1. What do you find on the chest X-ray?
2. What is the diagnosis?
3. What are the causes and clinical features?
4. What are the radiological features?
5. What is the differential diagnosis?

Answers on pages 101–153

Case 2.43

A 38-year-old patient presents with back pain and paraesthesia along the chest wall. On examination, there is tenderness in the lower dorsal spine. Multiple nodules are seen in the skin.

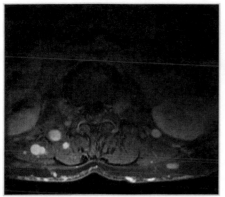
Fig 2.43a

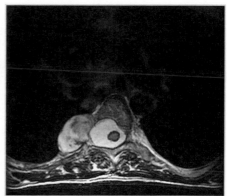
Fig 2.43b

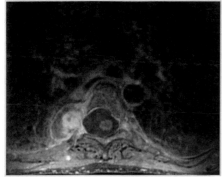
Fig 2.43c

1. What are the findings on MRI?
2. What is the diagnosis?
3. What are the most common location and the most common association?
4. What are the radiological features?
5. What are the complications and what is the differential diagnosis?

Answers *on pages 101–153*

Case 2.44

An 8-year-old girl presents with dyspnoea, fever and cough. Clinical examination showed tachypnoea. The heart sounds are shifted to the right side and the breath sounds are decreased on the right side.

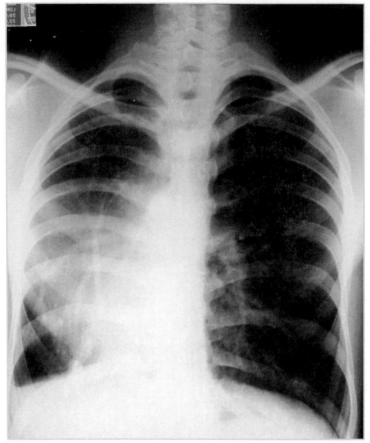

Fig 2.44

1. What do you see on the chest X-ray?
2. What is the diagnosis?
3. What are the causes and associations?
4. What are the clinical features?
5. What are the radiological features?

Answers on pages 101–153

Case 2.45

A 10-year-old Asian girl presents to the accident and emergency department (A&E) with high fever, cough with sputum, dyspnoea, cyanosis, respiratory distress and fatigue. On examination, she is febrile, tachypnoeic, with bilateral bronchial breathing and intercostal recession. Her chest X-ray was done for further evaluation.

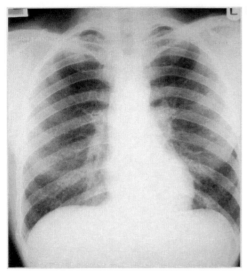
Fig 2.45a

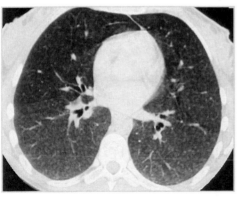
Fig 2.45b

1. What do you observe on the child's chest X-ray?
2. What do you see in this child's HRCT of the chest?
3. What is the diagnosis?
4. What are the clinical features and further tests required for confirmation?
5. What are the radiological features and how will you manage this child?

Answers *on pages 101–153*

Case 2.46

A 9-year-old boy was involved in a road traffic accident and was brought to A&E with dyspnoea, chest pain, haemoptysis and respiratory distress. On examination he was haemodynamically stable, tachypnoeic and had two rib fractures on the left side. Breath sounds were diminished on the left side.

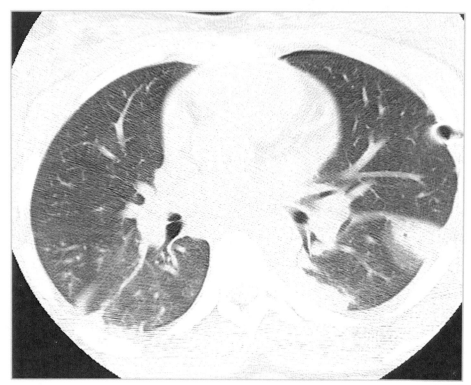

Fig 2.46

1. What do you see on the chest CT scan?
2. What is the diagnosis?
3. What is the differential diagnosis?
4. What are the radiological features and clinical course of this condition?

Answers on pages 101–153

Case 2.47

A 15-year-old girl with acute myeloid leukaemia underwent haematopoietic stem cell transplantation. On day 18 after transplantation, she presents with sudden onset of chest pain, dyspnoea and fever. On examination, she is febrile and tachypnoeic. There is bronchial breathing in the left upper lobe. Lab tests revealed neutropenia.

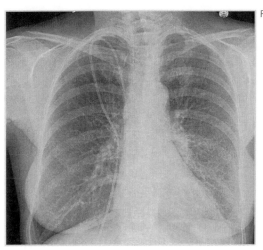

Fig 2.47a

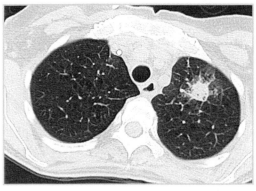

Fig 2.47b

1. What do you observe on the chest X-ray and CT scan?
2. What is the diagnosis?
3. What are the causes of this disease?
4. What are the other complications in patients with bone marrow transplantation?
5. What are the radiological features and differential diagnosis?

Answers *on pages 101–153*

Case 2.48

A 6-year-old girl with a chronic disease presents with dyspnoea and cough with productive sputum. On examination, bronchial breath sounds are heard bilaterally, more on the right side. A chest X-ray and CT scan were done.

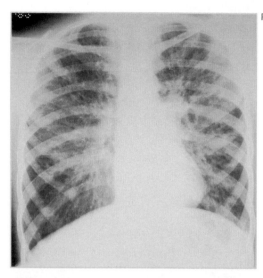

Fig 2.48a

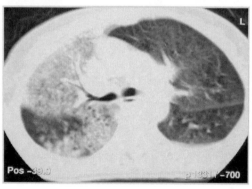

Fig 2.48b

1. What do you see on the chest X-ray and CT scan?
2. What chronic disease condition can you identify?
3. What is the aetiology and common diagnostic tests of this disease?
4. What are the respiratory complications of this disease?
5. What are the radiological features?
6. How is this disease scored?

Answers on pages 101–153

Case 2.49

A 17-year-old man presents with breathing difficulties and recurrent respiratory infections. On examination there are rhonchi in the right lung.

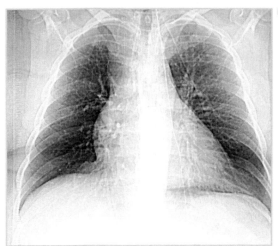

Fig 2.49a

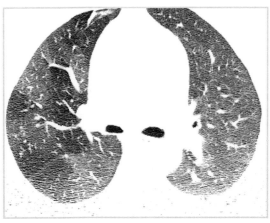

Fig 2.49b

1. What do you see on the chest film and CT scan?
2. What is the diagnosis?
3. What are the mechanism of development and causes of this disease?
4. What are the radiological features?
5. What is the differential diagnosis?

Answers *on pages 101–153*

Case 2.50

A 69-year-old woman presents with increasing dyspnoea and dry cough. She had a mastectomy 2 years ago for breast cancer.

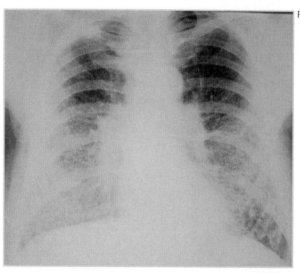

Fig 2.50a

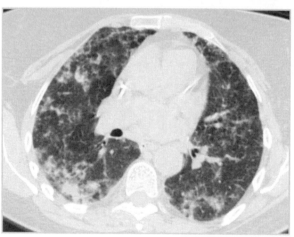

Fig 2.50b

1. What are the findings on the chest X-ray and scan?
2. What is the diagnosis?
3. What are the pathology and causes of this condition?
4. What are the radiological features?
5. What is the differential diagnosis?

Answers on pages 101–153

Case 2.1: Answers

1. The X-ray shows a large, thin-walled cavity in the right upper lobe, with an air–fluid level. There is also patchy consolidation adjacent to the cavity. The CT scan shows the cavitating lesion and surrounding consolidation.

2. Lung abscess.

3. Lung abscess is necrosis of pulmonary tissue and formation of cavities containing necrotic debris or fluid caused by bacterial infection. It is usually caused by anaerobic organisms, such as *peptostreptococcus, microaerophilic streptococcus, Bacteroides* and *fusobacerium*. Other causative organisms are *staphylococcus aureus, streptococcus pyogenes, streptococcus pneumoniase, klebsiella pneumoniase, hemophilius influenae, actinomyces, nocardia* and *gram negative bacilli*. Clinical features are fever, cough, decreased breath sounds, dullness to percussion, bronchial breathing and crackles. Digital clubbing can be seen. The organisms usually reach the lung by aspiration of orpharyngeal contents and are seen in poor dentition, alcoholics and seizure disorder. Haematogenous spread can occur. It can arise due to infection of an underlying bulla or lung cyst.

4. The X-ray shows an irregular cavitating lesion, usually in the lower lobes. The wall can be thin or thick walled. An air–fluid level may be seen. The surrounding lung shows patchy consolidation. Cavities secondary to aspiration are usually seen in the posterior segment of the upper lobe or superior segment of the lower lobe. The wall can be smooth or ragged. When it is nodular, carcinoma should be suspected. As the surrounding lung infection resolves, the wall thickness progresses from thick to thin and from ill defined to well circumscribed. There may be associated empyema. Infections with virulent organisms result in rapid progression to gangrene. CT is useful in identifying associated empyema and lung infarction.

5. The differential diagnoses for cavitating lesion are lung tumours (squamous, adenocarcinoma, lymphoma – a cavitating lung lesion in an older individual should raise suspicion), metastasis (squamous cell metastasis from the cervix, nasopharynx, oesophagus, sarcomas), collagen vascular diseases (Wegener's granulomatosis, rheumatoid arthritis, SLE), sarcoidosis, histiocytosis, infarction, other infections (TB, fungal, hydatid), traumatic lung cyst, large cystic bronchiectasis, bullae and bronchogenic cyst. It might be difficult to differentiate a large abscess from a large empyema. A lateral film helps in the differentiation. The size of the

empyema is different in anteroposterior (AP) and lateral views, but the abscess appears the same. Although the abscess forms an acute angle with the pleural surface, empyema forms an obtuse angle. CT is also helpful in differentiating empyema and lung abscess.

Case 2.2: Answers

1. The X-ray of the chest shows volume reduction, areas of consolidation, fibrosis and cavitations in the right upper lobe. A small area of shadowing is also noted in the medial aspect of the left upper lobe obscuring the aortic knob. The CT scan shows areas of nodular consolidation and small cavities in the posterior segment of the right and left upper lobe.

2. TB.

3. Pulmonary TB can be divided into primary and post-primary types. Primary TB is a disease of childhood and post-primary TB is a disease of adulthood. Post-primary TB is caused by reactivation of *Mycobacterium tuberculosis* infection or reinfection. TB evokes a granulomatous inflammatory response. Most of the lesions are located in the apex and posterior segments of the upper lobe. The superior segment of the lower lobe is also affected. It is more common in the right lobe. TB can be exudative, fibroproductive or cavitatory in nature.

4. The earliest changes in post-primary TB are patchy, ill-defined areas of consolidation, seen in the apical and posterior segments of the upper lobes. Cavitation is the hallmark of post-primary TB and is seen in 50% of individuals. The cavities are thick and irregular and become thin and smooth with treatment. The air–fluid level can be seen in the cavity and often indicates superinfection. Cavities are multiple and occur within areas of consolidation. Superimposed fungal ball infection can result in a crescent sign, which is caused by air entrapped in between the fungal ball and the wall. Cavities heal with scarring and emphysematous changes. The CT scan shows micronodules, consolidation and cavities. In airway spread/endobronchial disease, tree-in-bud opacities (resembling a branching tree with buds at the tips of its branches) are seen and are an indicator of active TB. In healing/healed TB areas of fibrosis and scars are seen. A thick-walled irregular cavity is seen as a result of expulsion of necrosis into the airways. Fibrosis causes volume loss, mediastinal shift and

fibrotic strands. Other findings are pleural thickening, pleural effusion, bronchopleural fistula and lymphadenopathy. Airway obstruction results in bronchial stenosis with resultant collapse, mucus plugging and obstructive pneumonitis. Tuberculous effusions are septated and may result in pleural thickening, calcification and bronchopleural fistulae.

5. Differential diagnoses for upper lobe fibrotic lesions are: post-radiation pneumonitis, silicosis, sarcoidosis, ankylosing spondylitis, eosinophilic granuloma, fungal infection and cystic fibrosis.

Case 2.3: Answers

1. The X-ray shows a cavity in the left upper lobe, with an intraluminal solid mass and a crescent of air between the wall and the solid lesion. The CT scan shows the cavity with an intraluminal solid lesion. There is air seen between the soft tissue and the wall of the cavity. A similar appearance is seen on the right side as well.

2. Fungal ball.

3. *Aspergillus fumigatus* is the causative organism. The fungus ball is produced by a mass-like collection of fungal hyphae matted with fibrin, mucus and cellular debris.

4. *A. fumigatus* colonises pre-existing cavities in immunologically normal patients. Cavities are seen in TB, sarcoidosis, cancer, bronchiectasis, pulmonary fibrosis, abscess, trauma, surgery, ankylosing spondylitis, neurofibromatosis and bullae.

5. The X-ray shows a cavitating lesion with an intraluminal solid lesion. The air crescent sign indicates a crescent-shaped airspace that separates the fungal ball from the non-dependent cavity. The fungal ball is gravity dependent within a spherical or ovoid, thin-walled cavity (Monad's sign). This can be demonstrated by taking X-rays in different positions; the position of the fungal ball changes with each position. The CT scan confirms the presence of an intraluminal gravity-dependent mass. Rim or scattered calcification can be seen. Pleural thickening and adjacent consolidation may be present.

6. The air crescent sign is produced by other intraluminal solid lesions such as invasive pulmonary aspergillosis, carcinoma and hydatid cyst. Rarer causes are tuberculoma, lung abscess, sarcoma, metastasis, adenoma, hamartoma, haematoma, thromboembolism and Rasmussen's aneurysm. In doubtful cases, biopsy or aspiration of the cavity is indicated to initiate treatment.

Case 2.4: Answers

1. The X-ray shows hyperinflated lungs, with loss of vascular markings and distortion of existing vascular markings. High-resolution CT (HRCT) shows extensive, dark, lucent areas in the lungs with multiple bullae.

2. Panacinar emphysema.

3. Emphysema is permanent, irreversible enlargement of airspaces distal to terminal bronchioles with destruction of the alveolar walls. The types are **centrilobular emphysema** (enlarged respiratory bronchioles, destruction of centrilobular septa surrounded by normal lung with sparing of distal alveoli, seen in people who smoke, usually in apical and posterior segments of the upper lobe and superior segment of the lower lobe), **panacinar emphysema** (involvement of entire acinus, with uniform destruction of all airspaces, associated with α_1-antitrypsin deficiency, more severe at the bases), **paracicatricial emphysema** (focal irregular emphysema caused by inflammation, infarction or infection) and **paraseptal emphysema** (involvement of alveolar ducts and sacs, and subpleural in distribution).

4. The radiological findings include hyperinflated lungs (the diaphragm seen below the seventh anterior rib), flat hemidiaphragm (< 1.5 cm distance between the line connecting the costophrenic and cardiophrenic angles and the top of the hemidiaphragm). The coronal diameter of the trachea is narrowed (sabre sheath trachea). In the lateral view, the AP diameter of the chest is increased (barrel chest) and there is increased retrosternal airspace (> 2.5 cm). The vascular markings are distorted and pruned. In late stages, with onset of cor pulmonale, the heart is enlarged and prominent pulmonary arteries are seen.

5. HRCT is not used in diagnosis, but is useful in planning for treatment. In centrilobular emphysema, there are dark areas of air density, with a central bright dot – the centrilobular artery. In panacinar emphysema, there is diffuse air attenuation, with distorted or absent vascular markings. HRCT is used to measure the lung volume and assess suitability of lung volume reduction surgery.

6. Pneumothorax can result from rupture of subpleural bullae. Respiratory failure and cor pulmonale are other serious complications. Emphysema is seen in α_1-antitrypsin deficiency (early presentation, bases involved and panacinar in type). Smoking, intravenous drug use, immunodeficiency syndromes, vasculitis, connective tissue disorders (cutis laxa, Marfan syndrome, Ehler–Danlos syndrome) and Salla syndrome are recognised causes of emphysema.

Case 2.5: Answers

1. The X-ray shows a homogeneous consolidation in the left midzone with an air bronchogram within it. There is no mediastinal shift and no blunting of the costophrenic angle. The CT scan of the chest shows a large area of consolidation in the lingula of the left lung, with surrounding ground-glass opacity.

2. Pneumonia: this is inflammation and consolidation of the lung tissue as a result of an infectious agent. Pneumonia developing 72 hours or more after hospital admission is called nosocomial pneumonia and outside the hospital setting community-acquired pneumonia.

3. In adults the most common cause of community-acquired pneumonia is pneumococci. Typical organisms in adults are *Strep. pneumoniae, H. influenzae* and staphylococci. Atypical pneumonias are caused by *Legionella, Mycoplasma* and *Chlamydia* spp. Nosocomial pneumonias are usually caused by Gram-negative organisms such as *Pseudomonas aeruginosa, Klebsiella pneumoniae, E. coli* and *Staphylococcus aureus*. In people with alcohol problems and those with altered mental status, anaerobic bacteria are responsible.

4. Predisposing factors are old age, debilitation, alcoholism, congestive cardiac failure, chronic obstructive pulmonary disease (COPD), multiple myeloma, hypogammaglobulinaemia and asplenia. Clinical features are blood-streaked rusty sputum and respiratory distress.

5. The usual radiological finding is an alveolar opacity, which is homogeneous and ill defined with an air bronchogram. The consolidation can be segmental or lobar. Extensive consolidation abutting the visceral pleura, confined to or extending beyond one lobe, is a characteristic finding of pneumococcal pneumonia. Anaerobes have a tendency to localise in the dependent portions. Community-acquired pneumonias cause less lung destruction and cavitation than organisms associated with bronchopneumonia and anaerobic lung infection. Effusions can be associated and occasionally empyemas are seen. Pneumatoceles are seen in staphylococcal infection. Occasionally pneumonias can present with just effusions, empyema or a bronchopneumonia-like pattern. Viral infections can present as bronchiolitis with a normal X-ray, bronchiolitis with parahilar or peribronchial opacities, atelectasis, or reticulonodular interstitial or hazy lungs. The differential diagnosis includes **aspiration pneumonia** – (has a characteristic distribution. In the supine position, it is seen in the upper lobe and superior segments of the lower lobes. In the upright position, it is seen in both lower lobes and associated with segmental and subsegmental atelectasis, interstitial fibrosis or inflammatory bronchial thickening and effusions), **pulmonary oedema, pulmonary haemorrhage, sarcoidosis, lymphoma, bronchoalveolar carcinoma and alveolar proteinosis**: HRCT can be used when the diagnosis is in doubt. The CT scan is also useful in the diagnosis of complications. Most pneumonias resolve quickly with antibiotic treatment and radiological changes improve within days with near or complete resolution in 2–3 weeks. Persistent or recurrent pneumonia should raise the suspicion of an underlying pulmonary abnormality.

6. Complications of pneumonia are pneumothorax, bronchiectasis, bronchiolitis obliterans, necrotising pneumonia, abscess, meningitis, endocarditis, septic arthritis, empyema, ARDS, respiratory failure and Swyer–James syndrome (small, hyperlucent lungs with decreased vascular markings). Antibiotics are administered depending on the organism.

Case 2.6: Answers

1. The chest X-ray shows volume reduction of the left thorax, mediastinal shift to the left side and veil-like opacification of the left lung. A subtle area of lucency is seen close to the aortic knuckle.

2. These are characteristic appearances of left upper lobe collapse.

3. The CT scan shows a triangular opacity in the left upper lobe indicating collapse. There is a convex smooth mass adjacent to the left main bronchus, which merges imperceptibly with the collapsed portion. This patient has bronchogenic carcinoma with collapse of the left upper lobe.

4. When the left upper lobe collapses the collapsed lobe and the oblique fissure moves forwards and the hilum is displaced upwards and the major fissure is displaced forwards. The lobe retains much of its original contact with the anterior chest wall. This produces a veil-like opacity over the left hemithorax, more dense towards the apex. The anterior mediastinal fat and trachea are displaced to the left side. The left diaphragm is moderately elevated. The lower lobe expands behind the collapsed left upper lobe. Hence, the aortic knuckle that is situated towards the back of the chest is clearly visible. Air is seen between the lung and aorta (Lufsichel's sign). In the lateral view, the collapsed lung is seen as a band of soft-tissue density retrosternally, with a sharp posterior margin caused by vertical oblique fissure. One of the most common causes of an obstructive atelectasis is a tumour mass located in the parahilar situation, producing a bulge in the contour of the collapsed lobe (the Golden S sign).

5. Lung cancer is the most common fatal malignant neoplasm in men. Aetiological factors are smoking, asbestos, arsenic, chromium, chloromethyl ether, mustard gas and genetic factors. Idiopathic pulmonary fibrosis, systemic sclerosis and TB increase risk of adenocarcinomas. Patients with central tumours present with wheezing, haemoptysis, cough, infection, laryngeal nerve palsy, pleural or chest wall pain, SVC obstruction, paraneoplastic syndromes (clubbing, hypertrophic osteoarthropathy, osteomalacia, Cushing's disease, hyponatraemia, neuromuscular dysfunction, myopathy, neuropathy, cerebellar degeneration, encephalomyelopathy). Common types are adenocarcinoma, squamous cell carcinoma, small cell carcinoma and large cell carcinoma. The CT scan is used for staging the tumour. Bronchoscopy, biopsy and staging CT scan of the chest and upper abdomen are performed. Chemotherapy, surgery or radiation is performed depending on the stage and histological type.

Case 2.7: Answers

1. The chest X-ray shows volume reduction of the lung bases. There are patchy reticular opacities in both lower lobes and the heart border is irregular. High resolution CT shows extensive thickening of the interlobular septa and honeycombing in both bases.

2. Usual interstitial pneumonia/idiopathic pulmonary fibrosis.

3. Interstitial pneumonias are divided into usual interstitial pneumonia, desquamative interstitial pneumonia, bronchiolitis-related interstitial pneumonia, non-specific interstitial pneumonia and lymphoid interstitial pneumonia. Usual interstitial pneumonia was previously called idiopathic pulmonary fibrosis, idiopathic interstitial pneumonia and cryptogenic fibrosing alveolitis. It is commonly seen in the fifth and sixth decades and is more common in men. Pathologically it is characterised by inflammatory cells, fibrosis, honeycombing and areas of normal lung tissue. Clinically, there is dyspnoea, non-productive couch, fatigue and clubbing. Velcro râles are heard in the end-inspiratory phase. Pulmonary function tests show a restrictive pattern and bronchoalveolar lavage shows lymphocytosis.

4. The X-ray shows bilateral, basal reticular or reticulonodular opacities. Honeycombing is seen in the later stages, where are there are multiple tiny cystic spaces. Volume loss is seen with a shaggy irregular heart margin and elevation of the diaphragm. In the early stages, HRCT is used to confirm the diagnosis. HRCT shows thickening of the interstitium, which is seen as thick interlobular septa. It is characteristically located in the peripheral subpleural regions of the lower lobes. Subpleural honeycombing, lines and bands can be seen. Traction bronchiectasis is seen as a result of fibrosis. In the early stages, ground-glass opacities can be seen caused by alveolitis, alveolar wall thickening or early fibrosis. The 5-year survival rate is 45%.

5. The common differential diagnoses for lower lobe fibrotic changes are usual interstitial pneumonia, desquamative interstitial pneumonia, asbestosis, connective tissue diseases (scleroderma, SLE, rheumatoid) and drug-induced lung disease (bleomycin, busulphan, cyclophosphamide, nitrofurantoin). Desquamative interstitial pneumonia is seen in a younger age group, located in middle and lower ones, and has a better prognosis and response with steroids.

Case 2.8: Answers

1. The X-ray shows a volume reduction of the right upper lobe, with tracheal deviation to the right side. There is a homogeneous area of consolidation in the right parahilar regions, on air bronchograms and a well-defined lateral margin.

2. Radiation pneumonitis.

3. Radiation pneumonitis is secondary to exposure of lungs to radiation. There are two types: **acute** and **chronic**. The acute type is seen 1–6 months after treatment with a peak at 3–4 months. The chronic type is seen 9–12 months after treatment.

4. The critical factors that increase the incidence are:

    (a) dose: it is seen if > 60 Gy given in 5–6 weeks or daily fraction > 2.7 Gy

    (b) fractionation of dose

    (c) lung volume irradiated > 25%

    (d) chemotherapy.

    Pathological changes occur in the first 24–48 hours, but these cannot be detected clinically or radiologically. Acute type peaks in 3–4 months. There is hyaline membrane formation, endothelial damage and arteritis. Regeneration begins at the peak of inflammation. Subsequently fibrosis starts, with progression for 12–18 months. Sclerosis of pulmonary vessels and bronchi leads to oligaemia and bronchiectasis

5. Acute radiation pneumonitis can be detected 6–8 weeks after the start of therapy. It has the appearance of a consolidation with an air bronchogram, but with well-defined, sharp margins conforming to the radiation portal field. In the earliest stages, ground-glass opacities can be seen. The changes are caused by depletion of surfactant, plasma exudation, and desquamation of alveolar and bronchial cells. It can be asymptomatic or produce couch, dyspnoea, fever and weakness, and usually persists for up to a month. The CT scan shows a discrete heterogeneous consolidation, with a sharp edge conforming to the radiation portal. Pleural effusions can be seen. During regeneration, the lung changes become more linear or reticular. The chronic type is caused by permanent damage to the alveolar and endothelial cells. The X-ray shows volume loss, opacity, fibrous strands, pleural thickening and pericardial effusion. The CT scan shows

the fibrosis with traction bronchiectasis, pleural thickening and volume loss with mediastinal shift. The acute stage is treated with steroids. The differential diagnosis for acute radiation pneumonitis includes all other causes of consolidation, such as infection, oedema, sarcoid. But the characteristic sharply defined margins and confinement to the radiation portal are pathognomonic. Differentiation between chronic radiation pneumonitis and recurrent tumour is essential. CT and MRI can be useful. Fibrosis will be of low signal in T1- and T2-weighted images, but tumour has low signal in T1- and high signal in T2-weighted images.

Case 2.9: Answers

1. There is homogeneous opacification of the right side of chest, which has been whited out. There is mediastinal shift to the left side, which is normal. In the CT scan, there is a collection with fluid density in the right hemithorax, and collapse of the underlying right lower lobe (seen medially as a dense opacity). There is no air in the pleural cavity. The mediastinum is shifted to the left side.

2. Pleural effusion. The differential diagnoses for a homogeneous opacification of lung are: consolidation (no mediastinal shift), collapse (mediastinal shift to same side), agenesis (mediastinal shift, compensatory inflation on opposite side), large pulmonary/pleural mass and radiation.

3. **Increased hydrostatic pressure**: congestive cardiac failure, constrictive pericarditis; **decreased colloid oncotic pressure**: cirrhosis, nephritic syndrome, hypothyroidism; **chylous effusion – infections**: empyema, parapneumonic effusion, TB, *Actinomyces* sp., hydatid amoebiasis, mycoplasmas; **tumours**: metastasis, lymphoma; **vascular**: PE; **abdominal diseases**: pancreatitis, oesophageal perforation, subphrenic abscess, abdominal tumour with ascites, bile fistula; **collagen vascular diseases**: juvenile rheumatoid arthritis, SLE, Wegener's granulomatosis, mixed connective tissue disease; **trauma, miscellaneous**: drugs, uraemia.

4. The characteristic features of exudates:

   (a) pleural fluid protein/serum total protein > 0.5

   (b) pleural fluid/serum lactate dehydrogenase (LDH) > 0.6

(c) pleural fluid LDH > two-thirds upper limit of normal, for serum LDH

(d) pleural fluid protein > 3 g/dl

(e) pleural fluid specific gravity > 1.016

(f) effusion has internal septations or loculations

(g) CT split pleura sign: enhancement of thickened pleural layers separated by fluid

(h) extrapleural fat thickening > 2 mm, with high density in the fat.

5. X-rays detect effusions when there is 300 ml fluid. Initially fluid collects in the subpulmonic space, which might not be seen well on the X-ray. Lateral decubitus view can detect 25 ml fluid. Ultrasonography can detect even smaller amounts and can differentiate effusion from consolidation. Transudates are clear, but exudates have septations or echogenic debris within it. Guided aspiration of fluid can be done for diagnosis or treatment. Subpulmonic effusions can be identified by a lateral peak of the diaphragm's dome, increased distance between the stomach bubble and lung, blunted posterior costophrenic angle and thin triangular mediastinal opacity. With increasing size of effusion, the costophrenic angles are blunted and there is homogeneous opacification of the lower lobes, with effacement of the dome of the diaphragm. There is a meniscus-shaped upper surface and associated collapse of the underlying lung. In massive effusion, the entire chest may be white, with mediastinal shift to the opposite side along with depression, flattening or inversion of the diaphragmatic dome. Loculated effusions can be drained under ultrasonic guidance.

Case 2.10: Answers

1. The X-ray shows multiple thin-walled cavities, of varying sizes in both upper zones. The CT scan shows thin-walled cavities in both the upper lobes. Surrounding consolidation is seen in the left upper lobe.

2. Wegner's granulomatosis.

3. Wegener's granulomatosis is an autoimmune disease characterised by systemic necrotising granulomatous destructive angiitis. The vasculitis affects medium- and small-sized pulmonary arteries, veins and capillaries, causing geographical necrosis and granulomatous inflammation. In the

lungs there are peribronchial granulomas and vasculitis. It is more common in males and seen in all age groups. Diagnosis is confirmed by cANCAs (cytoplasmic anti-neutrophil cytoplasmic antibodies) and lung or renal biopsy.

4. The earliest changes in the lungs are bilateral interstitial reticulonodular opacities in the bases. The characteristic appearance is multifocal, irregular nodules or masses, in the lower lobes, sparing the apices; eventually they cavitate, with thick walls and irregular shaggy lining. Multifocal consolidation can be seen. Pleural effusion and bronchial wall thickening may also be seen. CT shows peribronchovascular nodules. Large nodules show central cavitation, with feeding vessels entering the nodules. Pleurally based wedge-shaped infarcts are also seen. Clinical presentations are stridor, cough, haemoptysis, rhinitis, sinusitis and otitis media. Complications are airway stenosis, pulmonary haemorrhage and spontaneous pneumothorax.

5. The most common differential diagnosis is Churg–Strauss disease (shows pANCAs (perinuclear ANCAs), less severe renal and sinus disease, more cardiac involvement). Differential diagnoses for multiple cavitations in lungs are metastasis, TB, septic emboli, pseudomonas infection, bronchiectasis, lymphoma, multicentric bronchoalveolar disease, rheumatoid nodules, sarcoidosis and histiocytosis. Other clinical conditions to be excluded are SLE and subacute bacterial endocarditis.

6. The characteristic triad is respiratory tract granulomatous inflammation, systemic small vessel vasculitis and necrotising glomerulonephritis. Sinusitis, granulomatous mass in the nasal cavity with septal destruction, focal glomerulonephritis, migratory polyarthropathy, nodular skin lesions, coronary vasculitis and neuritis are other features. Complications are uraemia, hypertension and facial nerve palsy. Treatment is with steroids, cytotoxic agents and renal transplantation. Death is in 2 years as a result of renal or respiratory failure.

Case 2.11: Answers

1. The X-ray shows mediastinal widening with some trachial shift due to a large lobulated mass in the superior aspect of the mediastinum. The CT scan shows a lobulated mass in the prevascular space of the anterior mediastinum.

2. Thymoma.

3. Thymoma is the most common primary tumour in the anterior mediastinum. It arises from the thymus and is usually benign, although it can be malignant. It is commonly seen in the fifth and sixth decades. It can be predominantly epithelial, lymphocytic or biphasic. The nature of the tumour is determined by the presence or absence of spread beyond the capsule. Usually it is asymptomatic, but can present with features of mediastinal compression, cough, dyspnoea, chest pain, infection, hoarseness or dysphagia.

4. Myasthenia gravis is the most common association. Up to 55% of patients with thymoma have myasthenia gravis; 25% of patients with myasthenia gravis have thymomas (65% have thymic hyperplasia). Removal of a thymoma results in improvement of the myasthenia. Myasthenia can develop after surgical removal. Other associations are pure red cell aplasia, hypogammaglobulinaemia and Cushing syndrome.

5. Thymomas are commonly seen in the anterior mediastinum. The X-ray shows a round or oval, lobulated, sharply demarcated mass, resulting in a wide mediastinum. Amorphous or curvilinear calcification can be seen. In the lateral view, they are seen characteristically in the anterior mediastinum. Very rarely, they can be seen lower down in the mediastinum, adjacent to the heart. CT shows a homogeneous soft-tissue mass with lobulated margins, and homogeneous enhancement with areas of fibrosis, cysts, necrosis and calcification. Diagnosis can be confirmed by CT-guided biopsy. In malignant thymoma, the density is heterogeneous and the tumour extends along the pleural surfaces to reach the posterior mediastinum, diaphragmatic crus and retroperitonum. The differential diagnoses include other mediastinal tumours such as germ cell tumours, lymphoma, metastasis and retrosternal thyroid.

Case 2.12: Answers

1. The X-ray shows a lobulated mediastinal mass extending over the right hilar region which that is not obscuring the vascular structures, which are seen through the mass. There is also an enlarged right hilar node. The CT scan shows a lobulated mass in the anterior mediastinum, which is encasing the vascular structures and compressing and displacing the trachea to the left side.

2. Lymphoma: the clinical symptoms of head and neck swelling and oedema are produced as a result of compression of the SVC by the tumour.

3. Lymphoma is divided into Hodgkin's and non-Hodgkin's types. Hodgkin's lymphoma is more common in the thorax than non-Hodgkin's lymphoma at presentation. There are four types of Hodgkin's lymphoma: **lymphocyte predominant, lymphocyte depleted, mixed** and **nodular sclerosing**. Nodular sclerosing type is common in the mediastinum. Non-Hodgkin's lymphoma is classified into low-, intermediate- and high-grade lesions, according to the Working classification. According to the World Health Organization (WHO) classification, lymphomas are classified into B-cell, T-cell and natural killer (NK) cell tumours, Hodgkin's lymphoma and other minor groups.

4. In the chest, lymphoma commonly affects the anterior mediastinum, and pretracheal, hilar, subcarinal, axillary, perioesophageal, paracardiac, superior diaphragmatic and internal mammary nodes. Hodgkin's lymphoma affects the anterior mediastinum more whereas non-Hodgkin's lymphoma the posterior mediastinum.

5. The X-ray shows a lobulated anterior mediastinal mass. Mediastinal masses produce mediastinal widening. The location in the mediastinum can be determined by the relationship with the pulmonary vasculature and adjacent structures. If the pulmonary vasculature is seen through the lesion, the mass is in either the anterior or the posterior mediastinum. Middle mediastinal tumours obliterate pulmonary vasculature. In posterior mediastinal lesions, the paraspinal line is obliterated. The CT scan shows homogeneous, lobulated, lymph node masses. Calcification and necrosis are uncommon before treatment with radio- or chemotherapy. CT scans of the chest, abdomen and pelvis are indicated for staging the disease.

6. Germ cell tumour, thymoma, metastasis, retrosternal thyroid and aneurysm are the other differential diagnoses of anterior mediastinal disorders.

Case 2.13: Answers

1. The chest X-ray shows a round, well-defined, homogeneous mass in the periphery of the right lower lobe, with a crescent of air in the superior aspect. This is better seen in the lateral view.

2. Hydatid cyst of the lung.

3. Hydatid cysts are caused by the parasite *Echinococcus granulosus*. The primary host is sheep and humans are the intermediate host. Larvae develop in the duodenum, from where they penetrate the wall, enter blood vessels and travel to the liver and lungs. Clinical features are cough, haemoptysis, chest pain, fever, eosinophilia and positive Casoni's test. The lung is the second most common site after the liver. Hydatid cysts have two layers – the exocyst and the endocyst – within which daughter cysts are seen. The cysts grow rapidly and rupture into the lung and bronchi or rarely into the pleural cavity. Secondary infection can be seen.

4. Lower lobes are more commonly involved. Multiple and bilateral lesions are seen in 20–25%. Usually the lesions are very large and can range from 1 cm to 20 cm, and are well circumscribed round or oval masses. The various signs are:

(a) **crescent/meniscus sign**: a radiolucent crescent in the upper part of the cyst caused by rupture of the pericyst and air dissection between the pericyst and laminated membrane

(b) **mass within the cavity**: caused by membranes falling to dependent portion of cavity after expectoration of cyst fluid

(c) **air–fluid level**: rupture of all cyst walls with air entering the cyst

(d) **Cumbo's sign**: air–fluid level inside the endocyst and air between the pericyst and endocyst

(e) **serpent sign**: collapsed membranes inside the cyst outlined by air

(f) **waterlily sign**: collapsed crumpled membrane floating in the cyst fluid.

Calcification is not seen in the lung hydatid as a result of frequent respiratory movements. All these signs are well demonstrated on a CT scan. When there is secondary infection, the walls are thickened and differentiation from a bacterial lung abscess is difficult. Complications include abscess and rupture.

5. Differential diagnoses for a large peripheral mass in lung include: squamous cell carcinoma, large cell carcinoma, canon-ball metastasis, sarcoma, abscess and plasmacytoma.

Chest Answers

Case 2.14: Answers

1. The chest X-ray shows extensive, bilateral, coarse, reticular opacities and cystic changes, in the upper lobes.

2. *Pneumocystis jiroveci* pneumonia. The distribution of the disease in the upper lobes is a result of treatment with aerosolised pentamidine.

3. HIV. *Pneumocystis jiroveci* (formerly *P. carinii*) is a type of interstitial pneumonia seen in immunocompromised patients. It is caused by an obligate extracellular protozoon that produces trophozoites, which develop into cysts; these, in turn, produce eight daughter sporozoites, which are released at maturity and develop into trophozoites. The trophozoite attaches to cell membranes of type I alveolar cells, resulting in cell death and leak of proteinaceous fluid into the alveolar space. HIV, lymphoproliferative disorders and transplant recipients are common immunocompromised conditions.

4. The X-ray is occasionally normal. The characteristic features are perihilar, bilateral symmetrical, finely granular, reticular, interstitial or airspace infiltrates. This can progress to consolidation with an air bronchogram. Other features are nodules, cavitation, enlarged lymph nodes and pleural effusion. Cavities are seen in upper lobes, which may be thin or thick walled, regular or irregular. It usually responds to therapy with nebulised pentamidine or co-trimoxazole in 5–7 days. After prophylactic use of aerosolised pentamidine, the infection may be redistributed to the upper lobe. Shell-like calcifications and pneumothorax are also seen. CT shows a bilateral, asymmetrical, patchy mosaic appearance of a ground-glass pattern or bilateral linear/reticular markings. Characteristic features are air-filled spaces, which could be pneumatoceles (thin-walled space, without lobar predilection), thin-walled cysts or subpleural bullae. Associated features are lymphadenopathy, pneumothorax, nodules and cavities.

5. Diagnosis is confirmed with sputum collection, bronchoscopy, transbronchial, transthoracic/open lung biopsy. Differential diagnosis includes Kaposi's sarcoma, TB and MAI (*Mycobacterium avium-intracellulare*) infection.

Case 2.15: Answers

1. In the chest X-ray, the heart is located on the right side. There is also increased opacification of the right lower zone. The left lung appears normal

2. HRCT confirms the presence of dextrocardia. There are dilated bronchi in the right lower lobe. The bronchi are also thickened, with mucus plugging within them, and there are patchy opacities in the right lower lobe.

3. Kartagener syndrome.

4. Kartagener syndrome, also called immotile cilia syndrome, is caused by deficiency of dynein arms of cilia, which causes immobility of respiratory, auditory and sperm cilia, and is inherited in an autosomal recessive fashion. It is characterised by the triad of situs inversus, chronic sinusitis and bronchiectasis. The typical ciliary axoneme consists of two central microtubules surrounded by nine microtubular doublets. Each doublet has an A and a B subunit attached as a semicircle. A central sheath envelops the two central microtubules, which attach to the outer doublets by radial spokes. The outer doublets are interconnected by nexin links, and each A subunit is attached to two dynein arms that contain adenosine triphosphatase (ATPase) – one inner arm and one outer arm. The primary function of the central sheath, radial spokes and nexin links is to maintain the structural integrity of the cilium, whereas the dynein arms are responsible for ciliary motion. Clinically the patients have chronic mucoid rhinorrhoea, recurrent chronic sinusitis, recurrent otitis media, chronic bronchitis, recurrent pneumonia, bronchiectasis, obstructive lung disease, digital clubbing and infertility.

5. The radiological features are thoracic and abdominal situs inversus, bronchiectasis, sinus hypoplasia and mucosal thickening. A saccharine test and biopsy can be done to confirm ciliary dysmotility. Antibiotics are given for infections, tympanostomy done for otitis media, functional endoscopic sinus surgery for chronic sinus problems, and bronchodilators are given for obstructive lung disease.

Case 2.16: Answers

1. The chest X-ray shows a round, lobulated lesion in the right parahilar region, close to the right pulmonary artery. The CT scan shows a lobulated, tubular opacity in the anterior segment of the right upper lobe.

2. Bronchial atresia.

3. Bronchial atresia is an anomaly characterised by obliteration of the proximal lumen of segmental bronchus, with preservation of distal structures, probably secondary to insufficient blood supply to the bronchial bud during development, which results in blind termination of the bronchus. It is most common in the left upper lobe (apical and posterior segments), followed by segmental bronchi of the right upper lobe, middle lobe and, rarely, lower lobe. The bronchial tree proximal to the atresia is patent. Mucus secretions accumulate at the point of obstruction. Air enters the affected segment by collateral channels and causes air trapping. Clinical presentation is non-specific and can be asymptomatic, shortness of breath or cough. It can be associated with ASD, pericardial defects, left-sided IVC, congenital cystic adenomatoid malformation, partial anomalous venous drainage of the left upper lobe and sequestration.

4. Obstructed segment is seen as a lucent area on the X-ray. An area of mucus accumulation is seen as a tubular area with a branching pattern. A characteristic sign is the 'gloved finger' sign, which is characterised by branching tubular or finger-like opacities, originating from the hila and directed peripherally. The CT scan shows segmental overinflation. Mucoid impaction is seen as a tubular structure. Occasionally hyperinflation is not seen when the lesion is completely separated from other pulmonary lobes, preventing collateral ventilation from adjacent lung.

5. The most common differential diagnosis is a dilated pulmonary vascular structure, which can be easily differentiated by a CT scan. Other differential diagnoses are bronchogenic cyst and pulmonary sequestration. Acquired causes of mucoid impaction are bronchial hamartoma, lipoma, carcinoid and carcinoma. Non-obstructive causes of the gloved finger sign are allergic bronchopulmonary aspergillosis in asthmatic patients and cystic fibrosis. Overinflation of the left upper lobe can be caused by bronchial atresia, bronchogenic cyst in the aortic concavity and stenosed tracheal bronchus.

Case 2.17: Answers

1. The X-ray shows bilateral, enlarged and lobulated hilar nodes, and an enlarged right paratracheal node. The CT scan shows multiple nodules and consolidation in the central portions of the lungs and bilateral lymphadenopathy.

2. Sarcoidosis.

3. Sarcoidosis is characterised by the presence of non-caseating granulomas, made up of multinucleated giant cells, lymphocytes and fibroblasts with central necrosis. Stages of pulmonary sarcoidosis:
   Stage 0 – normal X-ray
   Stage I – mediastinal and hilar lymphadenopathy
   Stage II – lymphadenopathy and parenchymal disease
   Stage III – only parenchymal disease
   Stage IV – fibrosis.
   In sarcoidosis, hypercalcaemia and hypercalciuria are seen. The angiotensin-converting enzyme (ACE) levels are elevated and indicate the granuloma load in the body. The Kveim–Slitbach test is positive. When the lungs are involved, the vital capacity, functional residual capacity and total lung capacity are reduced.

4. The earliest change on the X-ray is lymphadenopathy. Garland's triad is characteristic of sarcoidosis and includes bilateral hilar adenopathy, right paratracheal node and aortopulmonary window node. The nodes are lobulated and have sharp margins. Egg-shell calcification is seen in 5–20%. The adenopathy decreases as the parenchymal involvement increases. Parenchymal involvement can present with small ill-defined nodules that are 6–7 mm or larger nodules of 10–50 mm, or consolidation with an air bronchogram. In the late stages fibrosis is seen. The disease distribution is in the mid and lower zones. HRCT is used for characterisation of the disease. It shows thickened peribronchovascular septa, with nodules and nodular septal thickening and centrilobular nodules. Honeycombing, fibrosis and traction bronchiectasis are seen in later stages.

5. Differential diagnoses of bilateral hilar adenopathy are TB, lymphoma and metastasis.

6. Complications are pneumothorax, cor pulmonale and fungal ball formation in cavities. In 60–80% of patients sarcoidosis is self-limiting. Treatment options in persistent cases include corticosteroids, non-steroidal anti-inflammatory drugs (NSAIDs), methotrexate, azathioprine, cyclophosphamide and chloroquine. Corticosteroids are used in cardiac involvement, neurological involvement, persistent hypercalcaemia, pulmonary fibrosis, severe erythema nodosum and uveitis.

Case 2.18: Answers

1. The chest X-ray shows dilated tubular structures with thick walls in the bases. The second picture is an HRCT scan. (HRCT imaging technique consists of obtaining 1- to 2-mm collimation scans at 10-mm intervals through the chest with a window level [WL] of –700 hounsfield units (HU) and a window width [WW] of –1000 HU). Thick-walled and dilated bronchi are seen. The bronchi are larger than the vessels adjacent to them.

2. Bronchiectasis.

3. Bronchiectasis is localised, irreversible dilatation of part of the bronchial tree. The three main types are **cylindrical, varicose** and **cystic**. In the cylindrical type, there is fusiform dilatation and tramlines (parallel lines corresponding to thickened, dilated bronchi). The varicose type is seen in destroyed lung and has a varicose tortuous appearance. The cystic type is seen in destroyed lung and has a saccular dilatation, with a string-of-cysts appearance. In HRCT, the internal bronchial diameter is greater than that of the adjacent artery. There is lack of bronchial tapering (the same diameter as the parent branch for > 2 cm). The bronchi are seen within 1 cm of costal pleura or abut the mediastinal pleura. Bronchial wall thickening is seen. A cystic cluster of thin-walled cystic spaces can be present, often with air–fluid levels (secondary infection). Indistinct central vessels are seen as a result of peribronchovascular inflammation/fibrosis. Atelectasis is not uncommon. Crowding of the vasculature can be seen as a result of volume loss caused by mucus obstruction of peripheral bronchi. In cylindrical bronchiectasis, bronchi coursing horizontally are seen as parallel lines, and vertically oriented bronchi are seen as circular lucencies that are larger than the adjacent pulmonary artery (signet-ring appearances). Varicose bronchiectasis is seen as non-uniform bronchial dilatation. Bronchial walls are thick with signet-ring signs. Areas of increased and decreased perfusion (oligaemia caused by hypoperfusion and compensatory hypertrophy in uninvolved segments) and attenuation are seen. Less common findings are tracheomegaly and enlarged

mediastinal nodes. Fluid-filled bronchi are revealed as tubular or branching structures when they course horizontally or as nodules when they are perpendicular to the plane of the CT scan section.

4. Causes of bronchiectasis: postinfective (childhood infections such as TB, atypical mycobacteria, measles, *Klebsiella*, *S. aureus*, *Mycoplasma pneumoniae*, pertussis, influenza, respiratory syncytial virus, herpes simplex virus, adenovirus, ABPA [acute bronchopulmonary aspergillosis]), cystic fibrosis, sequestration, neoplasm, inflammatory nodes, foreign body, aspiration, William–Campbell syndrome, Mounier–Kuhn syndrome, Kartagener syndrome, Young syndrome, Swyer–James syndrome, yellow nail syndrome, immunodeficiency, α_1-antitrypsin deficiency, traction secondary to fibrosis, lung and bone marrow transplants.

5. Differentiation of cystic bronchiectasis from cystic spaces of honeycomb lung can be difficult. Honeycombing does not have air–fluid levels. Emphysematous changes can be differentiated from bronchiectasis because they demonstrate expiratory air trapping.

Case 2.19: Answers

1. The chest X-ray shows a triangular opacity adjacent to the cardiac margin, wihch is causing loss of definition of the medial aspect of the right diagphragmatic dome, consistent with right lower lobe collapse. The CT scan shows a small, soft, tissue mass within the right lower lobe bronchus, with collapse of the distal lung.

2. Endobronchial mass, most likely neoplastic. In this case, a carcinoid tumour of the lung.

3. Carcinoid tumour is a slow-growing malignant tumour that arises from Kultchitsky's cells in the bronchial mucosa. Pathologically there are four types:
    Type I: classic type, centrally located, endobronchial, small, younger patient, females, well defined
    Type II: atypical carcinoid – less common, larger tumour, well-defined margin, older, male, metastasis seen
    Type III: large cell neuroendocrine carcinoma
    Type IV: small cell carcinoma – ill-defined margins with lymphadenopathy.

Ninety per cent are located centrally, unlike hamartomas, which are located peripherally. It is asymptomatic in 60%. Haemoptysis, cough, recurrent infections, wheezing, dyspnoea, pneumonia, hoarseness of voice and carcinoid syndrome (1%) may be seen.

4. Most of carcinoids present with an endobronchial nodule or obstructing mass, associated with atelectasis, obstructive pneumonitis, air trapping or mucoid impaction. They can extend extraluminally, producing a hilar or perihilar mass (iceberg lesion). The X-ray shows a central, peribronchial, perihilar mass. Calcification is seen in up to a third of patients. Secondary changes such as atelectasis, obstructive pneumonitis and air trapping can be seen and, in 15–20% of cases, they are seen peripherally as a solitary pulmonary nodule. The CT scan shows a solid mass, with or without calcification. There is good contrast enhancement, because the tumour is supplied by the bronchial circulation. Obstructive pneumonia and emphysema are seen as a result of bronchial obstruction. High uptake is seen in octreotide and depreotide scans, because of the presence of somatostatin receptors in the tumour.

5. Differential diagnoses for central tumours include bronchial carcinoma and lymph nodal mass. Other tumours such as hamartomas and metastasis should also be considered. When the diagnosis is in doubt, bronchoscopy with biopsy or percutaneous CT-guided biopsy would be of help.

Case 2.20: Answers

1. The chest X-ray shows volume reduction of the right lung. There is blurring of the right heart border, which is not clearly seen. In the lateral view, a wedge-shaped opacity is seen extending anteriorly from the hilum.

2. Right middle lobe collapse.

3. Collapse can result from any lesion that obstructs the right middle lobe bronchus or be a ventilation disorder. Persistent collapse in someone who smokes should raise the suspicion of a bronchogenic neoplasm. In young adults or older children, a mucus plug in asthma is a common cause that responds to physiotherapy. In children, a foreign body is the most common cause of obstruction. In postoperative patients, retention of secretions is a frequent cause. In ventilated patients, collapse occurs when the endotracheal tube is inserted distally into one bronchus that is ventilated,

but obstructs the other main bronchus. Obstruction can also be caused by lymphadenopathy, tumours, endobronchial tumours or granulation tissue.

4. The classic appearance of right middle lobe collapse is blurring of the right heart border, loss of volume of the right middle lobe and a triangular opacity adjacent to the heart border. The minor fissure is displaced inferiorly and medially. In the lateral view a wedge-shaped density extends from the hilum anteriorly and inferiorly, between the horizontal and oblique fissures. To confirm the diagnosis and to identify the underlying obstructing lesion, a CT scan can be done and will show the collapsed lung and any associated mass. The collapsed right middle lobe is seen as a triangular opacity against the right heart border with the apex pointing laterally.

5. The most common differential diagnosis is a right middle lobe consolidation, which also produces blurring of the right heart margin, but there is no volume reduction and no fissural displacement. Another differential diagnosis is fluid in the right horizontal fissure. In the lateral view, the fluid has convex margins.

Case 2.21: Answers

1. The chest X-ray shows a large pleural effusion on the right side, with no mediastinal shift. The CT scan shows a large pleural effusion, with multiple, nodular soft-tissue masses arising from the pleura.

2. Malignant mesothelioma

3. Malignant mesothelioma is a rare, malignant tumour of the serosal lining of the pleura, usually involving the parietal pleura and to a lesser extent the visceral pleura. It starts as pleural nodules, which coalesce to form a sheet of tumour encasing the lungs, extending into the fissures and eventually invading the chest wall, mediastinum and diaphragm. Predisposing factors are asbestos exposure (seen in > 50% of patients), TB, empyema and radiation. In asbestos exposure, crocidolite fibres are the most common cause. Of workers exposed to asbestos 10% develop malignant mesothelioma. The latent period is 20–45 years. It is seen in men aged 50–70 years. Histological types are epithelioid, sarcomatoid and biphasic. Mesothelioma is associated with hypertrophic pulmonary osteoarthropathy, peritoneal mesothelioma and the changes of asbestos exposure in the lungs.

4. The clinical features are cough, chest pain, coughing of asbestos bodies, weakness, fever and dyspnoea. Spread can be contiguous to the lung, chest wall, mediastinum, pericardium, diaphragm and peritoneum. Lymphatic spread is to the hila, mediastinum, and supraclavicular, axillary and cervical nodes. Haematogenous metastasis occurs to different organs. Associated pleural effusion is haemorrhagic, low in pH and low in glucose. Cytology of the effusion may reveal malignant cells. Pleural biopsy is required for confirmation.

5. The X-ray shows large pleural effusion or pleurally based, lobulated opacities or pleural thickening that extends into the fissures. There is no contralateral mediastinal shift, because encasement of the lung by tumour fixes the mediastinum. Rib destruction can be seen. Ultrasonography can differentiate effusion, thickening and mass. The CT scan shows pleural effusion. The volume of the lung is reduced with mediastinal shift, narrowed intercostal spaces and an elevated diaphragm. There is nodular pleural thickening, extending to the fissures and mediastinum. There is a large, lobulated, pleural mass, with destruction of the ribs. There might be spread to adjacent structures, including ascites. Calcified pleural plaques and underlying asbestosis can be seen.

6. Metastatic adenocarcinoma, benign mesothelioma, pleural fibrosis, fibrothorax and empyema are the differential diagnoses of pleural tumours. Metastatic adenocarcinoma is commonly seen in breast carcinoma and the appearances are similar, but there are no telltale signs of asbestos exposure, such as pleural thickening and plaques. Irregular, nodular thickening, involvement of the mediastinum and invasion of the adjacent structures enable differentiation from benign pleural thickening.

Case 2.22: Answers

1. The first chest X-ray shows well-defined, fine nodules, scattered in both upper and midzones. In the second X-ray the nodules are fewer. There is volume reduction in both lungs, with elevation of the hila and tenting of the diaphragm. There are bilateral, large, lobulated masses close to the paratracheal region. Emphysema is seen in the rest of the lung.

2. Coalworkers' pneumoconiosis with progressive massive fibrosis.

3. Coalworkers' pneumoconiosis (anthracosis) is an inhalational disease, caused by aggregates of coal dust (< 3 mm) which are taken by alveolar macrophages and deposited around bronchioles and alveoli. This results in the development of reticulin fibres associated with bronchiolar dilatation and bronchiolar artery stenosis. Pathologically they are different from the silicotic nodules through the absence of a hyaline centre and laminated collagen.

4. The X-ray shows small, well-defined, round, 5–10 mm opacities in the upper lobes. The nodules are seen only after 10 years of exposure, where they reach radiologically significant density. The nodularity correlates with the level of collagen, not the amount of coal dust. A reticular pattern can also be seen, similar to interstitial lung disease. The nodules become larger and more easily visible, with progression of the disease. Progressive massive fibrosis is a complication of coalworkers' pneumoconiosis and is seen in the posterior segment of the upper lobe or superior segment of the lower lobe. These are large (> 1 cm) opacities that are initially situated in the periphery of the lung, have a discoid contour (large in PA, flat in lateral view), with well-defined lateral borders and ill-defined medial margins. When this fibrosis develops, there is an apparent decrease in nodularity and the lesion progressively migrates towards the hila. Cavitation can be seen, and associated emphysema. A CT scan is useful in the early stages for diagnosis of small nodules and detection of complications.

5. Differential diagnoses are silicosis, baritosis, siderosis, metastasis and sarcoidosis.

6. Progressive massive fibrosis, chronic obstructive bronchitis, focal emphysema and cor pulmonale are the complications.

Case 2.23: Answers

1. The X-ray shows diaphragmatic pleural calcification. There is an amorphous area of geographical opacity in the pleura of the right lobe, which indicates a pleural plaque. There is also a lobulated mass in the perihilar region on the right side.

2. Asbestos exposure with diaphragmatic pleural calcification and pleural thickening. The complication seen in this patient is bronchogenic carcinoma, which is seen in the right perihilar region.

3. Asbestos exposure results in a wide spectrum of pulmonary abnormalities, including pleural disease. There are different types of asbestos fibres. The crocidolite fibres are associated with the largest numbers of pleural diseases. Asbestos exposure occurs in mining, milling, processing, insulation, shipbuilding, gaskets, brake linings, textile manufacturing and construction. The following are the various lung lesions encountered:

Pleural effusion: earliest abnormality

Focal pleural plaque: most common manifestation; hyalinised collagen in submesothelial layer of the parietal pleura

Pleural calcification: hallmark of asbestos exposure

Diffuse pleural thickening: thickening of parietal and visceral pleura causes restriction of pulmonary function

Round atelectasis: pseudotumour

Bronchogenic cancer: usually bronchoalveolar carcinoma, synergistic risk with smoking

Malignant mesothelioma.

4. Pleural plaque is the most common manifestation of asbestos exposure. It is often bilateral and multifocal and seen in the posterolateral midportion of the chest wall between the seventh and tenth ribs, in diaphragmatic aponeurosis, in the mediastinum and following rib contours. It spares the apices and costophrenic angles. Pleural calcification is the hallmark of asbestos exposure. Calcifications are seen in the chest wall, mediastinum, pericardium and diaphragm. Bilateral diaphragmatic calcifications with clear costophrenic angle are pathognomonic of asbestos exposure. Round atelectasis is a benign mass caused by asbestos and should be differentiated from lung cancer. It is seen in the posteromedial aspect of the lower lobe, and as a spiculated, peripheral, pleurally based mass, with associated pleural thickening. There are linear bands radiating from the mass to the lung parenchyma (crows' feet), which is characteristic. Bronchogenic carcinoma is the most important complication, and is seen as a spiculated mass in the lung. Extension to the lymph nodes and adjacent structures can be seen.

5. Pleural effusion at 8–10 years, pleural plaque 20 years, pleural calcification > 20 years, round atelectasis 20 years, bronchogenic carcinoma 25–35 years and malignant mesothelioma 20–40 years.

Case 2.24: Answers

1. The chest CT scan shows multiple areas of small cavitations in both the lungs and a small left pneumothorax.

2. Rheumatoid lung with necrobiotic nodules. One of the cavities on the left side has ruptured and there is a mild left pneumothorax.

3. Rheumatoid arthritis is an autoimmune disease, which is seen in women in the fourth and fifth decades. Arthritis precedes pulmonary changes in 90% and 90% have positive rheumatoid factor (90%). Rheumatoid lung is more common in males and can manifest in different ways:

    Pleural disease: most common manifestation, usually late, may antedate arthritis; bilateral pleural thickening and pleural effusion are seen

    Fibrosis: lower lobes, reticulonodular shadow, septal thickening and honeycomb lung

    Necrobiotic nodules

    Caplan syndrome: rheumatoid pneumoconiosis

    Bronchial lesions: bronchiectasis, bronchiolitis obliterans, bronchiolitis obliterans organising pneumonia, follicular bronchiolitis

    Pulmonary arteritis

    Cardiac: pericarditis, cardiac failure.

4. Rheumatoid nodule in the lung is a rare manifestation of rheumatoid arthritis. They are well-defined nodules in the lung, pleura or pericardium with a central zone of fibrinoid necrosis surrounded by fibroblasts. An X-ray shows well-defined multiple nodules, which vary in size from 5 mm to 7 cm. These wax and wane, paralleling the course of the subcutaneous rheumatoid nodules. They are more common in the bases. Cavitation can be seen with thick walls and smooth lining. This can result in haemoptysis or a pneumothorax. There is no calcification. Pleural effusion/thickening can be seen. Fibrosis is indistinguishable from idiopathic pulmonary fibrosis and manifests with ground-glass opacity, and subpleural interlobular and intralobular septal thickening. Air trapping is seen in bronchiolitis obliterans.

5. Sarcoidosis, Wegener's granulomatosis, metastasis, bronchiectasis, TB, histoplasmosis, pseudomonas infection, septic emboli and lymphoma are the differential diagnoses.

6. Caplan syndrome is a combination of rheumatoid lung and pneumoconiosis. It is a hypersensitive reaction to inhaled dust particles in rheumatoid lung. It is associated with joint manifestation and subcutaneous nodules. There are well-defined nodules, appearing in crops in the upper lobes and the periphery of the lung on a background of pneumoconiosis.

Case 2.25: Answers

1. The HRCT scan shows thickening of the interlobar septa with areas of honeycombing, in the subpleural region of both the lower lobes, more on the right side.

2. Scleroderma lung.

3. Scleroderma is a connective tissue disorder, characterised by increased production of collagen that causes exuberant interstitial fibrosis with atrophy and sclerosis. The lungs are involved in 100% of cases. It is commonly seen in the periphery of both lung bases. Clinical features are productive or dry cough, dyspnoea, haematemesis and restrictive lung function pattern.

4. The X-ray shows bilateral, basal, reticular or reticulonodular opacities. Honeycombing may be seen in the later stages, where are there are multiple tiny cystic spaces. Volume loss is seen with a shaggy irregular heart margin and elevation of the diaphragm. The HRCT scan is used to confirm the diagnosis. It shows thickening of the interstitium, which is seen as thick interlobular septa. It is characteristically located in the peripheral subpleural regions in the lower lobes. Subpleural nodules and ground-glass opacities are also seen. Subpleural honeycombing, lines and bands can be seen. In the early stages, ground-glass opacities can be seen, and alveolar opacities can be seen as a result of aspiration of gastrointestinal contents from a lax oesophageal sphincter. Dilated oesophagus filled with air may be seen.

5. The common differential diagnoses for lower lobe fibrotic changes are usual interstitial pneumonia, desquamative interstitial pneumonia, asbestosis, connective tissue diseases, drug-induced lung disease (bleomycin, busulphan, cyclophosphamide, nitrofurantoin). Complications are pulmonary arterial hypertension, aspiration pneumonia and lung cancer.

Case 2.26: Answers

1. The chest X-ray shows a large opacity in the right cardiophrenic angle. No mediastinal displacement is noted. The mass is obscuring the right dome of the diaphragm. Lateral view of the chest shows a homogeneous opacity protruding into the anterior aspect of lower thoracic cavity.

2. Morgagni hernia.

3. Morgagni hernia is caused by a defective development of septum transversum and herniation occurs through the space of Larrey which is an anteromedial parasternal defect. Morgagni hernia is common on the right side, since the heart prevents herniation on the left side. Although the defect is very small, omental fat, transverse colon and and liver may herniated. Symptoms depend on the size of the hernia and on the extension of the abdominal organs into the thorax, which may cause respiratory and bowel symptoms.

4. The X-ray shows an opacity in the right cardiophrenic angle. If there are bowel loops, these are clearly visualised. Barium study will confirm the diagnosis. A CT scan is useful in confirming the diagnosis and evaluating the herniated structures. Herniated fat is seen as a low-density structure, mimicking lipoma. Multiplanar reconstructions in the sagittal and coronal planes help in delineating the structures. Differential diagnoses for cardiophrenic angle mass are prominent cardiophrenic fat pad, pericardial cyst, bronchogenic cyst, lymph node, thymolipoma, varices, lymphoma, metastasis and aneurysm.

5. Traumatic diaphragmatic rupture is common on the left side and is located in the posterolateral portion of the diaphragm, medial to the spleen in a radial orientation.

Case 2.27: Answers

1. The chest X-ray shows bilateral, diffuse, opacification of the lung fields. The chest CT scan shows bilateral, diffuse, ground-glass shadowing and mosaic perfusion.

2. ARDS.

3. ARDS is a life-threatening acute respiratory distress, characterised by severe hypoxaemia, increased respiratory effort and widespread airspace consolidation. Causes are trauma, infection, drowning, disseminated intravascular coagulation (DIC), haemorrhagic/septic shock, inhalants, smoke, aspiration, narcotics , oxygen toxicity, radiation, pancreatitis, amniotic fluid/fat emboli and massive viral pneumonia.

4. In the first 12 hours, there are fibrin and platelet microemboli; in 12–24 hours interstitial oedema; in 24–48 hours capillary congestion, alveolar and interstitial oedema and haemorrhage, destruction of type I pneumocytes and atelectasis; in 5–7 days hyaline membrane formation, hypertrophy and hyperplasia of type II pneumocytes; in 7–14 days fibroblastic proliferation and collagen deposition, infection.

5. The radiological appearances depend on the stage and are variable:
   Exudative stage: interstitial oedema, perihilar opacification, alveolar opacities with air bronchogram, dependent atelectasis
   Proliferative stage: ground-glass opacities and thick septa
   Fibrotic stage: scarring, subpleural and intrapulmonary cysts.
   The X-ray is normal in the first 12 hours after onset of clinical symptoms. In 12–24 hours, patchy ill-defined opacities are seen and these progress in 24–48 hours to diffuse airspace opacities in all lungs. In 5–7 days consolidation becomes inhomogeneous as a result of resolution and focal areas of pneumonia are seen. In 7–14 days, reticular changes are seen caused by fibrosis. Differential diagnoses in the exudative stage are infections, cardiogenic oedema, aspiration and haemorrhage. Differential diagnoses in late stages include all the causes of pulmonary fibrosis.

6. Mechanical ventilatory assistance with positive end-expiratory pressure.

Case 2.28: Answers

1. The X-ray shows bilateral, perihilar, symmetrical, alveolar opacification. The CT scan shows ground-glass shadowing and alveolar opacities in the perihilar region. The heart appears normal.

2. Pulmonary haemorrhage, from Goodpasture syndrome.

3. Pulmonary haemorrhage can be diffuse or focal. Trauma, Bleeding diathesis, leukaemia, DIC (disseminated intravascular coagulation), pulmonary embolism, haemosiderosis, Goodpasture's syndrome, Wegner's granulomatosis, infections (Legionnaires, CMV, herpes, infectious mononucleosis, Rocky mountain fever, aspergillosis, mucormyocsis), drugs (Amphotericin B, mitomycin, cyclophosphamide, cytarabine, D pencillamine, anticoagulants), SLE, Henoch Schonlein purpura, hemosiderosis, metastasis (choriocarcinoma, renal cell carcinoma) and idiopathic pulmonary haemorrhage are the causes of diffuse pulmonary haemorrhage. Focal haemorrhage is caused by chronic bronchitis, bronchiectasis, pulmonary embolism, penetrating trauma, and trauma or localised infections. Pathologically, the red cells are cleared by alveolar macrophages and there are large numbers of haemosidern laden macrophages in alveolar spaces and interstitium. Recurrent haemorrhage results in mild interstitial fibrosis.

4. The X-ray shows bilateral, confluent, ill-defined, scattered areas of ground-glass opacities and alveolar opacities. Bilateral perihilar predominance is seen in diffuse haemorrhage, with relative sparing of the apices. The CT scan shows bilateral scattered, diffuse areas of ground-glass opacity/consolidation/nodules. The airspace opacity resolves in 2–3 days with replacement by interstitial opacities. The CT scan shows septal thickening.

5. Differential diagnoses for this appearance include pulmonary oedema, infection, lymphoma, sarcoidosis and alveolar proteinosis.

Case 2.29: Answers

1. The X-ray shows patchy, small calcifications scattered in both lungs.

2. Calcifications from varicella pneumonia.

3. Varicella pneumonia is seen in adults, with 75% seen in the third to fourth decades. Varicella infection is common in children, but complications are more common in adult infections. Clinically there are characteristic rashes and vesicles.

4. Acute varicella pneumonia may be seen as patchy consolidation or nodules in the lungs. Characteristic, tiny, 2–3 mm calcifications in the lungs are seen as a sequela of varicella infection. It takes years to develop calcifications and they are usually seen in the mid and lower zones.

5. Differential diagnoses of small nodules in lungs include miliary TB, histoplasmosis, metastasis from thyroid carcinoma/melanoma, silicosis, extrinsic allergic alveolitis, sarcoidosis, siderosis, tropical pulmonary eosinophilia and pneumoconiosis. Dense nodules are seen in haemosiderosis and microlithiasis, and pulmonary ossification in mitral stenosis.

Case 2.30: Answers

1. The chest X-ray shows a heterogeneous, patchy, alveolar opacification in both lower lobes. The CT scan shows patchy peribronchial alveolar opacities in the superior basal segment of the right lower lobe. (Changes in the left lower lobe are not shown in this picture.)

2. Aspiration pneumonia.

3. Aspiration pneumonia is caused by aspiration of gastric contents and is common in patients with neurological problems, people with alcohol problems and learning disabilities, recent general anaesthesia and oesophageal motility disturbances. The aspirated material causes obstruction of small airways or inflammatory changes in alveoli in dependent parts of the lung. Gram-negative bacteria, *Pseudomonas aeruginosa* and *Actinomyces* spp. are frequently isolated organisms. Chronic aspiration is seen in chronic underlying conditions such as pharyngeal pouch, oesophageal diverticula, oesophageal stenosis, tracheo-oesophageal fistula or neuromuscular disturbances. Fever, productive cough and choking on swallowing are clinical features.

4. Aspiration is common in the dependent portion of the lung. The most common locations are posterior segments of the upper lobes and superior basal segments of the lower lobes. The right middle and lower lobes are frequently affected. It can be bilateral.

5. The most common radiological pattern is that of a patchy bronchopneumonic infiltrate in the dependent portions of lungs. It can also produce lobar or segmental consolidation. Pneumonia, necrotising pneumonia and lung abscess are complications.

Case 2.31: Answers

1. The X-ray shows hyperexpanded lungs, which show multiple large cystic spaces. The CT scan shows hyperinflated lungs with numerous thin walled cystic spaces, replacing the lung.

2. Lymphangioleiomyomatosis.

3. Lymphangioleiomyomatosis is a rare disease occurring only in women of childbearing age and characterised by smooth muscle proliferation in lymphatic vessels, blood vessels and airways. Proliferation of spindle cells along the bronchioles results in air trapping and thin-walled cysts. Rupture of cysts causes pneumothorax. The disease can also involve the lymph nodes, resulting in enlarged nodes and chylous pleural effusion. Most patients die within 10 years of onset.

4. There is strong association with tuberous sclerosis, with up to 1/3 of women with tuberous sclerosis complex presenting with LAM. Chylous effusions, mediastinal and retroperitoneal lymphangioleiomyomatosis are associated. Pneumothorax is seen in 40%.

5. In lymphangioleiomyomatosis, the lung volume is normal or increased. The X-rays show a coarse reticular pattern. Cysts are thin walled and range in size from 0.5 cm to 6 cm, surrounded by normal lung parenchyma. The size of the cysts increases with disease progression. Diffuse lung involvement is seen even in mild disease. HRCT is useful in characterising the disease. Bronchovascular bundles are seen at the periphery of the cyst walls. Interstitial septal thickening and ground-glass opacities can also be seen. Associated findings are lymphadenopathy and chylothorax. Pneumothorax is a major complication, seen in 40% as a result of rupture of a cyst into the pleural space. Diagnosis is confirmed with open lung biopsy. Prognosis is bad as a result of pulmonary insufficiency. Lung transplantation has been successfully performed in patients with severe LAM (lymphangiomyomatosis).

6. Differential diagnoses of lymphangioleiomyomatosis include other cystic lung disorders such as tuberous sclerosis (with other associated findings such as cortical tubers, angiomyolipomas, epilepsy), neurofibromatosis (predominantly apical), histiocytosis (upper lungs, with sparing of costophrenic angles, initially nodules followed by cavitation), emphysema (cyst walls not seen, mosaic pattern, bronchovascular bundle seen centrally), bronchiectasis (thick bronchial walls) and honeycomb lung (small cystic spaces, volume reduction, fibrotic changes).

Case 2.32: Answers

1. The chest X-ray shows multiple, large masses in both lungs, of various sizes. The CT scan shows multiple pulmonary nodules.

2. Multiple pulmonary metastases

3. Most pulmonary metastases arise from common tumours, such as breast, colorectal, prostate, lung, head and neck, and renal cancers. The incidence of metastasis is high in vascular tumours such as renal cancers, bone sarcomas, choriocarcinomas, melanomas, testicular teratomas and thyroid carcinomas. Pulmonary metastases can be asymptomatic or present with dyspnoea. Sudden dyspnoea is usually the result of pleural effusion, pneumothorax or haemorrhage.

4. Usually, metastases are seen as multiple, pulmonary nodules, ranging in size from 3 mm to 15 cm. Nodules of same size originate at the same time, in a single shower of emboli. They are usually seen in the peripheral third of the lung. Smaller nodules have well-defined margins, but larger nodules have irregular margins. Differential diagnoses for multiple pulmonary nodules are:

Infective: TB, histoplasmosis, coccidioidomycosis, cryptococcosis, nocardia infection, measles, hydatid cysts, inflammatory pseudotumour, pseudolymphoma

Tumours: metastasis, lymphoma, hamartomas

Vascular: AV malformations, PEs, septic emboli

Collagen vascular: Wegener's granulomatosis, rheumatoid.

The differential diagnoses for solitary pulmonary nodules are granuloma, bronchogenic tumour, carcinoid, hamartoma, abscess, infection, infarct, etc. In a solitary pulmonary nodule, biopsy may be required to confirm the diagnosis.

5. Variations in presentation of metastasis:

Solitary pulmonary nodule: single nodule in lung which may require CT guided biopsy for the diagnosis.

Calcifying metastasis: osteosarcoma, chondrosarcoma, synovial carcinoma, treated testicular carcinoma

Cavitating: osteosarcoma, squamous cell carcinomas; can present with pneumothorax

Haemorrhagic: fuzzy margins, choriocarcinoma, sarcoma, other vascular tumours

Endobronchial metastasis: lymphoma

Airspace pattern, resembling infection: lymphoma

Sterilised metastasis: no change in size even after adequate chemotherapy, choriocarcinoma, testicular cancer

Benign tumours with metastasis to lungs: chondroblastoma, giant cell tumour

Pleural metastasis: lymphoma, breast

Fibrosis, necrosis, cyst: after treatment of metastasis.

Case 2.33: Answers

1. The chest X-ray shows bilateral, symmetrical, central, parahilar, reticulonodular opacities. There is no pleural effusion. HRCT shows bilateral areas of ground-glass opacity with superimposed, smooth, septal thickening, giving a crazy-paving appearance.

2. Alveolar proteinosis.

3. Alveolar proteinosis is a disease characterised by filling of alveolar spaces with periodic acid–Schiff (PAS)-positive proteinaceous material, rich in lipid. It is caused by an abnormality in production or clearance of surfactant. Most cases are idiopathic, but it is also associated with immunodeficiency, malignancies, chemotherapy and acute silicosis. It is common in men and peaks between 30 and 50 years. It presents with insidious onset of non-productive cough, dyspnoea and fever. It can be asymptomatic. Superimposed infection with *Nocardia* spp., *Mycobacterium avium-intracellulare* and *Pneumocystis jiroveci* can be seen. Treatment is removal of alveolar material with bronchoalveolar lavage (BAL). It can relapse and repeated lavage may be required.

4. In the X-ray, there is bilateral, patchy, diffuse/parahilar consolidation or ground-glass opacity, more severe in the bases. Dense consolidation amd reticulonodular opacities are rare. The appearances are difficult to distinguish from pulmonary oedema, but there is no cardiomegaly or pleural effusion. HRCT appearances are characteristic. There are bilateral areas of ground-glass opacity with smooth, interlobular, septal thickening, producing the characteristic crazy-paving appearance. These areas are sharply demarcated, giving a geographical appearance. It is bilateral and may be asymmetrical. The changes disappear after successful BAL.

5. Characteristic findings of alveolar proteinosis are geographical distribution of ground-glass opacity with smooth, interlobular, septal thickening producing the crazy-paving appearance, in a patient with subacute/chronic onset of symptoms. Differential diagnoses of crazy-paving appearance are ARDS, diffuse pulmonary haemorrhage, *Pneumocystis jiroveci*, sarcoidosis, non-specific interstitial pneumonia, organising pneumonia, mucinous bronchoalveolar carcinoma and lipoid pneumonia.

Case 2.34: Answers

1. Contrast enhanced CT scan of the chest shows a pleural fluid collection situated posteriorly on the right side. The two layers of the pleura encircling this collection are thickened and show contrast enhancement (split pleura sign).

2. Empyema.

3. Empyema is an infective pleural fluid collection. Common organisms are *Staphylococcus aureus,* Gram-negative bacteria or anaerobic bacteria.

4. There are three stages in the formation of empyema:

   Stage I: exudative phase – proteinaceous fluid is seen in the pleural space without infective organisms

   Stage II: fibrinopurulent phase – inflammatory cells accumulate and there is fibrin deposition on pleural surfaces

   Stage III: pleural fibrosis with recruitment of fibroblasts and capillaries, resulting in deposition of collagen and granulation tissue.

5. The X-ray shows a pleural fluid collection. Pleural fluid collection is seen as a homogeneous opacity in the lower zone, with a concave upper border (meniscus sign), and obliteration of the costophrenic angle and dome of the diaphragm. Ultrasonography helps to differentiate simple effusion and empyema. Simple pleural effusion is made up of clear fluid, but empyema shows internal echoes and loculations with thick pleura. The CT scan shows pleural fluid. The characteristic finding is a split pleural sign, where the pleural fluid collection is located between thickened and enhancing visceral and parietal pleura. Gas bubbles can be seen if the infection is with a gas-forming organism. Differential diagnoses are malignant effusion, mesothelioma, TB, rheumatoid disease and reactive mesothelial hyperplasia.

6. Empyema can be treated with percutaneous drainage under ultrasonic or CT guidance. The loculations can be broken up with fibrinolytics and antibiotics can be instilled through the drain tube. Persistent empyema requires decortication.

Case 2.35: Answers

1. Chest X-ray shows a thin rim of lucency between cardiac outline and pleura on the left side. There are streaky lucencies in the mediastinum. The lungs are hyperinflated. The CT scan shows lucent air situated around the heart in between the parietal pericardium and the mediastinal pleura.

2. Pneumomediastinum.

3. Bronchial asthma.

4. Pneumomediastinum can be caused by asthma, straining against a closed glottis (vomiting, weight lifting, parturition), chest trauma, alveolar rupture, oesophageal rupture, airway rupture, dental extraction, perforation of hollow viscus or spontaneous rupture. In asthma, after alveolar rupture, air tracks along the bronchovascular sheath and ruptures through the fascial sheath at the lung root into the mediastinum and extends to the fascial planes of neck, producing subcutaneous emphysema.

5. Pneumomediastinum is seen as streaky lucencies in the mediastinum, around the trachea, oesophagus and heart. **Continuous diaphragm sign** refers to air trapped posterior to the pericardium, producing lucency that connects both domes of the diaphragm. Air is seen in the azygo-oesophageal recess and pulmonary ligament. Air around the bronchi produces the double **bronchial wall sign**. Air around the major aortic branches produces a **tubular artery sign**. The **V sign** is produced by air between the mediastinal pleura and thoracic aorta or diaphragm. In children air outlines the thymus, which is called a **spinnaker or thymic sail sign**. Subcutaneous emphysema at the root of neck and upper trunk may be present.

6. Differential diagnoses are pneumopericardium, pneumothorax, pneumoperitoneum, anterior junction line, superior aspect of major fissure and the Mach band effect.

1. The CT scan shows a well-defined nodule in the posteromedial aspect of the left lower lobe. There are specks of calcification in the periphery of the nodule. In the centre of the lesion, there is an area of low density, equivalent to fat density.

2. Pulmonary hamartoma.

3. Pulmonary hamartoma is the most common benign tumour of the lung and is composed of normal lung tissue such as columnar/cuboidal/ciliated epithelium, fat, bone cartilage, muscle, vessels, fibrous tissue and calcification. It is usually seen in the periphery of the lung. It is seen in the fourth to fifth decades and is more common in males. Usually it is an incidental pick up on an X-ray or CT scan.

4. The X-ray shows a small, well-defined mass < 4 cm. The diagnosis can be made with confidence if the mass shows calcification or fat. A popcorn type of calcification is characteristic but seen only in 15%. The CT scan can confirm the diagnosis by showing fat and calcification. Fat is seen as a low-density area within the mass.

5. The most important lesion to be differentiated is a bronchogenic carcinoma. Lung cancers show ill-defined margins and are not calcified. Granulomas such as tuberculoma and histoplasmosis, carcinoid (more common centrally) and metastatic mucinous adenocarcinoma are the other lesions that can be confused with hamartoma.

6. **Carney's triad** consists of pulmonary chondroma, gastric epitheloid leiomyosarcoma and functioning extra-adrenal paraganglioma.
    (**Carney complex**: myxomas of heart and skin, lentiginosis, endocrine overactivity.)

Case 2.37: Answers

1. HRCT of the lung done in the expiratory phase shows a mosaic perfusion pattern. There are multiple areas of lucency along with dense bright areas within the lungs. The lucent areas represent areas of air trapping.

2. Bronchiolitis obliterans.

3. Bronchiolitis obliterans is caused by concentric fibrosis of submucosal and peribronchial tissue of terminal and respiratory bronchioles, resulting in bronchial narrowing or obliteration. The causes are infection (bacterial, mycoplasmal, viral), toxins (nitrogen dioxide, sulphur dioxide, ammonia, chlorine, phosgene, smoke), drugs (pencillamine, gold), collagen vascular disease, rheumatoid arthritis, chronic lung transplant rejection, bone marrow transplant with chronic graft-versus-host disease and idiopathic.

4. The chest X-ray can be normal or show hyperinflation with increased lucency and reduction of vascular markings. Bronchiectatic changes can be seen. The changes are bilateral. Unilateral changes with volume reduction are seen in the Swyer–James syndrome. In HRCT, the changes are focal areas of decreased lung density with small vessels (mosaic perfusion). This can be lobar, segmental or lobular. Air trapping is seen as the lucent areas in expiration. Bronchiectasis and tree-in-bud-shaped centrilobular opacities can be seen. Air trapping in expiration with normal inspiratory scans can be the only finding.

5. Other conditions that produce low density in the lungs are hypersensitivity pneumonitis, respiratory bronchiolitis and asthma. Tree-in-bud opacities can also be seen in cellular bronchiolitis, endobronchial TB, cystic fibrosis, fungal infections, panbronchiolitis, follicular bronchiolitis and endobronchial spread of tumour. Steroids are used in treatment of bronchiolitis.

Case 2.38: Answers

1. The X-ray shows a mass in the apical region of the right upper lobe with suspicion of underlying rib erosion. The CT scan confirms the presence of mass in the right upper lobe with destruction of the underlying rib.

2. Pancoast's tumour.

3. Pancoast tumour is lung tumour arising from the apex, also called superior sulcus carcinoma, thoracic inlet carcinoma or apical carcinoma. 5% of lung cancers occur in the lung apex. These tumours invade adjacent structures such as brachial plexus, sympathetic chain, subclavian artery and vein, ribs and vertebral bodies. Pancoast syndrome consists of pain in shoulder, radicular pain along C8, T1, T2 distribution and Horner's syndrome due to involvement of cervical sympathetic chain. Superior sulcus tumours are treated with combination of radiation and en bloc resection of tumour and adjacent chest wall in non small cell carcinomas (NSCLC.) Contraindications to therapy are – involvement of great vessels, extensive brachial plexus invasion, vertebral body/spinal canal, recurrent laryngeal nerve/phrenic nerve, mediastinal involvement, especially trachea or oesophagus and distant metastasis. Chemotherapy is the cornerstone of small cell carcinomas (SCLC) of lungs.

4. The chest X-ray shows a mass in the apical region or asymmetrical apical pleural thickening (> 5 mm difference). The CT scan confirms the presence of the mass and is useful for detecting the invasion of adjacent structures. MRI in the sagittal or coronal plane is more useful than CT in assessing chest wall invasion and extent, and the relationship to the great vessels and brachial plexus.

5. Differential diagnoses for apical mass/thickening: normal apical cap (< 5 mm thick, 10% of normal people, scars), extrapleural fat (obesity), Cushing syndrome, steroids, TB, neurogenic tumour, radiation fibrosis, mesothelioma, mediastinal haemorrhage, peripheral upper lobe collapse (in inflammatory conditions) and bronchial obstruction.

1. The X-ray shows a faint line in the anterior margin of the right lung, which separates a collapsed lung and a lucent lateral collection of free air within the right pleural cavity. Note: no vascular marking is noted within this area.

2. Spontaneous pneumothorax.

3. Pneumothorax can be **closed** (when the chest wall is intact), **open** (when there is a chest wound), which sucks air due to communication of the outside atmosphere or **tension** (check valve mechanism where air enters the pleural space, but cannot leave it). **Hydropneumothorax** presents with an air–fluid level. The causes of pneumothorax are spontaneous, trauma, iatrogenic, airway diseases (asthma, histiocytosis, tuberous sclerosis, cystic fibrosis), infections (lung abscess, necrotising pneumonia, bacterial, *P. jiroveci* pneumonia, TB), sarcoidosis, berylliosis, lung cancer, metastasis (osteosarcoma), connective tissue disorders (scleroderma, Marfan syndrome, Ehler–Danlos syndrome, rheumatoid), pneumoconiosis (silicosis, berylliosis), infarction and catamenial (during menstruation, endometriosis of diaphragm). Spontaneous pneumothorax is caused by rupture of subpleural blebs in the apical region. It is common in tall, young males who present with chest pain and dyspnoea. Recurrence is common in 30%, on the same or the opposite side.

4. In pneumothorax, there is an avascular, lucent collection of air, with a visceral pleural line demarcating it from collapsed lung. The most important diagnosis that should not be missed is a tension pneumothorax. In tension pneumothorax, there is a large pneumothorax, with inversion of the diaphragm, collapse of the lung, and displacement of the trachea and heart to the opposite side. A deep sulcus sign is seen as a result of a large costodiaphragmatic recess. An air–fluid level is seen in hydropneumothorax. The X-ray can be used in localising a small pneumothorax, quantifying a pneumothorax and following it up. If the pneumothorax is localised in the anteromedial location, there is an outline of the medial diaphragm under the cardiac shadow, with sharp delineation of the medial diaphragmatic contour. When there is subpulmonic pneumothorax, there is a hyperlucent upper abdomen, with a deep lateral costophrenic sulcus and visualisation of the inferior surface of the liver. In post-medial pneumothorax, a lucent triangle is seen with a vertex at the hilum, and a V-shaped base delineating the costovertebral sulcus.

5. Treatment of primary spontaneous pneumothorax includes observation, simple aspiration and chest tube placement. Secondary spontaneous pneumothorax and traumatic pneumothorax require chest tube placement. Iatrogenic pneumothorax is treated with observation or simple aspiration. Tension pneumothorax is a medical emergency and requires immediate needle decompression and chest tube placement. Treatment is with aspiration of tube drainage in severe cases. Observation is appropriate when pneumothorax is < 15% of chest volume. Pneumothorax > 35% volume requires a chest tube. Oxygen administration at 3–10 l/min increases the rate of pleural air absorption. Pneumothorax is resorbed at the rate of 1.25% per day. Recurrent pneumothorax may require pleurodesis.

Case 2.40: Answers

1. The chest X-ray shows a round mass in the right parahilar region, behind the right atrial shadow. The lungs are normal.

2. The CT scan shows a well-defined, hypodense, mediastinal cyst, which is seen just inferior to the carina and posterior to the left atrium. The margins of this lesion are well defined and there is no invasion of adjacent structures. There is no wall calcification.

3. Bronchogenic cyst. Differential diagnoses for cystic lesions include pericardial cyst, necrotic lymph node and lung abscess. The differential diagnoses for solid lesions include lymphoma and TB.

4. A bronchogenic cyst is a type of bronchopulmonary foregut malformation in which a supernumerary lung bud develops below the normal lung bud between week 26 and week 40 of gestation. Other diseases in this spectrum are sequestration, congenital cystic adenomatoid malformation and congenital lobar emphysema. The location and communication with the gastrointestinal tract depend on when in embryonic life the bud develops. Most malformations present clinically when they become infected.

5. The cysts are well defined, lined by columnar respiratory epithelium and filled with mucoid material. They are seen in the mediastinum in 85% (posterior > middle > anterior mediastinum) and in the lungs in 15%. The classic appearance is a well-defined round mass in the subcarinal or parahilar region. Intrapulmonary bronchogenic cysts are usually seen in the medial

third of the lung. The cysts are thin walled and can be fluid or air filled. Most of the cysts are asymptomatic. It can, however, produce fever and dyspnoea if infected and stridor or dysphagia as a result of mediastinal compression. CT shows a well-defined, non-enhancing cystic lesion, if the contents are mucoid. Calcification can be seen. On MRI, the cyst is usually bright in T2, but can be dark or bright in T1 depending on the content.

Case 2.41: Answers

1. The X-ray shows bilateral, parahilar, reticular opacities. HRCT shows bilateral, peribronchovascular, spiculated opacities.

2. Kaposi's sarcoma, involving the lungs.

3. Kaposi's sarcoma is a tumour, seen in 15–20% of HIV patients, that arises from primitive vascular tissues. It is the most common malignancy related to AIDS. It is more common in those who acquire AIDS through sexual contact. It is probably caused by infection with herpesvirus 8. Pulmonary involvement occurs in 20–50% of AIDS patients with Kaposi's sarcoma. It is usually preceded by cutaneous and visceral involvement. Pathologically, it is a patchy tumour, seen in the peribronchovascular interstitium in perihilar regions and pleura.

4. The chest X-ray shows bilateral, diffuse, patchy abnormalities. Coarse reticular opacities or ill-defined consolidation in perihilar regions or lower lobes is the characteristic appearance. Poorly defined nodules and ill-defined areas of consolidation are also seen. It is common in the bases. Thickening of the peribronchovascular interstitium in the bases is an early finding. Kerley lines, pleural effusions, and hilar and mediastinal adenopathy can be seen. In CT, thick peribronchovascular interstitium in the lung bases is seen. In advanced cases, flame-shaped, irregular, spiculated nodules are seen in the peribronchovascular regions. Peribronchovascular interstitial thickening, interlobular septal thickening, pleural effusion and lymphadenopathy can be seen.

5. Differential diagnosis in an immuno-compromised individual, includes infections and lymphoma. Characteristic finding of Kaposis sarcoma is irregular nodules, > 1 cm in peribronchovacular distribution. Diagnosis is established by the appearance in bronchoscopy. In cases of parenchymal Kaposi's sarcoma, transbronchial or open biopsies are necessary.

Case 2.42: Answers

1. The X-ray shows bilateral, multiple, dense nodules of varying sizes. There are patchy areas of fibrosis in the left upper zone.

2. Silicosis.

3. Silicosis is caused by inhalation of dust-containing silica (silicon dioxide), which is common in mining heavy metals and hard rocks. Pathologically the lungs are infiltrated with peribronchiolar nodules with layers of laminated connective tissue, more common in the upper lobes and parahilar regions. The risk of silicosis is related to the dose of exposure and is usually seen 10–20 years after exposure. Progression of the disease occurs many years after exposure. Simple silicosis causes few symptoms, but the development of complicated silicosis causes deterioration in lung function. Patients with silicosis have greater impairment than those with coalworkers' pneumoconiosis.

4. The characteristic findings on a chest X-ray are well-circumscribed nodules, measuring 10 mm, predominantly in the posterior upper lungs. Compared with coalworkers' pneumoconiosis, the nodules are larger, well defined and calcify in 10–20%. In HRCT, there are centrilobular/subpleural, symmetrical nodules in posterior and upper lobes. Hilar and mediastinal lymph nodes are enlarged in 30–40%. Egg-shell calcification of lymph nodes is a characteristic finding in silicosis. With progression, large opacities (progressive massive fibrosis) > 1 cm develop, as a result of conglomeration of silicotic nodules associated with fibrous tissue. They are usually seen in the periphery or midportion of upper lobes and gradually move to the centre to the hila, leaving emphysematous areas between them and the pleura. They are lenticular, paralleling the major fissure and oriented posteriorly. In CT, it is seen as a lenticular mass, associated with small nodules. Calcification, cavitation and necrosis can be seen.

5. Differential diagnoses of pulmonary nodules: TB, metastasis, sarcoidosis, coalworkers' pneumoconiosis. Differential diagnoses of egg-shell calcification: sarcoidosis, histoplasmosis, TB, scleroderma, amyloidosis and treated lymphomas.

Case 2.43: Answers

1. MRI of the chest shows a large mass in the right paravertebral region, which extends into the spinal canal, causing widening of the intervertebral foramen. There is widening of the spinal canal. There is mild enhancement of the mass in the post-contrast scan.

2. Spinal neurofibroma.

3. Neurofibroma is a nerve sheath tumour that is made up of neuronal elements containing Schwann cells, nerve fibres, fibroblasts and collagen. It is commonly seen at ages 20–30 years. In the spine, it is commonly seen in the intradural extramedullary location. It is more common at the cervical and thoracic levels. Other locations are in peripheral nerves. Spinal neurofibroma is a sign of neurofibromatosis type 1.

4. An X-ray shows neurofibromas as paraspinal masses when they are large. In the chest, the ribs are dysplastic and ribbon shaped. MRI shows a well-defined mass with a dumb-bell configuration, which widens the intervertebral foramen with scalloping or erosion of pedicles. In MRI the lesion is a homogeneous mass, isointense to muscle in T1 and hyperintense in T2. The target sign is characterised by a low signal centre in T2 caused by collagen and condensed Schwann cells. There is not much contrast enhancement. CT shows a homogeneous, hypodense, dumb-bell lesion that does not show contrast enhancement. Occasionally soft-tissue nodules are seen in the subcutaneous plane.

5. Cord compression can be seen in large tumours and malignant transformation is rare. The most common differential diagnoses are meningioma (not dumb-bell, hyperdense, contrast enhancement), metastasis, dermoid, lipoma, ependymoma and neurenteric cyst.

Case 2.44: Answers

1. Chest X-ray shows opacification and volume reduction of the right lung. There is dextroposition of the heart and there is herniation of over-inflated left lung to the right side. There is a long, linear band extending in a vertical direction in the right middle and lower lobes, to the level of the diaphragm which appears to be the right inferior pulmonary vein.

2. Scimitar syndrome: this is a combination of pulmonary hypoplasia and partial anomalous pulmonary venous drainage. In these patients, both the right pulmonary veins (superior and inferior) drain to the IVC via a descending vein coursing parallel to the right heart border. This condition is commonly associated with right lung hypoplasia of variable degrees.

3. Pulmonary hypoplasia contributes to 15–20% of neonatal deaths. It can be primary (10%) or associated with conditions that cause restricted lung growth or reduced breathing as a result of primary pulmonary malformation. Common causes include **oligohydramnios** (renal agenesis, urinary obstruction, prolonged rupture of membranes), **abnormalities causing compression of developing lung** (diaphragmatic hernia, pleural effusions or chondrodysplasia) or **disorders impairing fetal breathing** (anencephaly, neuromuscular disorders). It can be seen on antenatal ultrasonography. In bilateral pulmonary hypoplasia, the chest is bell shaped. The lungs may show normal appearance. Primary unilateral hypoplasia, also called hypogenetic lung, is often isolated and asymptomatic. Secondary hypoplasia is associated with diaphragmatic hernia, cystic adenomatoid malformation, oesophageal atresia and tracheo-oesophageal fistula.

4. Scimitar syndrome has variable presentation. Common presentations are dyspnoea, tachypnoea, respiratory distress, cyanosis, failure to thrive and cardiac failure. It can be asymptomatic. Clinical findings include shift in heart sounds and cardiac impulse to the right side and systolic murmur. Breath sounds may be diminished on the right side.

5. On X-rays, the normal lung is aerated and herniates with the mediastinum to the opposite side with no evidence of aerated lung in the opposite side. The CT scan confirms the appearance. In scimitar syndrome, there is hypoplasia of the right lower lobe with an associated abnormal pulmonary venous drainage, which drains into the IVC. This abnormal vein has the appearance of a scimitar on the chest X-ray. Differential diagnoses for this appearance are total collapse/consolidation of the left lung, lobectomy, hypoplasia and agenesis.

Case 2.45: Answers

1. The chest X-ray shows multiple small nodules in both lungs. There is no pleural effusion. The heart is normal.

2. The HRCT scan shows multiple, well-defined, tiny nodules in all the lobes.

3. Miliary TB: this is the widespread dissemination of *Mycobacterium tuberculosis* from haematogenous spread and is better described as acute disseminated TB. After exposure and inhalation of TB bacilli in the lung, a primary pulmonary complex is established and pulmonary lymphangitis and hilar lymphadenopathy develop. Mycobacteraemia and haematogenous seeding occur after the primary infection. After initial inhalation of TB bacilli, miliary TB may occur as primary TB or it may occur years after the initial infection

4. Classic miliary TB is defined as millet-like (1–5 mm) seeding of TB bacilli in the lung, as evidenced on the chest X-ray. This pattern is seen in 1–3% of all TB cases. Miliary TB may occur in an individual organ (very rare < 5%), in several organs or throughout the whole body (> 90%), including the brain. The infection is characterised by a large amount of TB bacilli, although it may easily be missed and is fatal if untreated. On postmortem examination, multiple TB lesions are detected throughout the body in organs such as the lungs, liver, spleen, brain and others. Up to 25% of patients with miliary TB may have meningeal involvement. In addition, miliary TB may mimic many diseases. Therefore, a high index of clinical suspicion is important to obtain an early diagnosis and ensure improved clinical outcomes. Signs and symptoms include weakness, fatigue, weight loss, headache, fever, cough, lymphadenopathy, hepatomegaly, splenomegaly and malaise. The erythrocyte sedimentation rate (ESR) is elevated and there can be leukopenia or leukocytosis. Cultures for mycobacteria are positive. Tuberculin testing is usually negative. Sputa for acid-fast bacilli and culture, tuberculin skin test and blood culture are needed for confirmation.

5. Classically, it appears as multiple, small, well-defined nodular opacities, 2–3 mm in size, throughout both lungs, but may also show patchy consolidation or reticulonodular opacities. The HRCT scan also shows tiny nodules diffusely scattered in the lung. Successful treatment allows the lung changes to resolve completely with no residual abnormality. Early empirical treatment is required to avoid death. For susceptible organisms,

this is carried out for 6–9 months and for meningeal involvement 9–12 months. Steroids are given for hypotension caused by adrenocortical insufficiency.

Case 2.46: Answers

1. The chest CT shows irregular areas of consolidation in the periphery of the left lower lobe. A chest tube is also noted.

2. Lung contusion: this is the most common manifestation of blunt trauma to the chest. Pathologically it is characterised by oedema and blood in the airspaces and interstitium. Clinically it presents with haemoptysis and is seen as early as 6 hours after trauma.

3. Pulmonary haemorrhage (larger area), infection, oedema (bilateral, batwing pattern), respiratory distress (diffuse) and fat embolism (takes 1–2 days) are the differential diagnoses.

4. The contusions are usually seen deep to the site of impact or contre coup. X-rays show irregular patchy or diffuse homogeneous consolidation. CT is more sensitive and shows non-segmental, coarse, ill-defined, amorphous opacification. There is no cavitation. There is subpleural sparing, of the 1–2 mm rim of lung tissue. Overlying rib fractures are seen. The opacity can enlarge for 48–72 hours and resolution begins from 48 hours. Complete resolution occurs in 2–10 days. Pneumothorax is a complication.

Case 2.47: Answers

1. The X-ray of the chest shows an area of heterogeneous opacification in the medial aspect of the left upper lobe. There are also patchy opacities in the left lower lobe. The CT scan of the left upper lobe shows an area of consolidation in the left upper lobe, with areas of ground-glass opacity surrounding it.

2. Fungal infection.

3. Fungal infections account for 25–30% of all pneumonias in bone marrow transplant recipients. Aspergillus infection is seen in 10% of all allogeneic bone marrow transplants. It can occur at any time after transplantation, but it is one of the most common infections in the early period. Risk factors for development are neutropenia in the early stages and steroid treatment for graft-versus-host disease in the later stages. Complications after bone marrow transplantation occur in specific phases. The pre-engraftment period (first 15–30 days), between stem cell transfusion and restoration of haematopoiesis, is characterised by severe pancytopenia. Early post-transplantation phase (30–100 days) begins after successful engraftment of donor stem cells and resumption of haematopoiesis. Although neutropenia resolves by this time, lymphocyte recovery lags behind. Late post-transplantation period (> 100 days) is characterised by normal lymphocyte level, but recovery of humoral immunity lags behind. Early complications in the lung are interstitial pneumonitis (infective and non-infective), infection, oedema, haemorrhage, thromboembolism, calcification and bronchiolitis obliterans.

4. Complications in other systems are:

   GIT and Hepatobiliary: graft-versus-host disease, neutropenic colitis, hepatic veno-occlusive disease, abscesses, post-transplantation lymphoproliferative disorder, hepatic regenerative nodules

   GUT: abscesses, haemolytic uraemic syndrome, papillary necrosis, renal vein thrombosis, nephrolithiasis, haematoma and haemorrhagic cystitis

   MSK: bone infarction, avascular necrosis

   CNS: infection, infarction, haemorrhage, therapy-induced toxic effects and recurrent malignancy.

5. On the X-ray, aspergillus infections are seen as peripheral pulmonary nodules. One of the characteristic signs is a hazy ground-glass opacity surrounding the nodule, which is caused by haemorrhage around central infarction as a result of vascular invasion of *Aspergillus* spp. The nodules cavitate when the neutrophil count recovers. Pleural effusions and lymphadenopathy are uncommon findings. Differential diagnoses are bacterial pneumonias (unusual in the early phase in spite of bacteraemia because of empirical use of broad-spectrum antibiotics), pulmonary oedema (prominent pulmonary vasculature, increased interstitial markings, and peribronchial thickening, perihilar shadowing, pleural effusions and airspace opacification), diffuse alveolar haemorrhage (patchy or diffuse airspace consolidation and ground-glass opacification), interstitial pneumonias (CMV, *P. jiroveci*, adenovirus, idiopathic causes – interstitial septal thickening, nodules, ground-glass opacities, patchy opacification).

Case 2.48: Answers

1. Chest X-ray shows bilateral diffuse reticular changes, which are predominantly seen in the central portions of the lung. There is bronchial wall thickening and dilatation. Some hyperinflation of the lung fields is noted. CT scan shows consolidation, particular on the right side, with some cystic spaces and some loss of volume of the right lung.

2. Cystic fibrosis.

3. Cystic fibrosis is an autosomal recessive disease, affecting chromosome 7, which has an incidence of 1/3000 in the Caucasian population. It is caused by an abnormality of CF transmembrane regulator (CFTR), which causes abnormal transmembrane transport of Na and Cl. It is diagnosed by the sweat test when the sweat Cl- > 60 mmol/ I (40–60 equivocal, < 40 is normal). In 2% of sufferers, sweat Cl- level will be normal. In such cases, DNA testing may provide the evidence of cystic fibrosis. When both these tests are normal, the diagnosis is made in some centres with measurement of voltage across the nasal epithelium of the patients.

4. Infection, inflammation, airway obstruction, bronchiectasis, respiratory failure and cor pulmonale are the respiratory complications of cystic fibrosis.

5. The lungs are normal initially, but abnormal chloride secretion results in viscid airway mucus. Infection, inflammation and airway obstruction cause progressive small and large airway disease. Bronchial wall thickening progresses to bronchiectasis and chronic airway disease causes hyperinflation. Initial changes are hyperinflation and peribronchial thickening. Progressive air trapping with bronchiectasis may be apparent in the upper lobes. With advancing pulmonary disease, pulmonary nodules resulting from abscesses, infiltrates with or without lobar atelectasis, marked hyperinflation with flattened domes of the diaphragm, thoracic kyphosis and bowing of the sternum develop. Pulmonary artery dilatation and RVH associated with cor pulmonale is usually masked by marked hyperinflation. Hilar enlargement can be a result of adenopathy or pulmonary hypertension with dilated central pulmonary arteries. Increasing cardiac size indicates cor pulmonale and prognosis is poor without transplantation. Pneumomediastinum and pneumothorax can occur. Lobar pneumonia is very rare in established cases and the chest X-ray does not reflect clinical changes in acute exacerbations.

6. There are many scoring systems. A commonly used scoring system is the Northern score. The lung is divided into upper and lower zones. Each zone is scored 0−4 based on radiological findings (1 − minimal increase in linear markings and/or nodular cystic lesions < 0.5 cm; 2 − more pronounced linear markings and/or more widespread nodular cystic lesions; 3 − prominent increase in linear markings, profuse nodular cystic lesions, large areas of collapse/consolidation; 4 − little or no area of normal lung). A further 0−4 points are allocated according to overall perception of severity. The maximum score is 20. This allows assessment of both acute changes and additional complications such as hilar adenopathy, cardiac size, hyperinflation and pneumothorax.

Case 2.49: Answers

1. The X-ray of the chest shows a small right lung, with increased lucency, compared to the contralateral side. The chest wall and left lung are normal. The CT scan shows lucent areas in the right lung, indicating air trapping and some reduction of pulmonary vascular markings.

2. Swyer−James syndrome.

3. Swyer−James syndrome is caused by post-infectious bronchiolitis in children, usually after viral infections such as respiratory syncytial virus, influenza, or mycoplasma, staphylococcal or streptococcal infections; this results in underdevelopment of the affected lung (arrested progressive growth, alveolarisation, resultant hypoplasia), which is smaller and more lucent as a result of overdistended alveoli and diminished arterial flow.

4. On X-rays the affected lung is smaller, with hyperlucency, and show air tapping on expiration. There is overexpansion of the opposite lung. Scarring or irregular vessels are seen. Fluoroscopy shows little change in volume of the involved lung with respiration. HRCT can be used to confirm the diagnosis. Areas of air trapping are demonstrated in the expiratory scans. Bronchi are pruned. A mosaic pattern or air trapping is seen.

5. Differential diagnosis: hypoplasia (from birth, whereas Swyer−James syndrome develops after severe childhood infection and over a period of time), emphysema (bilateral and overexpanded lungs) and pneumothorax (sudden onset, collapsed lung seen).

Case 2.50: Answers

1. The X-ray shows a diffuse, reticulonodular pattern in the mid and lower zones, bilaterally and prominance of hilar shadows. The CT scan shows bilateral interlobular septal thickening which is nodular and scattered alveolar opacities.

2. Lymphangitis carcinomatosis.

3. Lymphangitis carcinomatosis is an accumulation of tumour cells in the pulmonary interstitium. It usually follows tumour emboli and lymphatic obstruction, resulting in interstitial oedema and collagen deposition in the lung parenchyma. Primary tumours that cause lymphangitis are cancers of the lung, breast, stomach, thyroid, pancreas, larynx and cervix. Clinical presentation is dyspnoea, dry cough and haemoptysis.

4. The chest X-ray shows reticular or reticulonodular interstitial opacities, with septal lines. There is volume reduction of the lung. It is usually bilateral, but can be unilateral if the primary is lung cancer. Lymphadenopathy is seen in up to 50% of cases. The HRCT scan shows a smooth, thickened, polygonal, reticular network caused by thickened interlobular septa. Nodular thickening of interlobular septa and centrilobular nodules is seen. Pleural effusion is also a feature.

5. Usual interstitial pneumonia (lower zones, peripheral, no lymphadenopathy), sarcoidosis (more in upper and mid-zones, no polygonal structures, nodular thickening of interlobular septa and absence of pleural effusion) and extrinsic allergic alveolitis (upper zone predominance, no polygonal structures, pleural changes are rare) are the differential diagnoses.

3
GASTROINTESTINAL AND HEPATOBILIARY RADIOLOGY
QUESTIONS

Case 3.1

A 47-year-old woman presents with severe epigastric pain. On examination, epigastric tenderness was noted and the patient was tachycardic.

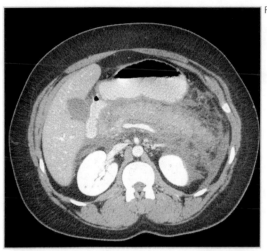

Fig 3.1a

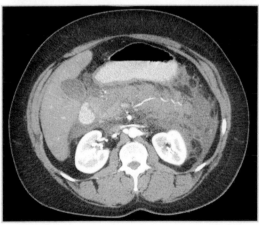

Fig 3.1b

1. What do you see on the first CT scan?
2. What is the diagnosis? What do you see on the follow-up CT scan?
3. What are the clinical features and lab abnormalities in this disease?
4. What are the common causes?
5. How is the disease staged? What is the optimal imaging test in evaluation of this disease?
6. How is this patient managed and what are the complications?

Answers *on pages 201–251*

Case 3.2

A 67-year-old woman presents with abdominal pain, haematemesis and weight loss. Clinical examination revealed a hard mass in the epigastric region.

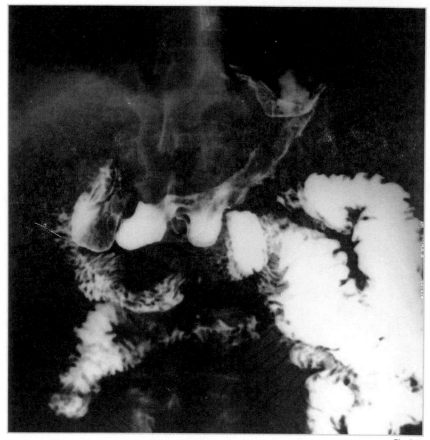

Fig 3.2

1. What do you see on the barium meal?
2. What is the cause of this appearance and what is the diagnosis?
3. What are the other causes of this appearance?
4. What are the radiological features?
5. What other investigations are required and what is the treatment?

Answers on pages 201–251

Case 3.3

A 12-year-old girl presents with colicky abdominal pain, nausea, vomiting and dyspepsia. On examination she is afebrile. There is no point tenderness in the abdomen. Bowel sounds are normal.

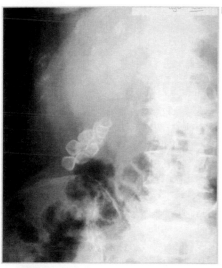
Fig 3.3a

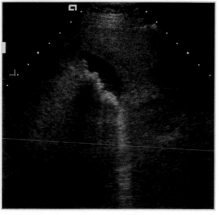
Fig 3.3b

1. What do you observe on the X-ray and ultrasound scan?
2. What is the diagnosis?
3. What is the aetiology of this disease?
4. What are the different types and what is the role of imaging?
5. What are the complications?

Answers *on pages 201–251*

Case 3.4

A 41-year-old man presents with severe haematemesis and jaundice. On clinical examination, his pulse was 120/min and blood pressure 100/70 mmHg. His liver was hard and nodular.

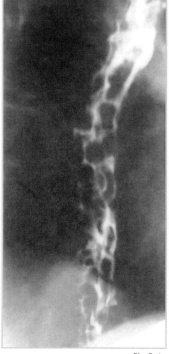

Fig 3.4a

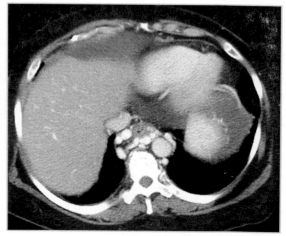

Fig 3.4b

1. What are the findings seen on a barium swallow and CT scan?
2. What is the diagnosis?
3. What are the types of process and what are the causes?
4. What are the radiological findings and the differential diagnosis?
5. What are the treatment and the role of radiology in management?

Answers *on pages 201–251*

Case 3.5

A 32-year-old man presents with epigastric pain, fullness and heartburn. Clinical examination revealed mild epigastric tenderness.

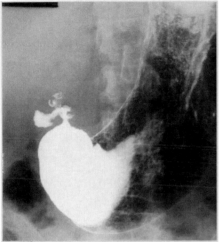
Fig 3.5a

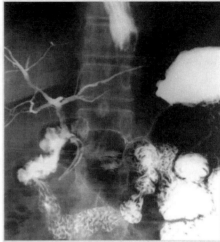
Fig 3.5b

1. What are the findings in barium meal pictures?
2. What is the diagnosis and what complication has developed?
3. What are the causes, predisposing factors and characteristic locations?
4. What are the radiological features and differential diagnosis?
5. What are the complications and the treatment?

Answers *on pages 201–251*

Case 3.6

A 37-year-old woman presents with dysphagia, coughing and vomiting.

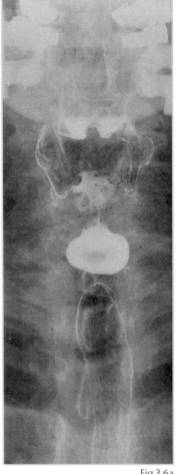

Fig 3.6a

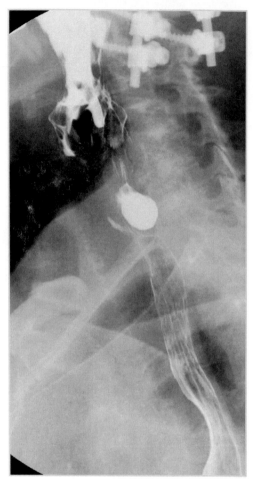

Fig 3.6b

1. What do you see on the barium swallow?
2. What is the diagnosis?
3. What are the clinical features and pathophysiology?
4. What are the radiological findings?
5. What are the variants of this disease?
6. What are the complications and treatment?

Answers *on pages 201–251*

Case 3.7

A 38-year-old presents with abdominal pain, vomiting and distension. On examination, the abdomen is distended and bowel sounds are not heard.

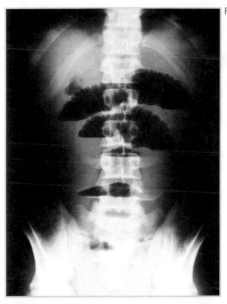

Fig 3.7a

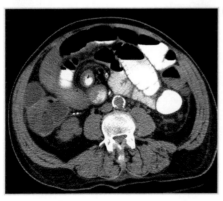

Fig 3.7b

1. What do you see on the plain X-ray of the abdomen and the CT scan?
2. What is the diagnosis?
3. What are the causes of this disease process?
4. What are the radiological findings in this disease?
5. What is the role of the CT scan?
6. What are the features of adynamic ileus?

Answers *on pages 201–251*

Case 3.8

A 57-year-old woman presents with chest pain, heartburn, dysphagia and vomiting.

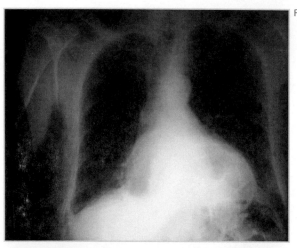

Fig 3.8a

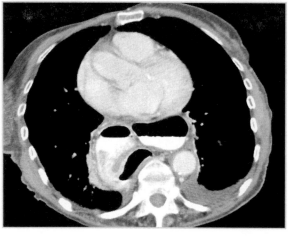

Fig 3.8b

1. What do you observe on the plain X-ray?
2. What do you observe on the CT scan and what is the diagnosis?
3. What are the types and radiological features?
4. What are the complications and treatment?
5. What is the radiological differential diagnosis?

Answers *on pages 201–251*

Case 3.9

A 57-year-old woman presents with jaundice, abdominal pain and abdominal distension. Clinical examination showed an enlarged liver and spleen.

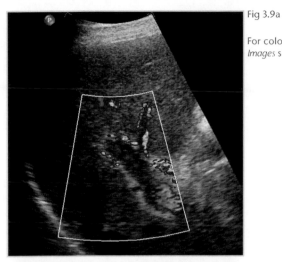

Fig 3.9a

For colour version, see *Colour Images* section from page 455.

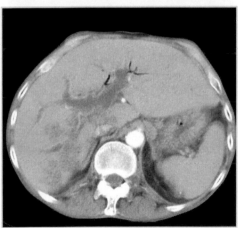

Fig 3.9b

1. What are the findings on ultrasonography and on the CT scan?
2. What is the diagnosis?
3. What are the common causes of this condition?
4. What are the radiological features?
5. What are the complications?

Answers *on pages 201–251*

Case 3.10

A 47-year-old woman presents with right upper quadrant pain, jaundice, body oedema and dyspnoea.

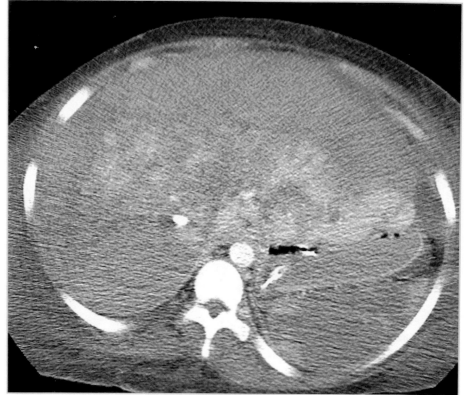

Fig 3.10

1. What are the findings on the CT scan?
2. What is the diagnosis?
3. What are the common causes of this condition?
4. What are the radiological features?
5. What are the treatment options?

Answers on pages 201–251

Case 3.11

A 29-year-old woman presents with abdominal pain, tenderness and fever. On examination, there is tenderness in the right upper quadrant.

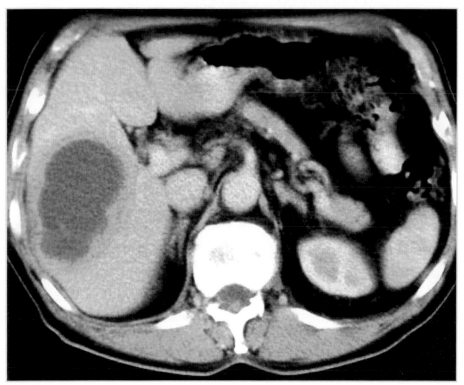

Fig 3.11

1. What do you find on the CT scan?
2. What is the diagnosis?
3. What is the aetiopathology of this disease?
4. What are the radiological features and differential diagnosis?
5. What are the complications and what is the role of radiology in treatment?

Answers on pages 201–251

Case 3.12

A 49-year-old man presents with jaundice, abdominal pain and abdominal distension. Clinical examination showed gynaecomastia, jaundice and vascular naevi in the skin. There was no abdominal mass.

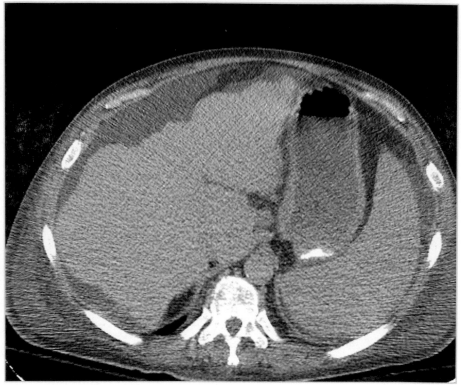

Fig 3.12

1. What are the findings on the CT scan?
2. What is the diagnosis?
3. What are the common causes of this condition?
4. What are the radiological features?
5. What are the complications?

Answers on pages 201–251

Case 3.13

A 47-year-old woman with diabetes presents with abdominal bloating and nausea. Clinical examination revealed hepatomegaly.

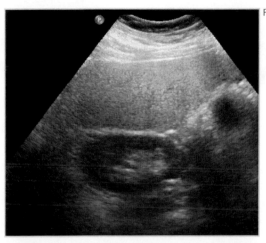
Fig 3.13a

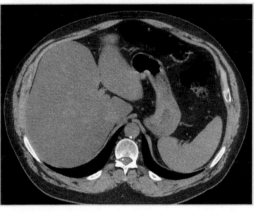
Fig 3.13b

1. What do you find on ultrasonography and on the CT scan?
2. What is the diagnosis?
3. What are the aetiological factors contributing to this disease?
4. What are the radiological features?
5. What is the differential diagnosis?

Answers *on pages 201–251*

A 67-year-old woman presents with weight loss and dysphagia for solid food. On examination she was anaemic. No mass was felt.

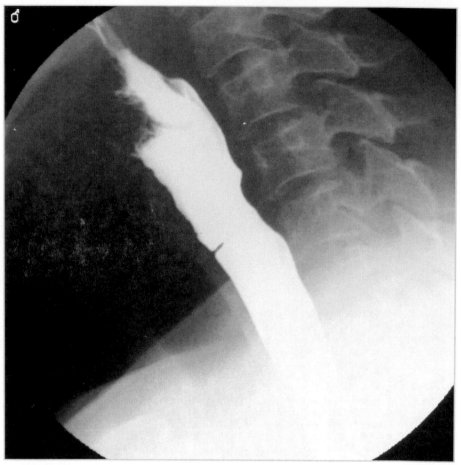

Fig 3.14

1. What do you find on the barium swallow?
2. What is the diagnosis?
3. What is the most common location of this disease?
4. What is the most important syndrome associated with this condition?
5. What are the complications and treatment?
6. What are the radiological features and differential diagnosis?

Answers on pages 201–251

Case 3.15

A 55-year-old man presented with dysphagia for solid foods, chest pain and weight loss.

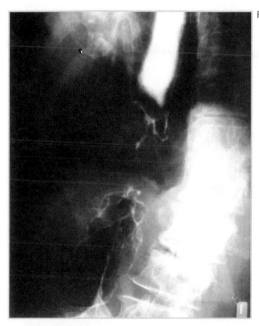

Fig 3.15a

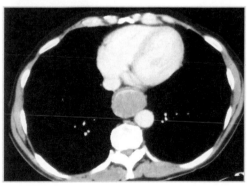

Fig 3.15b

1. What are the findings seen on barium swallow and on the CT scan?
2. What is the diagnosis?
3. What are the histological types and causes?
4. What are the clinical features and the routine investigations?
5. What are the radiological features?
6. What are the treatment and palliative options?

Answers *on pages 201–251*

Case 3.16

A 56-year-old woman presents with severe abdominal pain, fever and chills. Clinical examination showed severe tenderness and a mass in the right upper quadrant.

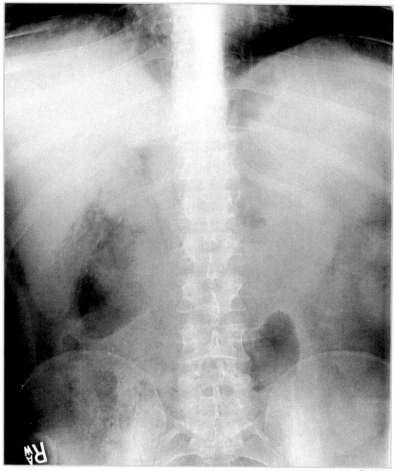

Fig 3.16

1. What do you see on the X-ray of the abdomen?
2. What is the diagnosis?
3. What is the predisposing factor for this condition?
4. What are the causative agents?
5. What are the types and radiological features?

Answers on pages 201–251

Case 3.17

A 54-year-old woman presents with weight loss and abdominal distension.

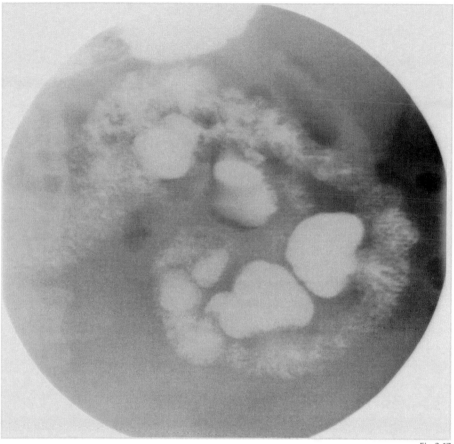

Fig 3.17

1. What do you find on the barium study?
2. What is the diagnosis?
3. What are the aetiology and common locations of this disease?
4. What are the radiological features?
5. What are the clinical features and complications?

Answers on pages 201–251

Case 3.18

A 65-year-old man presents with abdominal pain, vomiting and distension. Clinical examination revealed a paucity of bowel sounds.

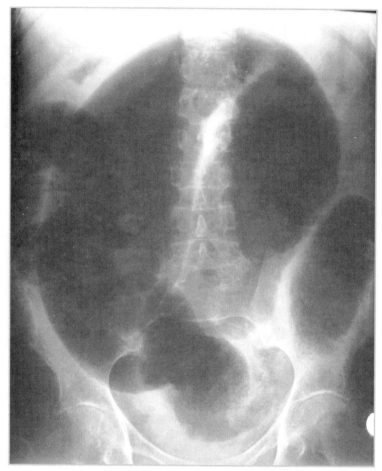

Fig 3.18

1. What do you see on the plain abdominal X-ray?
2. What is the diagnosis?
3. What are the aetiology and predisposing factors?
4. What are the radiological findings? What other investigations might be performed?
5. What are the complications and treatment?

Answers on pages 201–251

Case 3.19

A 54-year-old woman presents with dysphagia, heartburn, regurgitation and cough.

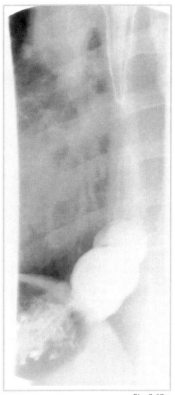

Fig 3.19a

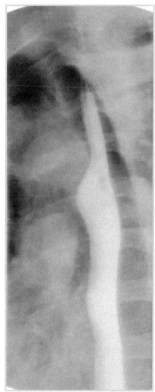

Fig 3.19b

1. What do you see in these pictures? The first picture was taken during swallowing of barium. The second image was taken after completion of drinking of barium.
2. What is the diagnosis?
3. What is the mechanism of development of this condition?
4. What are the radiological tests that are useful for diagnosis? What are the radiological findings?
5. What are the complications and the treatment of this disease?

Answers on pages 201–251

Case 3.20

An 11-year-old boy presents with severe abdominal pain, vomiting, nausea and tenderness. On examination, there is severe rebound tenderness in the abdomen. He is febrile and tachycardic.

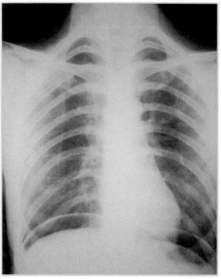

Fig 3.20a

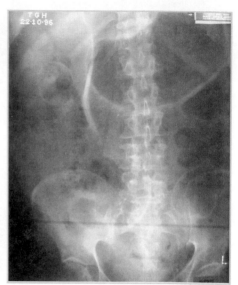

Fig 3.20b

1. What do you observe on the plain abdominal X-rays?
2. What is the diagnosis?
3. What are the radiological signs of this presentation?
4. What are the causes of this appearance?
5. What conditions may create difficulty in plain film diagnosis?

Answers on pages 201–251

Case 3.21

A 35-year-old woman presents with dysphagia for liquids and chest pain

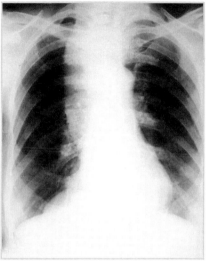

Fig 3.21a

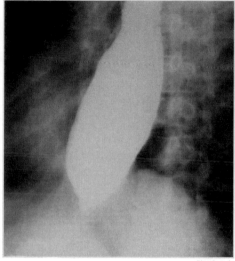

Fig 3.21b

1. What do you see on the chest X-ray and barium swallow?
2. What is the diagnosis? What is the pathophysiology of this disease?
3. What are the radiological findings and variants of this disease?
4. What is the most important differential diagnosis?
5. What are the complications and what is the treatment?

Answers *on pages 201–251*

A 29-year-old immunosuppressed patient develops dysphagia, chest pain and odynophagia.

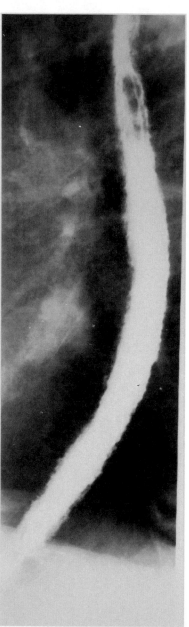

Fig 3.22

1. What do you observe on the barium swallow?
2. What is the diagnosis?
3. What are the predisposing factors and pathophysiology of this disease?
4. What are the radiological features?
5. What are the complications and treatment?
6. What is the differential diagnosis?

Answers on pages 201–251

Case 3.23

A 39-year-old man presents with severe chest pain after an endoscopic procedure for removal of a foreign body.

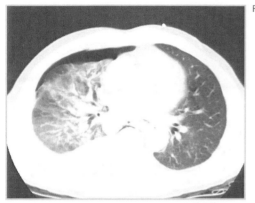
Fig 3.23a

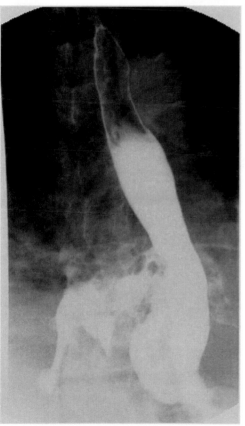

Fig 3.23b

1. What do you observe on the CT scan and contrast swallow?
2. What is the diagnosis?
3. What are the predisposing factors, common locations and clinical features?
4. What are the radiological features?
5. What are the complications and treatment of this disease?

Answers *on pages 201–251*

Case 3.24

A 17-year-old girl presents with abdominal pain, loss of weight and loose stools with blood and fever. On examination she is febrile. There is tenderness in the right iliac fossa. The bowel sounds were normal.

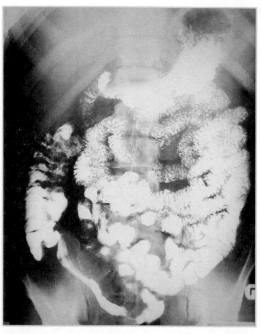

Fig 3.24a

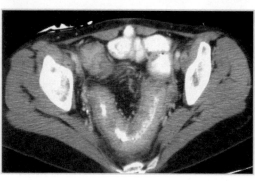

Fig 3.24b

1. What are the findings in the first picture?
2. What do you observe on the abdominal CT scan?
3. What is the diagnosis?
4. What are the clinical features, complications and treatment?
5. What are the radiological features and differential diagnosis?

Answers *on pages 201–251*

Case 3.25

A 31-year-old woman presented with epigastric pain, worse after eating, vomiting and fullness

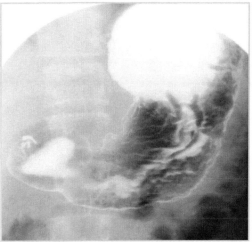

Fig 3.25a

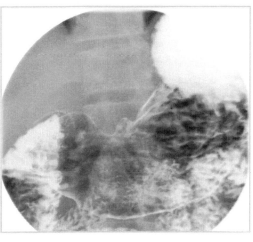

Fig 3.25b

1. What are the findings in the barium meal pictures?
2. What is the diagnosis?
3. What are the causes?
4. What are the predisposing factors?
5. What are the radiological features and differential diagnosis?
6. What are the complications and treatment?

Answers on pages 201–251

Case 3.26

A widely travelled 31-year-old business man presents with intermittent abdominal pain and weight loss. Clinical examination is unremarkable. Abdomen is soft and tender.

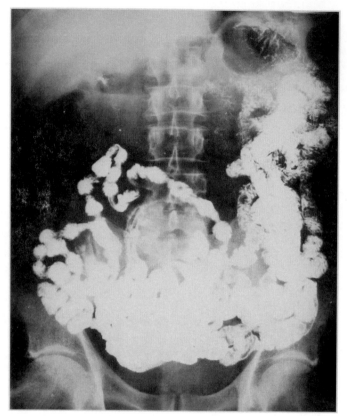

Fig 3.26a

1. What do you find on the barium follow-through study?
2. What is the diagnosis?
3. What are the causative agent and pathophysiology?
4. What is the most common location in the bowel?
5. What are the complications?

Answers on pages 201–251

Case 3.27

A 48-year-old woman presents with abdominal distension and pain.

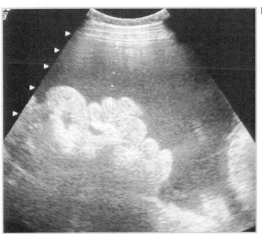
Fig 3.27a

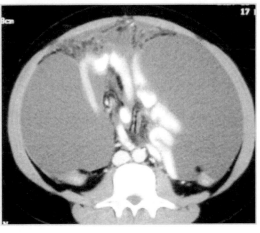
Fig 3.27b

1. What do you see on ultrasonography and on the abdominal CT scan?
2. What is the diagnosis?
3. What are the causes?
4. What are the radiological features? How do you differentiate benign and malignant subtypes of this condition?
5. What is the pathophysiology of this condition? What is the earliest location of this condition?
6. What is the role of radiology in diagnosis and treatment?

Answers *on pages 201–251*

Case 3.28

A 71-year-old man presents with fatigue, abdominal pain and rectal bleeding.

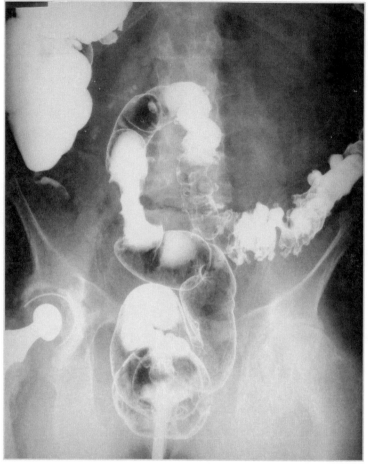

Fig 3.28

1. What do you see on the barium enema?
2. What is the diagnosis?
3. What are the chronic conditions that increase the risk of this disease?
4. What are the investigations that are used in early diagnosis of this disease and what are the common locations?
5. What is the role of radiology in disease at this stage?
6. What are the complications and what is the differential diagnosis?

Answers on pages 201–251

Case 3.29

A 28-year-old man with relevant family history presented with rectal bleeding and anaemia.

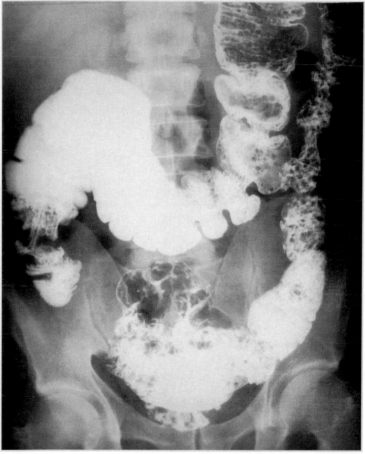

Fig 3.29

1. What are the findings from the barium enema?
2. What is the diagnosis? What syndrome does the patient have?
3. What are the radiological features? What are the different pathological types?
4. What is the risk of malignancy? What is the management of this condition?
5. What are the other clinical conditions with similar radiographic change?

Answers *on pages 201–251*

Case 3.30

A 73-year-old man presents with sudden onset of severe abdominal pain and abdominal distension. Clinical examination shows decreased bowel sounds. The patient is hypotensive, tachycardic and acidotic.

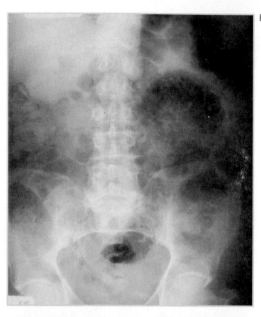

Fig 3.30a

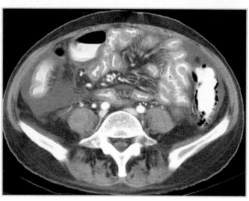

Fig 3.30b

1. What are the findings on the X-ray and CT scan?
2. What is the diagnosis?
3. What are the radiological features and causative factors of this condition?
4. What are the differential diagnoses?

Answers on pages 201–251

Case 3.31

A 37-year-old woman presents with diarrhoea, abdominal bloating and loss of weight. Clinical examination revealed mild tenderness in the right upper quadrant.

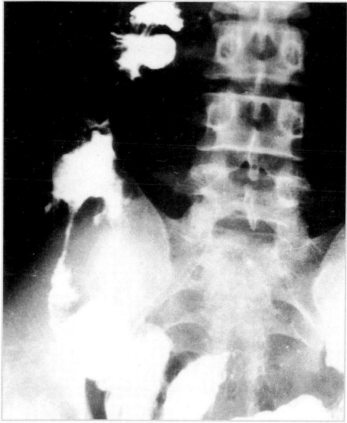

Fig 3.31

1. What are the findings from the barium study?
2. What is the diagnosis?
3. What is the aetiopathology of the disease? What are the various types?
4. What are the radiological features?
5. What is the differential diagnosis?

Case 3.32

A 55-year-old man presented with left lower quadrant pain and tenderness. He had a barium enema 1 month ago.

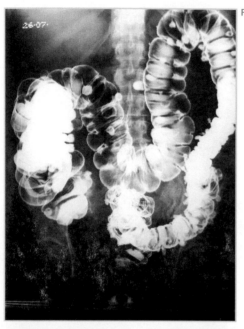

Fig 3.32a

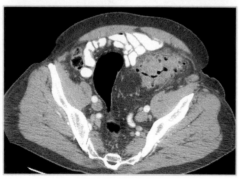

Fig 3.32b

1. What do you see on the barium enema and CT scan?
2. What is the diagnosis?
3. What are the predisposing factors?
4. What are the complications?
5. What are the radiological features and differential diagnosis?
6. What is the treatment?

Answers *on pages 201–251*

Case 3.33

A 63-year-old woman presents with jaundice, abdominal pain and loss of weight. A percutaneous transhepatic cholangiogram is performed.

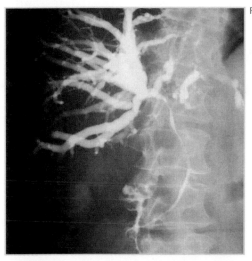

Fig 3.33a

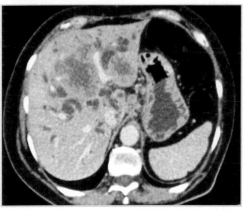

Fig 3.33b

Gastrointestinal Questions

1. What do you see on the cholangiogram and CT scan of abdomen?
2. What is the diagnosis?
3. What are the predisposing factors, types and common locations?
4. What are the radiological features?
5. What is the differential diagnosis and what is the treatment?

Answers on pages 201–251

Case 3.34

A 56-year-old man, with a history of cirrhosis secondary to hepatitis B, presents with right upper quadrant pain and jaundice. His liver function test is markedly abnormal. On examination, a non-tender, firm mass was felt in the right upper quadrant.

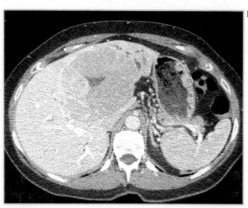
Fig 3.34a

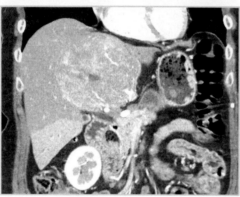
Fig 3.34b

1. What do you see on the CT scan?
2. What is the diagnosis?
3. What are the predisposing factors and clinical features?
4. What are the radiological features?
5. What is the differential diagnosis?
6. What is the management of this condition? What is the role of radiology in management?

Answers on pages 201–251

Case 3.35

A 36-year-old woman presents with jaundice, fever and abdominal pain.

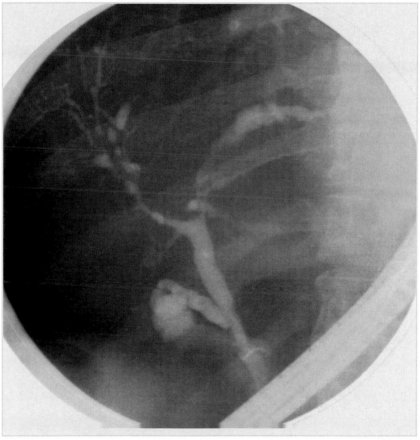

Fig 3.35

1. What do you observe in this test?
2. What is the diagnosis?
3. What is the most important disease that is associated with this condition?
4. What are the radiological findings?
5. What are the major complications?
6. What is the differential diagnosis?

Answers *on pages 201–251*

Case 3.36

A 31-year-old woman presents with bloating, steatorrhoea and bone pain. On clinical examination, there is abdominal distension, with decreased bowel sounds, but no mass was palpated. Multiple skin lesions are noted on the scalp of the patient.

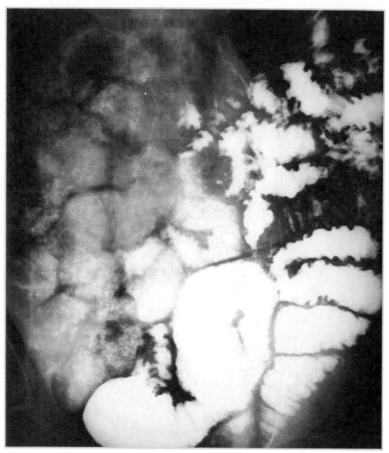

Fig 3.36

1. What are the findings on the barium follow-through?
2. What is the diagnosis? What are the clinical features?
3. What are the radiological findings?
4. What is the differential diagnosis?
5. What are the complications and treatment?

Answers on pages 201–251

Case 3.37

A 67-year-old woman presents with fatigue and rectal bleeding.

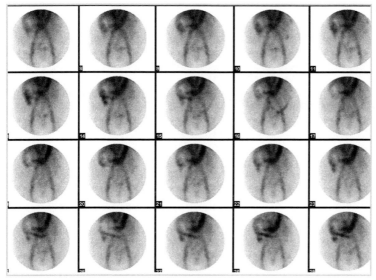

Fig 3.37a

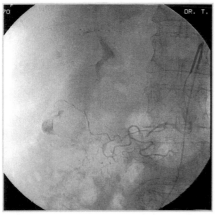

Fig 3.37b

1. What is the first investigation and what are the findings?
2. What is the second investigation and what are the findings?
3. What is the diagnosis?
4. What are the other causes for this clinical condition?
5. What are the investigations used in diagnosis?
6. What is the role of radiology in treatment?

Answers on pages 201–251

A 9-year-old boy presented with severe abdominal pain and rectal bleeding. On examination, she was haemodynamically stable. Tenderness was elicited in the lower abdomen.

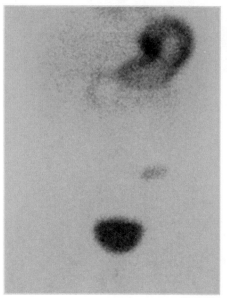

Fig 3.38a

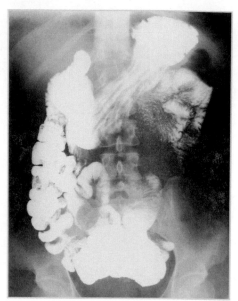

Fig 3.38b

1. What is the test on Fig 3.38a? What are the findings in this patient?
2. What is the diagnosis?
3. How is this scan done?
4. What is the aetiology of this condition? What are the clinical features and treatment?
5. What do you see on the second picture, which was taken after a week? What are the complications?

Answers on pages 201–251

Case 3.39

A 16-month-old baby presents with diarrhoea, rectal bleeding and incessant cry. X-ray and ultrasonography of the abdomen were performed.

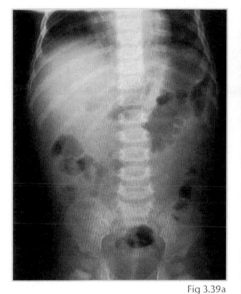

Fig 3.39a

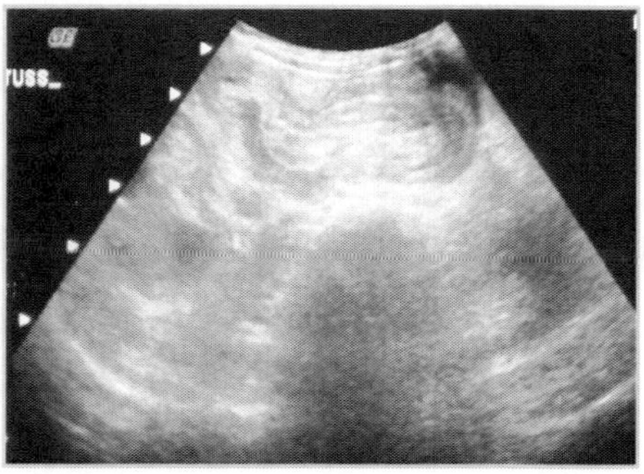

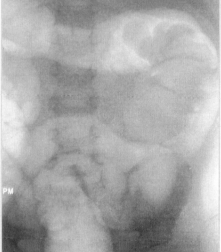

Fig 3.39b

Fig 3.39c

1. What do you observe on the plain X-ray and ultrasonography?
2. What is the diagnosis?
3. What are the clinical features?
4. What are the radiological features?
5. What do you see on the third picture and what is the management of this patient?

Answers *on pages 201–251*

Case 3.40

A 37-year-old woman presented with abdominal pain, fever, weight loss and bloody diarrhoea. On examination she has tenderness in the lower abdomen.

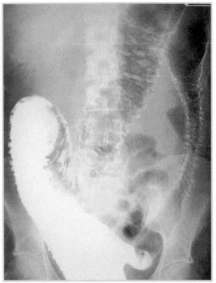
Fig 3.40a

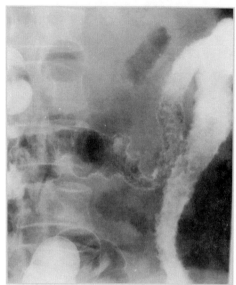
Fig 3.40b

1. What are the findings on the barium enema?
2. What is the diagnosis and what complications do you observe?
3. What are the clinical features and the characteristic locations?
4. What are the radiological findings and the differential diagnosis?
5. What are the complications and the risk of malignancy?
6. What is the treatment?

Answers on pages 201–251

Case 3.41

A 43-year-old woman presents with abdominal pain, diarrhoea and weight loss. On examination, there is mild tenderness in the epigastric region and a cystic mass is palpated.

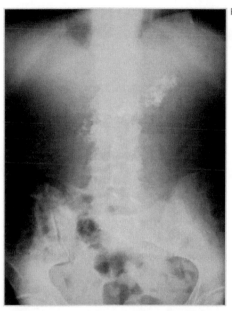

Fig 3.41a

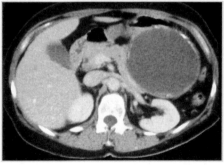

Fig 3.41b

1. What do you see on the X-ray and CT scan of the abdomen?
2. What is the diagnosis?
3. What is the classification of this disease? What are the causes?
4. What are the imaging features?
5. What are the complications and the most important diagnostic dilemma?
6. What is the role of radiology in treatment?

Answers *on pages 201–251*

Case 3.42

A 38-year-old woman presents with abdominal pain, diarrhoea and vomiting. She also complains of episodes of flushing and falls. A barium meal was performed. A CT scan was also performed a few days later, immediately after an ERCP.

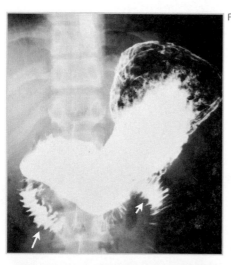
Fig 3.42a

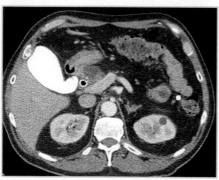
Fig 3.42b

1. What are the findings from the barium study (arrows) and on the CT scan?

2. What is the diagnosis?

3. What are the pathology and the pathophysiology of this disease?

4. What are the radiological features?

5. What are the complications and treatment?

Answers on pages 201–251

Case 3.43

A 43-year-old man who underwent bone marrow transplantation for leukaemia presents with severe itching, skin rash, nausea, vomiting and diarrhoea. Clinical examination revealed a diffuse rash. His abdomen is diffusely tender, but no mass was palpated.

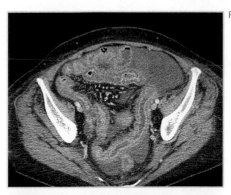
Fig 3.43a

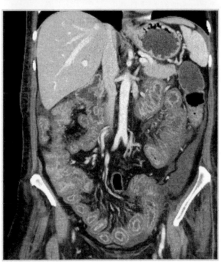
Fig 3.43b

1. What do you observe on the abdominal CT scan?
2. What is the diagnosis?
3. What are the clinical features and pathophysiology of this disease?
4. What are the radiological features?
5. What are the differential diagnosis and the treatment?

Answers *on pages 201–251*

Case 3.44

A 37-year-old woman presents with a chronic, systemic disease, with diarrhoea and abdominal pain. Clinical examination showed decreased bowel sounds. A barium meal follow-through examination was performed.

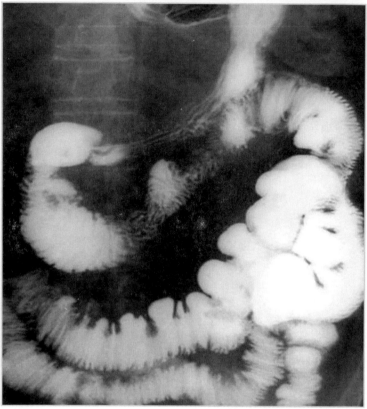

Fig 3.44

1. What are the findings in this 1½ hour film of barium follow-through examination?

2. What is the cause of this appearance? What is the cause of diarrhoea and bone pain?

3. What are the clinical features and other complications of this condition?

4. What are the radiological features?

5. How will you manage this patient?

Answers on pages 201–251

1. The initial CT scan shows an enlarged pancreas, which in turn shows normal enhancement with contrast. There is a small area of non-enhancement in the head. There is fluid around the pancreas, which is extending anterior to both kidneys, especially on the left side.

2. Acute pancreatitis. In the second CT scan, the entire gland is dark and shows no areas of enhancement, implying development of pancreatic necrosis.

3. Epigastric or right upper quadrant pain/tenderness, nausea, vomiting, fever, hypotension, tachycardia, tachypnoea, jaundice and decreased bowel sounds are the clinical features. Raised amylase and lipase are the common abnormalities seen in acute pancreatitis. Other abnormalities include raised WBC, altered liver function tests and abnormal electrolytes.

4. Alcohol and biliary stone are the most common causes of acute pancreatitis. Other causes include medications, hyperlipidaemia, trauma, carcinoma, pancreas divisum, cardiopulmonary bypass, infections and peptic ulcer disease.

5. Pancreatitis is graded and staged using Ranson's criteria, APACHE II and CT severity index. CT grading of pancreatitis (scores given in parentheses):

   Grade A: the pancreas appears normal

   Grade B: pancreas is enlarged and oedematous (1)

   Grade C: inflammation extends to peripancreatic tissue (2)

   Grade D: one fluid collection, without abscess (3)

   Grade E: multiple fluid collections or pancreatic abscess (4).

   Grades of necrosis 2 < **30%;** 4 **30–50%;** 6 > **50%**. The combined score of CT grading and necrosis is calculated and the severity depends on the score. The CT scan is done in non-contrast, arterial and venous phases. Areas of necrosis do not enhance in arterial phase and this is an important prognostic indicator. Usually, acute pancreatitis is a clinical diagnosis. The CT scan is used when the diagnosis is indeterminate or for evaluation of complications. Ultrasonography is done for the assessment of gallstones.

6. The management of acute pancreatitis includes no oral intake, nasogastric intubation, parenteral nutrition, analgesics, antibiotics, fluids and electrolyte replacement. Collections are drained under CT guidance. Pancreatic phlegmon, pancreatic necrosis, pancreatic abscess, pseudocyst, pseudoaneurysms, haemorrhagic pancreatitis, pancreatic ascites, biliary obstruction and thoracopancreatic fistula are the local complications. Fat necrosis, hypocalcaemia, ARDS, pleural effusion, consolidation, acute circulatory failure and acute renal failure are the systemic complications.

Case 3.2: Answers

1. Barium meal shows a severely contracted stomach, with fixed narrowing of the lumen, which does not show any peristalsis. This did not shows any change in configuration on delayed images (not shown here).

2. This appearance is called linitis plastica or leather bottle stomach and is caused by diffuse infiltration of stomach submucosa by a scirrhous gastric carcinoma.

3. Gastric cancer is the most common cause of a linitis plastica appearance. Other causes of this radiological appearance are chronic gastric ulcer with severe spasm, lymphoma, pseudolymphoma, metastasis, TB, Crohn's disease, syphilis, histoplasmosis, actinomycosis, toxoplasmosis, corrosives, radiation, hepatic chemoembolisation, sarcoidosis, amyloidosis, eosinophilic gastritis and polyarteritis nodosa.

4. The characteristic appearance on a barium meal is a leather bottle stomach, which is a diffusely narrowed stomach with wall thickening, and no change in configuration with peristalsis. The morphological types of gastric carcinoma are ulcerative, polypoid, scirrhous, superficial spreading and multicentric.

5. Further investigations are endoscopy and biopsy to confirm the diagnosis and a CT scan to assess the extension to the perigastric soft tissue, adjacent organs, lymphadenopathy, liver metastasis and distal metastasis. Treatment options are surgery and chemotherapy. The selection of the surgical procedure depends on the location of the tumour, the growth pattern seen on biopsy specimens and the expected location of lymph node metastases. For proximal third gastric cancer, an extended

gastrectomy, including the distal oesophagus, is performed. Middle third cancer requires total gastrectomy. Distal third gastric cancers undergo total gastrectomy if biopsy shows 'diffuse-type' carcinoma and subtotal gastrectomy if the biopsy reveals 'intestinal-type' adenocarcinoma.

Case 3.3: Answers

1. X-ray of the abdomen shows multiple, laminated opacities in the right upper quadrant. In US scan, there are multiple, echogenic (bright) opacities within the lumen of the gall bladder, with distal shadowing. The wall of the gall bladder is not thickened and there is no fluid collection around the gall bladder.

2. Cholelithiasis.

3. Causes of cholelithiasis in children: sickle cell disease, hereditary spherocytosis, other haemolytic anaemias, cystic fibrosis, malabsorption, Crohn's disease, total parenteral nutrition, intestinal resection and choledochal cyst. Calculi in neonates are caused by: haemolytic anaemia, infection, parenteral nutrition, dehydration, starvation, phototherapy, biliary atresia, short gut syndrome and furosemide.

4. Calculi can be cholesterol stone or pigment stone. Pure cholesterol stones are radiolucent and are not seen in X-ray. In CT, they are hypodense and float in contrast enhanced bile. A mixture of cholesterol and calcium carbonate stones are laminated and opaque in plain films (20%). Pigment stones (30%) are denser than bile. In X-ray, 85% of stones are lucent and 15% are opaque. Of the lucent stones 85% are cholesterol and 15% are pigment. Of the opaque stones, 67% are pigment stones and 33% are cholesterol stones. Calcium phosphate is deposited centrally in cholesterol stones and calcium carbonate is deposited peripherally around cholesterol. In ultrasound, the gallstones might appear to float. This is either due to pure cholesterol stones or gas containing stones or rise in specific gravity of bile. Gas containing stones result from dehydration of older stones with internal shrinkage and nitrogen gas filling (Mercedes Benz sign). The role of imaging is to establish the diagnosis, detect the state of intra and extrahepatic bile ducts and detect the complications of cholelithiasis.

5. Complications of gallstones are acute cholecystitis, chronic cholecystitis, perforation, abscess, porcelain gallbladder and carcinoma. Acute

cholecystitis is seen as thick-walled, oedematous gallbladder with pericholecystic fluid collection. Chronic cholecystitis has thick walls. In perforation, the gallbladder wall is irregular, stones might be seen outside the gallbladder and there is gas in the peritoneum. Focal fluid collections can be seen outside the gallbladder.

Case 3.4: Answers

1. Barium swallow shows smooth, longitudinal filling defects in the thoracic oesophagus. The CT scan shows tortuous enhancing lesions surrounding the distal oesophagus, which appears thickened.

2. Oesophageal varices.

3. Oesophageal varices are plexus formed by dilated subepithelial veins, submucosal veins and venae comitantes of vagus nerves outside muscularis. There are two types: **uphill varices** carry collateral blood from the portal vein via the azygos vein to the SVC; **downhill varices** carry blood from the SVC via the azygos into the IVC/portal vein and is seen in the upper oesophagus. Uphill varices are the most common and caused by cirrhosis, splenic vein thrombosis, obstruction of hepatic veins/ IVC and marked splenomegaly. Downhill varices are caused by obstruction of the SVC distal to entry of the azygos vein as a result of lung cancer, lymphoma, goitre, mediastinal tumours or mediastinal fibrosis. In normal people, the anterior branch of the oesophageal vein is connected to the left gastric vein. The posterior branch is connected to the azygos and hemiazygos veins, which are the veins commonly involved in oesophageal varices.

4. Barium swallow is often used in diagnosis. Thin barium is used and images are acquired with the Valsalva manoeuvre/deep inspiration or left anterior oblique projection with the patient in a recumbent position. Varices are seen as thickened folds, with tortuous radiolucent filling defects. Occasionally varices are incidentally discovered on CT scans. The oesophageal wall is thickened and there are right- and left-sided soft-tissue masses around the oesophagus, which enhance in serpiginous fashion. The common differential diagnoses are varicoid carcinoma of the oesophagus (fixed appearance, no variation with Valsalva manoeuvre) and candidiasis (irregular ulcerations).

5. Oesophageal varices with bleeding are treated with resuscitation and endoscopic sclerotherapy/variceal banding. Surgical procedures are portosystemic shunt and devascularisation or liver transplantation in advanced liver disease. Interventional radiology is useful in management of severe bleeding. Percutaneous transheptic embolisation of gastro-oesophageal varices is done by catheterisation of the gastric collaterals that supply blood to the varices through the transhepatic route. An TIPSS (transjugular intrahepatic portosystemic shunt) is used if the medical and endoscopic treatment fails.

Case 3.5: Answers

1. The barium meal shows deformed and irregular duodenal cap. The second picture shows contrast in the biliary tree.

2. Duodenal ulcer. In the second picture, barium is seen entering the biliary tree, indicating a choledochoduodenal fistula.

3. Predisposing factors are NSAIDs (cyclo-oxygenase or COX-I inhibition, which decreases protective prostaglandins), steroids, *Helicobacter pylori* infection (increased gastric acid production by cytokines, immunological response against duodenal mucosa secondary to bacterial colonisation in gastric metaplasia induced by high acid, proteases, urease), smoking, alcohol, caffeine, diet, Zollinger–Ellison syndrome, mastocytosis, chemotherapy, radiation and cocaine use. Of duodenal ulcers 95% are seen in the bulbar region and are more common in the anterior wall; just 5% are seen in the post-bulbar region with most in the medial wall above the papilla. Ulcers in the post-bulbar region, especially beyond the ampulla and in the jejunum are suspicious of Zollinger–Ellison syndrome caused by gastrinomas.

4. Barium meal is sparingly used nowadays because the diagnosis is made by endoscopy. In early stages, a round or oval ulcer is seen in the duodenal bulb. Kissing ulcers are seen as ulcers opposite to each other in the anterior and posterior walls. Giant ulcers are large and measure > 2 cm. Most of the ulcers present with deformity of the duodenal bulb. The deformity can be a cloverleaf deformity or an hourglass stenosis. Differential diagnoses for duodenal narrowing and deformity are TB, strongyloidiasis, Crohn's disease, sprue, malignancy, pancreatitis, pancreatic carcinoma and trauma.

5. Complications are obstruction, perforation (anterior wall), bleeding (posterior wall) and penetration with sealed perforation. Duodenal ulcer is the most common cause of bowel perforation. Pneumoperitoneum is seen on a plain X-ray. A CT scan of the abdomen can be used to confirm and find the location of the perforation. Leak of air and contrast can be demonstrated from the site of the duodenal ulcer. Fistula can develop to the bile duct. Treatment depends on the aetiology and presentation. *Helicobacter pylori*-induced ulcers receive an eradication therapy regimen. For ulcers caused by NSAIDs, the drugs are discontinued and proton pump inhibitors (PPIs) used. Bleeding ulcers are treated with endoscopic therapy (cautery/adrenaline [epinephrine]/argon plasma coagulation). H_2-receptor antagonists and PPIs are also used. Failure of endoscopic therapy for bleeding, recurrent bleeding and perforation is an indication for urgent surgery. Vagotomy with pyroplasty or antrectomy is done in patients who are refractory/intolerant to or non-compliant with medical management.

Case 3.6: Answers

1. Anteroposterior view of barium swallow shows a focal collection of barium in the lower part of neck. Lateral view shows a large outpouching filled with barium, extending posteriorly from the lower part of hypopharynx. This is seen above the level of a contracted cricopharynx.

2. Pharyngeal pouch.

3. Pharyngeal pouch or Zencker's diverticulum is a pulsion diverticulum, where the pharyngeal mucosa herniates posteriorly between cricopharyngeus and the inferior pharyngeal constrictor muscles (Kilian's dehiscence) as a result of failure of coordination between the relaxation of cricopharyngeus during swallowing and contraction of the pharyngeal wall. Clinical features are dysphagia, regurgitation, aspiration and halitosis. It is common in men of old age.

4. Barium swallow is the diagnostic procedure of choice. The pouch can be of any size. When it is very small, it might be obscured by the barium pool and delayed images are required to notice stasis of contrast. Large pouches are seen in lateral views and in AP views after the barium has passed through the rest of the oesophagus. When the pouch is very large, it might displace the oesophagus laterally and extends distally towards the thoracic inlet. A prominent cricopharyngeal impression is also seen.

5. Lateral pharyngeal pouches are persistent protrusions of the lateral pharyngeal wall at sites of anatomical weakness such as the posterior thyrohyoid membrane and tonsillar fossa after tonsillectomy. They are seen as hemispherical protrusions in the upper hypopharynx above the thyroid cartilage. On lateral views, the pouches are seen as ovoid barium collections anteriorly in the upper hypopharynx.

6. Squamous cell carcinoma is associated in 0.5–1.5%. Bezoars, tracheal fistula, vocal fold paralysis, cervical osteomyelitis and retained foreign body are complications. Hiatus hernia, laryngocele, oesophageal web, oesophageal spasm/stenosis, achalasia and gastric ulcers are also associated. Small asymptomatic pouches do not require treatment. Surgery is indicated when the diverticulum is large and complications develop. Surgical options are diverticulectomy with cricopharyngeal myotomy or diverticulopexy with myotomy or endoscopic division of the diverticular wall.

Case 3.7: Answers

1. The plain X-ray shows dilated loops of small bowel with air-fluid levels in the central part of the abdomen. There is no gas in the colon. The CT scan shows dilated loops of small bowel.

2. Small bowel obstruction.

3. Adhesions, hernia, tumours, volvulus, intussusceptions and gall stone ileus are common causes of obstruction in adults.

Classification based on disease process:

Congenital – Atresia, duplication, stenosis of small bowel, midgut voluvus, Meckel's diverticulum, meconium ileus.

Extrinsic (Extramural) – Adhesions, hernia, volvulus, extrinsic neoplasm compressing small bowel.

Intraluminal – Foreign bodies, intussusception, intrinsic tumours such as polyps.

Intramural – Tumours, strictures, inflammatory (Crohns's disease, backwash ileitis, etc), ischaemia, radiation, haemorrhage (trauma, Henoch Schonlein, anticoagulants)

4. The X-ray is the mainstay in diagnosis. In a normal abdomen, there might be gas in three to four variable shaped loops < 2. 5 cm in diameter. In obstruction, there are dilated loops of small bowel. Jejunal loops have frequent and high valvulae conniventes. Ileum has spared or absent valvulae conniventes. Normal small bowel loops are centrally placed and show valvulae conniventes. Large bowel loops are in the periphery and show haustrations. Erect films show distended small bowel loops (> 3 cm) with air–fluid levels. There is little or no gas in distal small bowel. A stepladder appearance is seen in a lower obstruction. String-of-beads appearance is seen with air entrapped in the valvulae in obstruction. Occasionally the bowel loops are completely filled with fluid and there is no gas in the abdomen. The point of obstruction is identified if there is a sudden transition from a dilated to a non-dilated loop. Water-soluble contrast can be orally administered and follow-up films are done after 3 and 24 hours. In complete small bowel obstruction , there is no passage of contrast after 3–24 hours. In low-grade small bowel obstruction there is some flow of contrast distal to the obstruction with visualisation of folds. In high-grade obstruction, there is a delay in the arrival of contrast, which is diluted and hence the folds are not clearly seen.

5. The CT scan is used for diagnosis of obstruction (dilated small bowel loops > 2.5 cm: small bowel faeces sign – gas bubbles mixed with particulate matter proximal to obstruction) detecting the level of obstruction and presence of other intraperitoneal lesions.

6. Adynamic/paralytic ileus is a derangement that impairs proper distal propulsion of intestinal contents. Common causes are postoperative, pain, peritonitis, perforation, peptic ulcer, pancreatitis, appendicitis, hypokalaemia, pregnancy, pyelonephritis and pneumonia. In adynamic ileus, dilated small and large bowel loops are seen, but the small bowel distension decreases on serial films. There is delayed, although free, passage of contrast material through the bowel.

Case 3.8: Answers

1. The plain X-ray shows a large opacity behind the heart, with an air–fluid level. The lungs are normal.

2. The CT scan shows herniation of the stomach and oesophagogastric junction into the thorax. Note the stomach lying in the posterior mediastinum. This is a case of hiatus hernia.

3. Hiatus hernia is herniation of the stomach through the oesophageal hiatus. There are two types: sliding and rolling. The **sliding type** is the most common, where the oesophagogastric junction is in the chest and is caused by rupture of the phrenico-oesophageal membrane with repetitive stretching on swallowing. The **rolling type** (paraoesophageal) is a rare type (1%), where the stomach is displaced into the chest, with the oesophagogastric junction in the abdomen. On the plain X-ray, retrocardiac soft-tissue opacity or opacity with an air–fluid level might be seen. Barium swallow is used for further evaluation. In a sliding hiatus hernia, the oesophagogastric junction and part of the stomach are located above the diaphragm. The distance between the B ring and the oesophageal hiatus is > 3 cm. Tortuous oesophagus is seen joining eccentrically with the hiatus. Within the hiatus, thick folds are seen (more than six) with reflux oesophagitis. In rolling hernia, the oesophagogastric junction is seen in the abdomen and a portion of stomach is seen in the thorax. On the CT scan, the diaphragmatic hiatus is > 15 mm, stomach is seen in the chest, with thick walls and there is increased fat around oesophagus as a result of fat herniation.

4. Volvulus, incarceraton, obstruction, perforation, gastroesophageal reflux, reflux oesophagitis, Barrett's oesophagus and carcinoma are the complications. Gastric ulcer is seen in the lesser curvature in rolling hernia. Saint's triad is a combination of hiatus hernia with reflux, diverticulosis and gall stones. Duodenal ulcer is also associated. Medical treatment of reflux due to hiatus hernia is by lifestyle modification, H_2 receptor antagonists and proton pump inhibitors. Surgical treatment with Nissen's total fundoplication or Toupet's partial fundoplication gives good result. The gastric fundus is wrapped or plicated around the inferior part of the oesophagus, restoring the function of the lower oesophageal sphincter. The procedure can be done laparoscopically.

5. Radiological differential diagnosis for gas filled opacity in lower chest are – congenital diaphragmatic hernia, basal lung abscess, empyema, cavitating tumors, post surgical pull through anastomosis between soesophagus and stomach and congenital intrathoracic stomach.

Case 3.9: Answers

1. On Doppler ultrasonography, there is no flow in the right portal vein, which is filled with an echogenic lesion within it. In the contrast-enhanced CT scan, the portal vein is expanded and there is non-enhancing hypodense material within it.

2. Portal venous thrombosis.

3. Portal venous thrombosis is caused by cirrhosis with portal hypertension, tumour spread (hepatocellular carcinoma [HCC], cholangiocarcinoma, pancreatic carcinoma, gastric carcinoma, metastasis), trauma, neonatal sepsis, umbilical vein catheterisation, surgery, splenectomy, hypercoagualable state, blood dyscrasias and portal phlebitis (pancreatitis, appendicitis and ascending cholangitis).

4. Ultrasonography shows echogenic material in the portal vein, which is distended. Portosystemic collateral vessels are seen. Extensive collateral formation around an occluded portal vein is called cavernomatous malformation of the portal vein. Doppler ultrasonography shows no colour flow within the portal vein. When the thrombus is caused by malignancy, pulsatile flow can be seen within the thrombus. The hepatic artery's resistive index is reduced. The CT scan shows low density of the affected segment as a result of oedema/fibrosis. After contrast administration, wedged-shaped enhancement may be seen in the affected segment as a result of increased arterial flow. The portal vein has a low density surrounded by high-density contrast. MRI shows the thrombus, which is hyperintense in T1 and T2. CT or MRA shows the filling defect within the lumen of the portal vein.

5. Complications of portal venous thrombosis are cavernous transformation, hepatic infarction and bowel infarction. Other complications would result from portal hypertension such as splenomegaly, ascites, renal failure, hepatopulmonary syndrome, etc.

Case 3.10: Answers

1. A post-contrast CT scan shows prominent enhancement of the centre of the liver, with poor enhancement of the periphery. There is hepatic enlargement and some ascites.

2. Budd–Chiari syndrome: this is caused by hepatic venous outflow obstruction, which results in elevated sinusoidal pressure, causing delayed or reversed portal venous flow, ascites and altered hepatic morphology. There are three types:

   Type I – occlusion of the IVC ± hepatic veins

   Type II – occlusion of major hepatic veins ± the IVC

   Type III – occlusion of small centrilobular veins.

3. Hypercoagulable states (pregnancy, contraceptive pills, thrombocytosis, paroxysmal nocturnal haemoglobinuria, polycythaemia rubra vera), idiopathic, trauma, radio- and chemotherapy, tumour, membrane/diaphragm, constrictive pericarditis, right heart failure and right atrial tumour are the causes of Budd–Chiari syndrome. Clinical features are right upper quadrant pain, dyspnoea, oedema, jaundice and elevated liver function tests.

4. Features of ultrasonography are hepatosplenomegaly, ascites and gallbladder thickening. Non-visualisation or narrowed hepatic veins, thrombus in hepatic vein, loss of phasicity in the hepatic vein, a dilated portal vein and collateral circulation are the features in Doppler ultrasonography. The CT scan shows hepatomegaly and diffuse low density. The hepatic veins are narrowed or thrombosed. Contrast enhancement is patchy. A flip-flop pattern of contrast enhancement is seen. In early arterial phase after contrast, there is enhancement of the centre and poor enhancement of the periphery and, in delayed scans, there is good enhancement of the periphery and poor enhancement in the centre. Mottled hepatic enhancement is also seen. The caudate lobe shows normal enhancement, because it is supplied directly from the IVC. MRI also shows patchy enhancement

5. Diagnosis can be confirmed by inferior venocavography and wedged hepatic venography. Medical treatment includes control of ascites with diuretics, salt restriction, anticoagulation and thrombolytic therapy. Membranes or stenosis can be treated with balloon dilatation, under fluoroscopic guidance. Refractory cases are treated with TIPSS (transjugular intrahepatic portosystemic shunt). Liver transplantation is required for advanced cases.

Case 3.11: Answers

1. The CT scan shows a large hypodense lesion in the right lobe, which is surrounded by a thick, contrast-enhancing rim.

2. Liver abscess.

3. Liver abscess could be pyogenic or amoebic. *E. coli,* aerobic streptococci, *S. aureus* and anaerobic bacteria cause pyogenic liver abscess. Amoebic abscess is caused by *Entamoeba histolytica.* The infection can be by ascending cholangitis (obstructive biliary disease), portal phlebitis (appendicitis, colitis, diverticulitis), infarction (sickle cell disease, embolism), direct spread from adjacent infections (cholecystitis, peptic ulcer, subphrenic abscess), trauma (rupture, wounds, biopsy, surgery), indwelling catheters or cryptogenically (45%). Amoebic abscess is common in the posterosuperior segment of the right lobe. Pyogenic abscess is usually solitary and in the right lobe. There is preferential distribution of blood flow in the liver. The blood that flows from the superior mesenteric vein is distributed to the right lobe and from the splenic vein to the left lobe. Amoebic abscess usually spreads from primary infection in the ileocecal junction. Hence its common appearance in the right lobe.

4. Ultrasonography shows a hypoechoic lesion with a well-defined rim and internal debris or septations. The CT scan shows a hypodense, loculated cavity with a thick wall, which enhances. Gas can be seen within the cavity. A cluster of abscesses indicates biliary spread. MRI shows a low signal in T1 and a high one in T2 with rim enhancement. Multiple abscesses are seen in 10% (usually biliary rather than haematogenous spread). Differential diagnoses include hepatic cysts, haematoma, hydatid cyst, polycystic kidney disease, cystic metastasis (gastric, ovarian), necrotic hepatoma, large haemangioma and biliary cystadenoma. The most important factor in diagnosis is a large hypodense/hypoechoic lesion with rim enhancement, in contrast-enhanced CT/MRI scan.

5. Complications are septicaemia, rupture into the subphrenic space/ peritoneal cavity/pleural cavity/pericardium, empyema and biliary obstruction. Amoebic abscess can rupture into the colon, right adrenal gland or bile ducts. Liver abscesses are treated with antibiotics. Large abscesses are drained percutaneously under radiological guidance.

Case 3.12: Answers

1. The CT scan of the abdomen shows a shrunken liver, with irregular, nodular margins. There is moderately large ascites. There is some splenic enlargement.

2. Cirrhosis. This is characterised by diffuse parenchymal necrosis, regeneration and scarring with distorted hepatic architecture. Cirrhosis can be micronodular (< 3 mm), macronodular (3–15 mm) or mixed.

3. Causes of cirrhosis are alcoholism, hepatitis, drugs, haemochromatosis, haemosiderosis, sclerosing cholangitis, cystic fibrosis, veno-occlusive disease and prolonged cardiac failure. Uncommon causes are Wilson's disease, α_1-antitrypsin deficiency, autosomal recessive polycystic kidney disease, glycogen storage disease, tyrosinaemia, familial and cryptogenic causes.

4. Ultrasonography shows a shrunken liver with nodularity. The right lobe and medial segment of the left lobe are atrophied, but the caudate lobe and lateral segment of the left lobe are hypertrophied. In the early stages, the liver may be enlarged. The internal architecture of the liver is distorted. Other features are gallbladder thickening, ascites, portal hypertension, splenomegaly and omental thickening. The CT scan shows nodularity, hypodensity, patchy enhancement, portal venous dilatation and portosystemic collaterals. Oesophageal varices and other shunts caused by portosystemic collaterals can be seen. MRI is used for confirming diagnosis and for HCC. Regenerative nodules are hypointense in T2-weighted MRI as a result of the presence of iron. Dysplastic nodules are iso- or hyperintense in T1 as a result of the presence of fat. HCC is a variable signal in T1 and hyperintense in T2, and shows early enhancement in the arterial phase and washout in the portal venous phase.

5. The most important complication in cirrhosis is the development of HCC. Regular follow-up imaging of cirrhotic patients is indicated, to detect early development of HCC, regenerative nodules and dysplastic nodules. Follow-up is ideally done with a four-phase CT scan or MRI, which has non-contrast, arterial, portal and delayed phase images. Early HCCs are bright in the arterial phase, show early washout of contrast and become hypodense in portal and delayed images. Other complications are portal hypertension, ascites, cholangiocarcinoma, variceal bleeding, hepatorenal syndrome, spontaneous bacterial syndrome and hepatic encephalopathy.

Gastrointestinal Answers

Case 3.13: Answers

1. Ultrasound shows a diffusely bright liver. CT scan shows a diffusely dark liver, when compared to spleen. (The normal liver is brighter than spleen). The blood vessels are seen as bright structures, within the liver parenchyma.

2. Fatty liver.

3. Fatty liver (steatosis) is a condition in which large vacuoles of triglyercide fat accumulate in the cytoplasm of hepatocytes. The progression of disease is microvesicular → macrovesicular → steatohepatitis → cirrhosis. Fatty liver can be divided into alcoholic liver disease caused by excessive fat consumption and non-alcoholic liver disease caused by insulin resistance and metabolic syndrome:

   Metabolic: glycogen storage disease, α_1-antitrypsin deficiency, abetalipoproteinaemia, acute fatty liver of pregnancy, lipodystrophy, Wilson's disease, haemochromatosis, cystic fibrosis, dysmorphic syndromes

   Nutritional: obesity, malnutrition, total parenteral nutrition, starvation, gastric bypass, jejunoileal bypass, severe weight loss, bacterial overgrowth

   Drugs and toxins: steroids, amiodarone, methotrexate, valproate, diltiazem, hepatotoxins, antiretroviral therapy, tamoxifen, radiation

   Inflammatory: hepatitis B and C, inflammatory bowel disease, HIV.

4. On ultrasonography of a normal liver, the echotexture is homogeneous, equal or slightly more than the renal cortex and spleen; the walls of the intrahepatic vessels are sharply demarcated and posterior aspects of the liver clearly seen. In fatty liver, the echogenicity of the liver is more than that of the renal cortex/spleen, visualisation of the vascular walls is difficult and there is loss of definition of posterior aspects of the liver and diaphragm. On CT scans, normally the liver is slightly brighter than the spleen, because of the glycogen within it, and the vascular structures are seen as dark areas. In a fatty liver, however, the liver appears dark (< 40 HU) and is of lower density than the spleen (at least 10 HU less). The vasculature appears bright against the fat-containing liver. In focal fatty infiltration, focal areas of low density are seen. In MRI, fatty liver appears brighter than normal in T1- and T2-weighted images. A special sequence called chemical shift imaging can confirm the diagnosis. Loss of signal in the opposed phase indicates fatty liver and this can be quantified by the degree of signal loss. Imaging cannot

differentiate simple steatosis from advanced steatohepatitis. Liver biopsy under ultrasonic guidance is useful for assessing the histological severity. **Variants**: Occasionally there is **focal fat deposition** or diffuse fat deposition with **focal sparing**. These might be confused with mass. These lesions have fat content, no mass effect on vessels and other structures and a geographical configuration, are seen in characteristic locations (adjacent to falciform ligament/ligamentum venosum, porta hepatica, gallbladder fossa) and show contrast enhancement similar to normal liver. Fat can also be deposited in multifocal locations, around portal veins and subcapsular location.

5. Differential diagnoses for focal fatty liver infiltrative HCC, hypovascular metastasis, lymphoma, ischaemic/mucinous metastasis, and for diffuse fatty liver chemotherapy, diffusely infiltrative tumour, early cirrhosis and hepatitis.

Case 3.14: Answers

1. Barium swallow shows a shelf-like mucosal indentation arising from the anterior wall of the upper part of the cervical oesophagus and protruding within the lumen, which is filled with barium.

2. Oesophageal web.

3. Oesophageal web is a 1–2 mm mucosal membrane, covered by squamous epithelium protruding into the oesophageal lumen, which produces circumferential narrowing. It is seen in the cervical oesophagus usually at the level of the cricopharyngeal sphincter. It is less common in thoracic oesophagus. It is pathologically characterised by hyperkeratosis and chronic inflammation of submucosa. It is common in middle-aged females. Occasionally it can be multiple.

4. Paterson–Kelly syndrome (Plummer–Vinson syndrome) is a combination of iron deficiency anaemia, stomatitis, glossitis, kollonychia, dysphagia and thyroid disorder.

5. The most important long-term complication is a high risk of upper oesophageal and hypopharyngeal carcinoma. Treatment is with iron replacement for anaemia, balloon dilatation or bougeinage. The web may or may not improve with iron replacement.

6. Barium swallow shows a shelf-like indentation in a fully distended oesophagus, arising at right angles from anterior oesophageal wall, 1–2 mm thick. Differential diagnosis is a stricture, which is thicker and circumferential.

Case 3.15: Answers

1. The barium swallow shows an irregular stricture at the distal part of the oesophagus, causing almost complete obstruction with holding of barium proximally. The proximal oesophagus is not significantly distended. The CT scan confirms the presence of a concentric soft-tissue mass in the oesophageal wall, which is occluding its lumen.

2. Oesophageal cancer.

3. Squamous carcinoma is seen in the mid-third of the oesophagus and adenocarcinoma in the distal third. Predisposing factors for squamous cell carcinoma are smoking, alcohol, Plummer–Vinson syndrome, achalasia, caustic strictures, chronic hot liquid ingestion, nitrosamines, poor oral hygiene and tylosis palmaris. Barrett's oesophagus associated with chronic reflux oesophagitis is the common predisposing factor of adenocarcinoma.

4. Dysphagia for solids initially but later solids and liquids, pain, weight loss, haematemesis, hoarseness and respiratory symptoms are the clinical presentations of oesophageal cancer. Routine blood tests, endoscopy, endoscopic ultrasonography, bronchoscopy for carcinoma in the mid-third of the oesophagus, CT of the thorax and upper abdomen, and a bone scan are investigations used for diagnosis and staging of oesophageal cancer.

5. Barium swallow is often the initial test used in diagnosis. Oesophageal cancer is often seen as an irregular stricture with loss of normal mucosal pattern, with different degrees of occlusion of lumen. Presence of shouldering at the site of stricture and eccentric soft tissue filling defect points towards carcinoma. However, from barium study it is not always possible to differentiate benign from malignant strictuire. Impaction of food particles at the site of stricture makes the task more difficult and endoscopic diagnosis is needed. Extension outside oesophagus, invasion of adjacent structures such as trachea, bronchi, aorta and mediastinum,

regional lymphadenopathy in thorax and abdomen, liver and pulmonary metastasis are assessed by CT scan. Tumour staging is better done with endoscopic ultrasound. **Tis** – carcinoma in situ, **T1** – invasion of lamina propria/submucosa, **T2** – muscularis propria, **T3** – adventitia, **T4** – adjacent organs, **N1** – regional lymph nodes, **M1** – distal metastasis, celiac lymph nodes in lower oesophageal tumours, non regional nodes in mid oesophageal tumour and cervical nodes in upper oesophageal tumour.

6. Transhiatal or transthoracic oesophagectomy with gastric pull-through is done to manage resectable oesophageal tumours. Other options are the Ivor Lewis procedure (laparotomy and posterolateral right thoracotomy), the McKeown procedure (anterolateral right thoracotomy, laparotomy and cervical anastomosis) and the left thoracoabdominal approach. Bypass surgery provides an alternative food passageway when the oesophagus is completely obstructed by cancer. Expandable metallic stents can be inserted under fluoroscopic guidance through the diseased stenotic segment. Radiotherapy, laser ablation and photodynamic therapy are other palliative options.

Case 3.16: Answers

1. The X-ray shows an ovoid gas filled structure in the subhepatic area in the right upper quadrant, in the shape of the gallbladder. Foci of air are also noted in the wall of the gallbladder. No air is seen in the hepatic ductal system. Bowel gas pattern appears normal.

2. Emphysematous cholecystitis. This is an acute infection of the gallbladder caused by gas-forming organisms.

3. Pathogenesis of emphysematous cholecystitis involves four factors: vascular compromise (atherosclerotic stenosis or occlusion, resulting in impaired viability), gallstones (seen in 30–80%, impaction in neck causes oedema predisposing to necrosis), impaired immunity (diabetes in old age) and infection with gas-forming organism.

4. Causative organisms include *Clostridium* spp., *E. coli*, *Klebsiella* spp., enterococci and anaerobic streptococci. Although the intramural gas observed in patients with emphysematous cholecystitis seems to result from gas-forming bacteria, whether these bacteria represent the primary cause of the disorder or are secondary invaders remains unclear. It is common in men in the fifth and sixth decades. Clinical features are right upper quadrant pain/tenderness, fever, chills, flank pain, lethargy, confusion, enlarged tender gallbladder and diminished bowel sounds in peritonitis.

5. The X-ray shows gas in the gallbladder wall, and gas may also be seen in the lumen in the non-dependent portion. It can extend to the pericholecystic tissues and extrahepatic ducts. On ultrasonography, gas can completely obscure visualisation of the gallbladder lumen. Gas in the wall shows the typical ring-down/comet-tail artefact with bright shadows. The CT scan shows thickened gallbladder wall with gas, which may extend to the pericholecystic tissues. Due to occlusion of cystic duct from oedema or impaction with stone, gas rarely extends into the bile ducts. Differential diagnosis for gas in the biliary tree is biliary enteric fistula, after endoscopic retrograde cholangiopancreatography (ERCP)/ sphincterotomy or cholangitis with gas-forming organisms. Treatment is with emergent cholecystectomy or percutaneous drainage and decompression, followed by interval excision of the gallbladder.

Case 3.17: Answers

1. The barium follow-through shows multiple barium-filled outpouchings from the wall of the small bowel, which has mucosal pattern of jejunum.

2. Jejunal diverticulosis.

3. Jejunal diverticulosis is a pulsion diverticulum caused by increased intraluminal pressure and herniation of mucosa. It is seen in the mesenteric border of the bowel at the entrance of vasa recti. It is more common in the proximal jejunum. Ileum is involved in 15% and the overall incidence is 2%. It is more common in men aged over 40. It can be associated with scleroderma, visceral myopathy and neuropathy. There is an association with Ehler–Danlos syndrome.

4. Plain abdominal X-ray shows air–fluid levels in the diverticula. The barium follow-through shows trapped barium, which might stay after the barium has cleared from the rest of the bowel. The diverticulum is not filled with barium if there is a narrow neck, inflammation or stagnant secretions in the pouch. The size of the diverticulum ranges from a few millimetres to many centimetres. Complications such as perforation and abscess formation may produce, a mesenteric mass, displacing the bowel loops. The diverticula can also be incidentally seen in other imaging studies such as ultrasonography or a CT scan.

5. Clinical features are abdominal pain, flatulence, diarrhoea, steatorrhoea, malabsorption and vitamin deficiency. Complications are diverticulitis (inflammation is uncommon as a result of the fluid nature of the small bowel contents and broad opening), perforation, abscess, blind loop syndrome caused by bacterial overgrowth, haemorrhage and obstruction resulting from enteroliths. Jejunal diverticulosis is a common cause of pneumoperitoneum. Small openings in the wall of the diverticulum may allow the passage of air, but not intestinal contents.

Case 3.18: Answers

1. The X-ray shows a huge distended loop of sigmoid colon, arising from the pelvis and extending to the left upper quadrant under the dome of the diaphragm. There are no haustra in the dilated colon and the walls are thick.

2. Sigmoid volvulus.

3. Sigmoid volvulus is the most common volvulus in the gastrointestinal tract. The cause is an unusually narrow attachment of the root of the sigmoid mesentery to the posterior abdominal wall, resulting in close proximity of the two limbs of the sigmoid colon, making it vulnerable to twisting. The loop can be rotated any degree, although 360° is the most common type. It is common in elderly, neurological and psychiatric patients. Chronic constipation, high roughage diet and lead poisoning are predisposing factors.

4. Plain film appearances are usually characteristic for the diagnosis of sigmoid volvulus. A distended sigmoid colon is seen (inverted U shape), with the limbs of the sigmoid loop directed toward the pelvis and the apex extending to the left dome of the diaphragm. **Coffee bean sign** – distinct midline crease due to gas in sigmoid colon surrounding thickened edematous walls. The colonic haustra are lost, walls are thickened and there might be air fluid levels. If the loop is full of fluid, it might be seen as a soft tissue density lesion. In the supine film, a dilated sigmoid reaching the level of transverse colon (**northern exposure sign**), is a reliable sign of voluvus. In subacute or recurrent cases, barium or CT scan can be done, but is not necessary. Barium shows '**Bird of Prey**' sign, which is the tapered hook like end of the barium column at the site of twisting. '**Twisted tape**' sign refers to the mucosal pattern at the site of twist. CT scan shows the '**Whirl sign**' which is due to twisted mesentery formed by afferent and effect loops.

5. Obstruction, ischaemia and perforation are the complications. In patients with no ischaemia or perforation, sigmoidoscopic decompression of the rectum can be attempted. Sigmoidopexy is done for those with recurrent volvulus and complications, as an elective procedure. Sigmoid resection should be performed when it can be done safely.

Case 3.19: Answers

1. This is a videofluoroscopic barium swallow. The first picture, taken during swallowing shows free flow of barium into the gastric fundus from the lower oesophagus. In the second film, done in supine position, barium is seen filling the oesophagus retrogradely from the stomach.

2. Gastro-oesophageal reflux disease.

3. Gastro-oesophageal reflux is reflux of the stomach contents into the lower oesophagus, which is not equipped for handling the acid overload. Normally the reflux is prevented by the lower oesophageal sphincter, phrenico-oesophageal membrane, the length of the subdiaphragmatic oesophagus and the gastro-oesophageal angle of His. Reflux results when these defence mechanisms are overcome. The factors that determine the consequences of reflux are the frequency, volume and content of reflux, adequacy of reflux mechanism and resistance of tissue.

4. Videofluorosopic examination with barium is used for evaluation of the gastro-oesophageal reflux. Barium is administered with the patient in a supine or prone position. When the barium has passed through the oesophagogastric junction into the stomach, the reflux is assessed. Normally reflux of barium is assessed in the right posterior oblique position. Provocative manoeuvres can be used for bringing out reflux, and include coughing, Valsalva manoeuvre, deep respiratory movements, swelling, saliva/water or anteflexion in the erect position. A water siphon test can be used with a combination of barium and water, which induces reflux in the prone position when drunk with a straw. Another test is the radionuclide reflux test, where an isotope is mixed with orange juice and oesophageal counts are measured. Oesophageal manometry and measurement of the oesophageal pH are also useful. Reflux is demonstrated by the above-mentioned manoeuvres. Associated hiatus hernia is seen, which can be a sliding or mixed type of hernia. When reflux oesophagitis develops, it is seen in the lower third to half of oesophagus. There is segmental narrowing, granular mucosa, ulcers/erosions, superficial ulceration, prominent mucosal folds, incompetent sphincter, tertiary peristaltic contractions and transverse ridges of oesophagus (felinisation).

5. Complications of reflux: motility disorder, stricture, Barrett's oesophagus, reflux oesophagitis, carcinoma, iron deficiency anaemia, aspiration pneumonia, Mendelson syndrome and pulmonary fibrosis. Mild reflux is managed by lifestyle changes (reducing weight, avoiding smoking/alcohol/chocolates/ citric acid, sleeping 3 hours after last meal, elevation of head end of bed) and medications (H_2-receptor antagonists, PPIs, prokinetic agents). Surgery is indicated when there is no response to medications or complications develop. Laparoscopic fundoplication is preferred to open surgery.

Case 3.20: Answers

1. There is air under the domes of the diaphragm. There is also air outlining the falciform ligament. The X-ray done in the supine position shows clear visualisation of the bowel wall, as a result of air outlining either side of it.

2. Pneumoperitoneum resulting from hollow viscus perforation.

3. The X-ray findings: in an erect film, air collects under the diaphragm. In supine views, the diagnosis may depend on subtle findings:

Rigler's sign: air on both sides of bowel (indicates > 1000 ml gas)

Football sign: large pneumoperitoneum outlining the entire abdomen

Tell's triangle sign: air among three loops of bowel

Inverted V sign: outlining of both lateral umbilical ligaments

Outlining of medial umbilical ligaments, falciform ligament

Urachus sign: outlining of middle umbilical ligament

Doges' cap sign: triangular collection in Morrison's pouch

Falciform ligament sign: linear lucency

Ligamentum teres sign: vertical, slit/oval area between ribs 10 and 12

Ligamentum teres notch: V-shaped inverted, under the liver

Cupola sign: gas below central tendon of diaphragm

Visualisation of diaphragmatic muscular slips.

---

4. Causes of pneumoperitoneum:

Trauma: blunt/penetrating

Iatrogenic: post-laparotomy (absorbed in 1–24 days, air after 3 days is suspicious), laparoscopy, endoscopy, enema tip injury, intussusception reduction

Gastrointestinal tract disorders: hollow viscus perforation, perforated appendix, foreign body, inflammatory bowel disease, obstruction, tumours, imperforate anus, Hirschsprung's disease, meconium ileus

Ruptured pneumatosis of small and large bowel

Idiopathic perforation in pre-term infants

Extension from chest

Gas-forming peritonitis

Introduction through female genital tract.

---

5. **False positive**: other gas-filled structures such as diverticulum, Chiladiti syndrome (hepatic flexure interposition between liver and diaphragm), diaphragmatic hernia, abscess, subdiaphragmatic fat, omental fat between liver and diaphragm, basal atelectasis, irregular diaphragm, pneumothorax. **False negative**: erect X-ray should be taken 5 min after keeping the patient in an erect position, otherwise it may be negative. Lateral decubitus films may be acquired for confirmation. Ultrasonography can be used to detect air.

Case 3.21: Answers

1. Chest X-ray shows an elongated soft tissue shadow in the right paravertebral region, with a clear lateral margin, extending from the root of neck to the lower thorax. This has a mottled appearance and represents a dilated oesophagus with food residues and fluid. Barium swallow shows proximally dilated oesophagus with smooth, tapered narrowing of the distal oesophagus and hold up of barium in the proximal oesophagus.

2. Achalasia cardia. This is failure of relaxation at the level of the lower oesophageal sphincter and failure of peristalsis. Most of the cases are idiopathic and caused by abnormality of the Auerbach plexus or a defect in the dorsal nucleus of the vagus. Chagas' disease is another known cause.

3. The X-ray shows a dilated oesophagus with air in it. A gastric bubble is not visualised. A paratracheal opacity is seen as a result of the fluid-filled oesophagus. Patchy alveolar opacities are seen as a result of aspiration pneumonitis. The barium swallow shows a grossly dilated oesophagus with food debris and air. Absence of peristaltic contractions in the upper oesophagus and secondary peristaltic waves are seen. There is symmetrical narrowing of the distal oesophagus, with a bird-beak deformity.
    Hurst's phenomenon is temporary transit through the cardia when the hydrostatic pressure of the barium column is more than the pressure of the oesophageal sphincter. There might be sudden emptying after ingestion of warm water and carbonated beverage. The sphincter relaxes after amyl nitrate inhalation. There is a variant called **rigorous achalasia**, in which there are peristaltic waves; this is an early stage of achalasia.

4. Differential diagnoses: **secondary achalasia** produced by tumours (asymmetrical tapering, irregular mucosa, normal peristalsis, separation of gastric fundus from diaphragm), and **benign peptic stricture**. Differential diagnoses for air in oesophagus on a plain X-ray are normal variant, achalasia, scleroderma, stricture, tumour, post-laryngectomy, intubation, thoracic surgery, mediastinitis.

5. There is increased risk of development of oesophageal carcinoma (2–7%). Oesophagitis and aspiration pneumonia are other complications. Calcium channel blockers, anticholinergic agents, nitrates and opioids are used to relax the smooth muscle of the distal oesophagus and lower oesophageal sphincter. Botulinum toxin works by inhibiting release of acetylcholine from presynaptic terminals. Pneumatic balloon dilatation or surgical cardiomyotomy (Heller's) are used to relieve achalasia cardia. Surgery can be performed by open or laparoscopic methods.

Case 3.22: Answers

1. The barium swallow shows a shaggy outline of the oesophagus with multiple, extensive ulcerations along its entire length, giving it an irregular contour.

2. Candida oesophagitis.

3. Candida oesophagitis is seen in immunosuppressed individuals such as those with HIV, leukaemia and chronic diseases. Patients on immunosuppressive therapy for renal/hepatic/pancreatic/cardiac transplant are also vulnerable. Use of steroids, chemotherapy, radiotherapy and antibiotics are predisposing factors. It is also seen patients with poorly controlled diabetes, inadequate nutrition, drug and alcohol abusers. Patients with sluggish oesophageal motility such as scleroderma, achalasia, strictures and after surgeries such as fundoplication are prone to developing this. Candida albicans is an opportunistic fungal infection. It produces creamy white plaques covering friable erythematous mucosa. Clinically there is dysphagia, odynophagia, chest pain and oral thrush. It is commonly seen in the upper half of the oesophagus. In HIV patients, oesophageal candidiasis is an AIDS defining clinical condition.

4. Barium swallow shows a cobblestone appearance in the early stages as a result of mucosal nodularity. Longitudinal plaques are also seen. The characteristic appearance is a shaggy outline of the oesophagus, which has an irregular serrated contour caused by a combination of ulcers, plaques, erosions, pseudomembranes and haemorrhage. The lumen is narrowed in the later stages and there are tertiary peristaltic contractions. Strictures are rare. Intramural diverticulosis may be seen. Double-contrast swallow is the most sensitive investigation. Endoscopy can also be performed.

5. Complications are stricture, systemic candidiasis and gastric bezoar. Treatment is with antifungal medications such as ketoconazole or fluconazole. Therapeutically unresponsive patients will require endoscopic biopsy for confirmation of diagnosis.

6. Differential diagnoses: reflux oesophagitis, superficial spreading carcinoma, varices, artefacts, herpes oesophagitis, glycogen acanthosis, caustic ingestion, Barrett's oesophagus, pseudodiverticulosis and papillomatosis.

Case 3.23: Answers

1. The CT scan shows air in the mediastinum and a right-sided hydropneumothorax with collapse of the right lung. The contrast swallow shows leakage of contrast into the mediastinum, from the lower oesophagus.

2. Oesophageal perforation.

3. Oesophageal perforation is seen commonly after iatrogenic injury (endoscopy, stricture dilatation, bougie, surgery, intubation), spontaneous rupture (Boerhaave's syndrome – rupture of distal oesophagus after an episode of vomiting) and chest trauma. The common locations of perforation are the cervical and upper thoracic oesophagus. The left posterolateral wall of the distal oesophagus, just superior to the gastro-oesophageal junction, is another common location of perforation. Chest pain, dysphagia, odynophagia, sepsis and hypotension are clinical features. Surgical emphysema may be present in the neck and chest wall.

4. X-ray findings in oesophageal rupture are – extensive pneumomediastinum, subcutaneous emphysema, left pleural effusion and left lower lobe atelectasis. Extrapleural air in lower mediastinum between parietal pleura and diaphragm is called V sign of Naclerio. Medastinal widening indicates development of mediastinitis. The diagnosis and site of rupture is confirmed with a water soluble contrast swallow, which shows the leak in 90% of patients. If the leak is not demonstrated with a contrast swallow and the clinical suspicion is high, dilute barium solution can be given to demonstrate the leak. CT scan performed immediately after contrast ingestion can also demonstrate the leak. CT also shows mediastinal air, haematoma, oesophagal wall thickining, pleural effusion and lung changes secondary to aspiration.

5. Small oesophageal perforations cause mediastinitis, mediastinal abscess and SVC obstruction due to fibrosis. Large perforations give rise to marked systemic disturbance with cardiovascular collapse. Boerhaave's syndrome usually requires surgical repair because the tear is large. Small localized perforations are managed conservatively.

Case 3.24: Answers

1. The first study is a small bowel study with barium. There is a long abnormal segment of terminal ileum, which is narrowed with focal areas of ulcerations. This segment did not show any peristaltic movement and is rigid. There are proximally dilated small bowel loops.

2. The CT scan shows diffuse circumferential wall thickening of the terminal ileal loops. There is increased density of fat in the adjacent mesentery and retroperitoneum, suggestive of inflammatory change. Minimal dilation of loops of ileum proximal to this lesion is noted.

3. Crohn's disease of the small bowel (terminal ileum).

4. Crohn's disease is a chronic inflammatory disease of the bowel with discontinuous, asymmetrical involvement of the gastrointestinal tract. Diarrhoea, rectal bleeding, abdominal pain, weight loss, anaemia, joint pain, growth failure and delayed puberty are clinical features. Complications are fistula, sinus, abscess, perforation, toxic megacolon, hydronephrosis and adenocarcinoma in the ileum. Fatty liver, liver abscess, gallstones, cholecystitis, sclerosing cholangitis, urolithiasis, hydronephrosis, amyloidosis, cystitis, ankylosing spondylitis, erosive arthritis, avascular necrosis, osteomyelitis, septic arthritis and abscesses are other complications. Treatment consists of 5-aminosalicylic acid (aspirin) preparations, antibiotics such as metronidazole, corticosteroids, immunosuppressants (methotrexate, 6-mercaptopurine, azathioprine, antibodies to tumour necrosis factor [TNF]-α). Surgery is performed when medical therapy fails and complications develop.

5. A barium meal shows involvement of the terminal ileum in the form of thickened and nodular folds, aphthous ulcers, cobblestone mucosa. There is rigidity of small bowel loops with wide separation of the loops. Post-inflammatory polyps, mucosal granularity and pseudodiverticula can be seen. Pathologically Crohn's disease is characterised by transmural involvement and granulomas. A CT scan shows homogeneous thickened walls or a double-halo configuration (lumen surrounded by oedematous hypodense mucosa and soft-tissue density muscularis and serosa). There are skip lesions of asymmetrical bowel wall thickening. A characteristic feature on CT is the creeping fat sign where there is massive proliferation of mesenteric fat that separates the bowel loops. Dilated bowel loops, sinus, fistula, adenopathy and abscesses are other features. Radiological differential diagnoses of small bowel Crohn's disease are TB (involvement

of caecum, pulmonary TB), infection with *Yersinia* spp. (resolution in 3–4 months), radiation enteritis, lymphoma (no spasm, nodular/aneurysmal), actinomycosis, carcinoid and eosinophilic gastroenteritis.

Case 3.25: Answers

1. The barium meal shows a smooth, oval, mucosal projection extending outside the gastric contour, from the distal part of the lesser curvature.

2. Gastric ulcer.

3. Gastric ulcer is caused by a disrupted mucosal barrier as a result of either *Helicobacter pylori*, which results in increased susceptibility to gastric juice, or increased secretion of gastric acid.

4. Gastric ulcer disease is the result of peptic ulcer disease, gastritis, Zollinger–Ellison syndrome, steroids, stress, Cushing's ulcer (caused by cerebral disease), Curling's ulcer (caused by burns), uraemia, NSAIDs, leiomyoma, pseudolymphoma and granulomatous disease. The most common location of a gastric ulcer is in the lesser curvature of the gastric antrum a few centimetres from the pylorus. The ulcer is located close to the oesophagogastric junction as a result of a hiatus hernia. It is seen in the gastric cardia in older patients.

5. Radiological diagnosis is best achieved with double contrast barium meal. The ulcer can be round oval or linear. It has a **niche**, which is a small projection of barium outside the gastric contour. The **ulcer crater** is a round or oval barium collection with a smooth border. **Hampton line** is 1 mm lucency around the orifice of the ulcer niche. **Ulcer collar** is a smooth thick lucency between the niche and gastric lumen. **Ulcer mound** is a smooth, sloping tissue mass surrounding the bending ulcer. Smooth folds radiate toward the ulcer mucosa. The radiological differentiating points between a benign and malignant gastric ulcers are – malignant ulcer is usually seen in the greater curvature, does not project beyond the gastric margin, eccentrically located within tumour, shallow ulcer with width greater than depth, nodular floor, with abrupt transition between normal and abnormal mucosa, shouldered edges around ulcer, nodular irregular folds radiating towards the ulcer, rigidity, lack of distensibility, irregular soft tissue mass. Carman meniscus sign (crater with convexity of crescent towards gastric wall) and Kirklin meniscus (radiolucent elevated

border) are seen in malignancies. The differential diagnosis for narrowing and deformity seen in benign gastric ulcer are -- malignancy, TB, chronic granulomatous disease, histoplasmosis, sarcoidosis, syphilis, Crohn's disease, caustic ingestion, eosinophilic gastritis and radiation.

6. Malignant change in gastric ulcers have been well documented. Other complications are obstruction, deformity, perforation, bleeding, penetration and fistula to adjacent organs. Gastrocolic fistula usually extends to the transverse colon. Treatment includes proton pump inhibitors and antibiotics against *H. pylori* and in a small group of patients by surgery (gastrectomy or vagotomy with pyloroplasty and excision of ulcer). It is essential to perform endoscopic histology to rule out malignancy, before commencing treatment.

Case 3.26: Answers

1. The barium follow-through examination of the small bowel shows a long linear filling defect within the proximal jejunum.

2. Ascariasis infection of the small bowel.

3. *Ascaris lumbricoides* is a roundworm that causes infection of the small bowel. Infection spreads to humans by ingestion of contaminated soil containing eggs of the parasite. The eggs hatch in the duodenum, and the larvae penetrate the venules and lymphatics, reaching the lungs, from where they pass to the bronchial tree and are swallowed into the gastrointestinal tract, where they mature into adult worms. The worm is endemic in tropical countries.

4. Ascariasis is common in the jejunum. The ileum and duodenum are also affected. Clinical features are intermittent abdominal colic, haematemesis, jaundice, pneumonitis and appendicitis. The barium follow-through shows a 15–40 cm long tubular filling defect in the small bowel. Occasionally, barium can be seen within the alimentary canal of the worm, giving a characteristic linear structure within the lucent worm. Clusters of worms produce a whorled appearance. Similar appearances are seen on ultrasonography and a CT scan. In ultrasonography, the worms are seen as non-shadowing, mobile/non-mobile, linear, echogenic structures within the bowel lumen. The worm's alimentary canal can be seen. A 'target' sign can be seen, with a central bright dot separated by a hypoechoic area from

peripheral, hyperechoic rim. When there is a large clump of worms, they can be seen on a plain X-ray as a large, inhomogeneous soft-tissue density with fuzzy borders, outlined by bowel gas.

5. Complications are perforation, obstruction, peritonitis and appendicitis. Differential diagnoses are tumours, polyps and foreign bodies. The worms can enter the bile ducts and produce cholangitis, abscess, granuloma and stones.

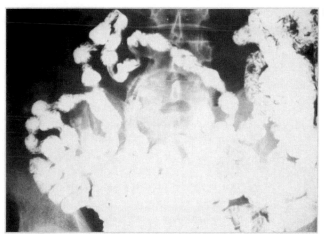

Fig 3.26b

Magnified view of the small bowel, showing ascariasis.

Case 3.27: Answers

1. Ultrasonography of the abdomen shows a large clear fluid collection in the peritoneal cavity, with centrally floating bowel loops. The CT scan shows fluid collection in the peritoneal cavity, with floating contrast filled bowel loops.

2. Ascites. This is an abnormal accumulation of intraperitoneal fluid.

3. Common causes of ascites are related to:

   Portal hypertension – Cirrhosis, hepatic outflow obstruction, congestive cardiac failure, constrictive pericarditis, Budd Chiari syndrome.

   Malignancy – Intraperitoneal primary tumor or peritoneal metastasis

   Renal – chronic renal failure, nephrotic syndrome.

Inflammatory/ Infective-Peritonitis, pancreatitis, TB, Fitz Hugh Curtis syndrome, filariasis

Endocrine – Myxoedema, Meig's syndrome, ovarian stimulation syndrome.

Miscellaneous – Trauma

4.   On the X-ray, the abdomen is distended, with bulging flanks and centrally placed bowel loops. The peritoneal flank stripe is thickened. The space between the properitoneal fat and the gut is > 3 mm, with medial displacement of the lateral liver margin (Hellmer's sign) and medial displacement of the ascending and descending colon. A white-out appearance of the abdomen is seen. The radiological changes are seen only when the fluid is > 500 ml. Ultrasonography is very sensitive and can detect 5–10 ml of fluid. On ultrasonography a transudate is seen as a clear collection and an exudate has internal echoes or internal septations. On a CT scan, even small quantities of fluid are detected. The density of the collection can indicate the nature. Occasionally it might be possible to differentiate benign and malignant ascites. Benign fluid collection is usually clear, but occasionally shows septations or loculations; the bowel loops are free floating and the gallbladder wall appears thick. Benign ascites is seen primarily in the greater sac and not in the lesser sac. Malignant ascites is highly echogenic with internal debris and loculations. The bowel loops are fixed and the gallbladder wall is not thickened. Associated masses indicate malignancy. Malignant ascites is seen proportionally in the greater and lesser sacs. The presence of coarse internal echoes indicates blood and fine internal echoes are caused by chyle.

5.   Fluid from the supramesocolic compartment extends along the shelves on the mesenteric side of the small bowel loops and drops into the inframescolic compartment and then into the pelvis. From the pelvis, the fluid flows along the paracolic gutters. The fluid in the right paracolic gutter extends all the way to the right subhepatic spaces, but, on the left, is limited by the phrenicocolic ligament. In a supine patient, the earliest site of fluid collection is Morrison's pouch (hepatorenal). The most dependent part of the pelvis is the pouch of Douglas. High-density acscites indicates haemoperitoneum, infection or malignancy. Trauma, TB and ovarian/ appendiceal tumour (pseudomyxoma) are causes of high-density ascites.

6.   Fluid is aspirated under ultrasonic guidance for diagnostic and therapeutic purposes. Ultrasonic guidance enables aspiration from even small collections, and helps avoid vascular structures, bowel loops and bladder. Therapeutic paracentesis is performed in refractory or tense ascites. Albumin 5 g should be supplemented for each litre aspirated over 5 litres. TIPSS is useful in refractory ascites.

Case 3.28: Answers

1. The barium enema shows a narrowing of the distal sigmoid colon, with overhanging edges, the characteristic apple-core lesion. Several diverticula are also noted in the proximal descending colon.

2. Carcinoma of the sigmoid colon.

3. Of colorectal carcinomas, 93% arise from a pre-existing adenoma. A patient with one adenoma has a 10% chance of having a colorectal carcinoma in 15 years. Predisposing factors are a past history of adenoma/carcinoma, dysplasia, family history, inflammatory bowel disease (ulcerative colitis, Crohn's disease), history of endometrial, ovarian or breast carcinoma, irradiation and ureterosigmoidstomy, polyposis syndromes such as familial adenomatous polyposis (FAP), Cowden's disease, juvenile polyposis and hereditary non-polyposis colon cancer (HNPCC) syndrome (Lynch syndrome)

4. Colonoscopy is the preferred diagnostic tool in suspected cases of colonic cancer. However, double contrast barium enema is used for screening patients who present with altered bowel habits or rectal bleeding. Double contrast enema has a sensitivity of up to 97% for detection of polyps > 1 cm. Polyps which are broad, sessile with irregular margins are suspicious for malignancy. Virtual colonoscopy is as effective in diagnosing early polyps, especially in older patients who cannot be put through the rigorous barium enema. Air is insufflated in the colon and CT scan images are acquired in the prone and supine position. Computer reconstructions results in images similar to colonoscopy with ability to fly through the colon, Endoscopy is the other procedure routinely used for colonic bleeding, but caecum is not visualised on some cases and fails to detect 10% of small polyps. The commonest location is the rectosigmoid region. Other locations are descending colon (10%), transverse colon (12%), ascending colon (8%) and caecum (8%) Colonic cancers can be fungating polypoid, annular ulcerating, saddle type or scirrhosing. Calcification is seen in mucinous carcinoma (in primary, peritoneal/hepatic metastasis). Histologically they can be adenocarcinoma, mucinous carcinoma, squamous or adenosquamous carcinoma. Left sided lesions are annular and present early with obstruction, but right sided lesions are polypoidal and present late with chronic anaemia.

5. Barium enema is used to diagnose these lesions and for finding

synchronous lesions in other segments of colon. CT can be used for staging the tumour. Tumour can be seen as a poypoidal mass or a circumferential thickening of the rectum. When the tumour extends outside the colon, there is surrounding pericolonic stranding. Lymph nodes, hepatic and lung metastasis are assessed. Apple core appearance is produced by an annular ulcerating carcinoma, due to tumour growing along the lymphatic channels which parallel the circular muscle fibers of the inner layer of muscularis propria. The tumour is seen as annular constriction with overhanging edges. Ultrasound is often used as a screening tool for liver metatases.

6. Complications of colonic cancer are obstruction, perforation, abscess, fistula, intussusception, pneumatosis and psseudomyxoma peritonei. Lymphoma and colonic endometriosis can also produce apple core appearance. Less common causes are chronic Crohn's disease/ulcerative colitis, ischemic colitis, infections (lymphogranuloma venereum, tuberculosis,amoeboma) and benign tumours (villous adenoma). Strictures and oedema in colonic diverticulitis may mimic carcinoma and they can also coexist in same patient. Carcinoma in a segment of colonic diverticular disease may present as a stricture than a mass.

Case 3.29: Answers

1. Barium enema shows the entire colon studded with multiple small polyps. This is more prominently seen in the descending colon. The transverse colon and ascending colon are filled with barium, which is masking the change. Large polypoidal filling defects are also noted in the sigmoid colon.

2. Colonic polyposis. The patient has familial adenomatous polyposis. FAP is an autosomal dominant disease with 80% penetrance, characterised by tubular/villotubular adenomas carpeting the entire colon. There is a family history and the symptoms start in the third to fourth decades, with abdominal pain, weight loss, diarrhoea and bloody stools.

3. Barium enema or colonoscopy is used for diagnosis. Barium enema shows the entire colon carpeted with polyps, 2–3mm in size with maximal size of 2 cm. Polyps are occasionally seen in stomach and small bowel. Pathologically, there are 4 distinct types of colonic polyps – inflammatory

(polyps in chronic ulcerative colitis), hyperplastic or metaplastic (most rectal polyps, no malignant change), hamartomatous (juvenile polyp, Peutz Jegher's polyp) and neoplastic (adenomas- tubular, tubulovillous and villous, all with malignant potential). Adenomas consist of 10% of all colonic polyps, 90%of them are small and less than 1.5 cm. Risk of malignant conversion increases with villous adenomas (cauliflower appearance), sessile and larger size adenomas (> 2cm).

4. FAP is associated with hamartomatous polyps in the stomach and adenomas in the duodenum. Malignant transformation of polyps is seen, with increasing incidence with age. The risk is 12% by 5 years, 30% by 10 years and 100% by 20 years. Usually carcinoma presents at 20–40 years. Periampullary carcinoma is also associated. Drugs used for treatment are sulindac and celecoxib. Flexible sigmoidoscopy is done every 1–2 years. Prophylactic colectomy is done once polyps are detected and the patient is old enough or advanced features develop. After development of colonic carcinoma, a permanent ileostomy, endorectal pull-through pouch or Kock's pouch (distal ileum formed into a one-way valve by invagination of bowel at the skin site) are indicated.

5. Differential diagnoses include other polyposis syndromes:

    Gardner syndrome: FAP, osteomas, desmoid tumours, thyroid cancer, cysts. Colonic polyps have similar malignant potential as FAB.

    Peutz–Jegher syndrome: hamartomatous polyps, mucocutaneous lesions, minimal risk of malignancy documented.

    Cronkhite–Canada syndrome: hamartomas, pigmentation, nail destruction, cancers

    Cowden syndrome: hamartomas, papillomas, keratoses, breast/thyroid carcinoma

    Juvenile polyposis

    Ruvalcaba syndrome: hamartomas, penis pigmentation, macrocephaly

    Turcot syndrome: brain tumours (medulloblastoma, glioma)

    Lynch syndrome: HNPCC syndrome

    Ulcerative colitis: pseudopolyps (inflamed mucosa on background of denuded mucosa), filiform polyps (postinflammatory, projection of submucosa covered by mucosa on all sides)

    Lymphoid hyperplasia

    Lymphosarcoma.

1. X-ray shows small bubbles of gas in the wall of sigmoid colon and distal descending colon. In the CT scan, the descending colon has bright oral contrast within its lumen. There is gas in the wall of the descending colon, surrounding the oral contrast. (Compare this with the loop located anteriorly on the right side, which has bright contrast within it, but has a thin wall without gas in it.) There is some free fluid in the peritoneal cavity there is thickening of small bowel loops.

2. Pneumatosis coli caused by ischaemia.

3. Pneumotosis intestinalis is presence of gas in the intestinal wall. The gas usually collects in the subserosa, followed by submucosa, muscularis and is common in the mesenteric side. The collection can be microvesicular, in the lamina propria or linear/curvilinear type with streaks parallel to the bowel wall. X-ray shows small locules in bowel wall. CT scan shows wall thickening, gas in bowel wall, gas in retroperitoneum, peritoneum, gas in portal vein and mesenteric vein. Bowel ischemia can be acute/chronic mesenteric ischemia, focal segmental ischemia or colonic ischemia. Most of them are caused by arterial disease (occlusive/non-occlusive, thrombotic/emboli). Acute occlusion is usually embolic/thrombotic and is seen in elderly patients, especially those with cardiovascular diseases. Chronic ischemia is due to atherosclerosis. Superior mesenteric artery is more commonly involved. X-rays show bowel wall gas and thumbprinting due to bowel oedema. CT scan shows bowel wall thickening, absence of enhancement and gas in the bowel wall/mesentery/portal veins. With modern multidetector CT scanners, the thrombus can be seen within the contrast enhanced vessels. CT angiography is very accurate in diagnosing the cause of bowel ischemia. Bowel ischemia requires emergent surgical resection.

4. The most common and the most serious cause is bowel ischemia, where gas enters into bowel wall due to damaged mucosa. Other causes are bowel obstruction, intestinal trauma, infection, inflammation and graft versus host disease. Air in bowel wall can arise from the lungs, due to alveolar rupture and extension along bronchovascular bundles to mediastinum and retroperitoneum. COPD, cystic fibrosis and trauma are the other causes.

Case 3.31: Answers

1. The barium study shows a long irregular stricture of the terminal ileum, with ulceration. The ileocaecal valve and the proximal caecum are also irregular and the caecum has been lifted up out of the right iliac fossa.

2. TB of the small bowel.

3. Mycobacterium tuberculosis reaches the small bowel by ingestion of sputum or haematogenous spread of infected with cow milk containing mycobacterium bovis. Clinical features are weight loss, night sweats, abdominal pain, nausea and vomiting. TB of the small bowel can be an **ulcerative** form or **hypertrophic** form. The ulcerative form has ulcers with long axis perpendicular to intestinal axis. It is associated with pulmonary TB and caused by swallowed TB bacilli. In hypertrophic form, thickening of bowel is seen and is caused by ingestion of TB, usually from milk. Tuberculous peritonitis can be **wet** type (exudative ascites), **dry** type (caseous with adhesion) or **fibrotic fixed** (omental cake).

4. Tuberculosis of small bowel commonly occurs in the ileocaecal area, due to abundant lymphoid tissue in this location, along with relative stagnation of intestinal contents. The earliest sign is called **Fleishner sign**, where the ileocaecal valve is patulous and there is narrowing of terminal ileum. **Steirlin sign** is rapid emptying of the narrowed terminal ileum into short obliterated cecum. Ileocaecal valve is thick. The typical ulcers are oriented transversely in the small intestine, with elevated margins (deep fissures plus large shallow linear/stellate ulcers). In advanced cases, there is napkin ring type of stenosis of the terminal ileum, with a conical, shrunken caecum, elevated out of the right iliac fossa due to retraction of the mesocolon. CT shows circumferential thickening, ulcers, thick valve, soft tissue stranding, lymph node masses and peritoneal disease. The bowel wall thickening is concentric or eccentric. Skip areas of bowel wall thickening, bowel narrowing and dilatation can occur in other parts of small bowel in addition to the ileocaecal involvement.

5. Crohn's disease, infection with *Yersinia* spp., amoebiasis, carcinoma, lymphoma, radiotherapy and ischaemia are the differential diagnoses. The characteristic appearances of an ileocaecal junction help in differentiating TB from these lesions.

Gastrointestinal Answers

Case 3.32: Answers

1. The barium enema shows extensive diverticular disease in the whole of the left colon and sigmoid. The CT scan shows a thickened sigmoid colon, and few diverticula. There is soft-tissue stranding adjacent to the sigmoid colon.

2. Sigmoid diverticulosis with diverticulitis.

3. Decreased faecal bulk, caused by a diet high in refined fibre and low in roughage, is believed to be the cause of sigmoid diverticula. Overactivity of the sigmoid smooth muscle secondary to high intracolonic pressure results in herniation of mucosa and submucosa through the muscle layers. This is most common in the sigmoid colon because it is the narrowest colonic segment with the highest pressure. The herniations occur along the natural openings created by vasa recta or nutrient vessels in the wall of the colon.

4. Complications are diverticulitis and bleeding. Complications of diverticulitis are abscess, perforation, obstruction and a fistula to bladder/vagina/small bowel.

5. Diverticula are seen as outpouchings arising from the colon. They might be seen on a plain X-ray if there is barium remaining from a previous exam. Barium shows the diverticula as barium-filled outpouchings. Lateral diverticula are seen between the mesenteric and antimesenteric teniae on the opposite sides. Diverticulitis is best diagnosed with a CT scan with contrast. The wall of the sigmoid colon is thickened, diverticula are thickened, and air is trapped as a result of neck thickening and increased soft-tissue density in the pericolonic soft-tissue causing stranding. Abscesses are seen as fluid collections with rim enhancement. Fistulous tracks and obstruction can be noted. The most important radiological differential diagnosis of the diverticulitis is carcinoma. Diverticulitis involves a long segment and is associated with diverticula. Tumours have shorter segment involvement, heaped-up margins and ulcerated mucosa. Another differential diagnosis is colitis, which involves a long length of colon and has ulcerations in the early stages.

6. Diverticulosis does not require treatment. Diverticulitis is treated with broad-spectrum antibiotics. Surgery is indicated when complications develop or there is no response to medical treatment. Percutaneous drainage of abscesses is done under CT or ultrasonic guidance.

Case 3.33: Answers

1. Cholangiogram shows dilatation of the intrahepatic tributaries of the right and left hepatic ducts. There is a filling defect at the confluence of the right and left hepatic ducts, beyond which only a small amount of contrast has passed. CT scan shows a hypodense, poorly enhancing mass at the junction of right and left hepatic ducts, with proximal intrahepatic ductal dilatation.

2. Cholangiocarcinoma.

3. Inflammatory bowel disease giving rise to sclerosing cholangitis, (10 times increased risk), gallstones, primary sclerosing cholangitis, clonarchis infection, choledochal cyst, biliary atresia, biliary hamartoma, congenital hepatic fibrosis, Caroli's disease, autosomal dominant polycystic disease, recurrent pyogenic choangitis, choledochoenteric anastomosis, α_1-antitrypsin deficiency and thorotrast exposure are predisposing factors. Cholangiocarcinoma is an adenocarcinoma arising from epithelium of the small intrahepatic bile duct with a prominent desmoplastic reaction; mucin and calcification can be seen. Pathologically, cholangiocarcinoma can be exophytic, diffuse infiltrative or a polypoid mass. Histologically, it can be a well, moderately or poorly differentiated ductal tumour, of papillary, mucinous or signet-ring type. Rarely it can be mucoepidermoid, adenosquamous or cystadenocarcinoma. The lesion can be extra- or intrahepatic. In the extrahepatic duct, the common location is in the distal common biliary duct (CBD). Intrahepatic locations are rarer than extrahepatic locations and can be seen hilar, central or in a peripheral location distal to second-order branches.

4. Ultrasound detects dilated bile ducts and level of obstruction, but ultrasonic appearance of the mass is non specific and shows a homogenous or heterogenous area with fibrosis and occasional calcifications. CT scan and MRI are the most useful imaging examinations. CT scan show a singe, homogenous round or oval hypodense mass with irregular margins. On contrast administration, in the early stages, there is a moderate rim enhancement and in delayed images there is clearing of the rim and there is progressive and delayed enhancement of the central parts due to the fibrous component in the tumour. MRI shows the lesion as hypointense in T1. In T2 the rim is hyperintenese due to viable tumour and central is hypointense due to fibrosis and shows delayed enhancement. Angiography can show avascular, or hypovascular lesion. Occasionally it is hypervascular. Local spread to portal vein or involvement of hepatic artery may be seen.

5. The main differential diagnosis is hepatocellular carcinoma. Hepatoma is usually associated with a cirrhotic liver. The characteristic appearance with CT/MRI is early arterial enhancement of the whole tumour. The density of enhancement decreases with time and the tumour is less dense than the liver in delayed images (washout). In cholangiocarcinoma, however, the enhancement characteristics are different because of the presence of fibrous tissue. The centre of the tumour is full of fibrous tissue and the viable tumour is found only in the periphery. So the viable periphery enhances in early stages and washes out, but the central fibrotic portion does not enhance in early stages and enhances only in late scans. The tumour is very aggressive. It spreads along the duct, and infiltrates liver substance and regional lymph nodes. Only < 20% are resectable. Where it is possible, radical resection of liver tissue with affected bile ducts is the accepted treatment.

Case 3.34: Answers

1. There is large mass with central areas of necrosis in the left lobe of the liver. The left portal vein is not clearly seen.

2. Hepatocellular carcinoma.

3. Alcohol, hepatitis B, hepatitis C, haemochromatosis, aflatoxin, biliary cirrhosis, androgenic steroids, oral contraceptives, thorotrast and porphyria cutanea tarda are predisposing factors. It is more common in the Far East, Asia and sub-Saharan Africa. Pruritus, jaundice, splenomegaly, variceal bleeding, cachexia, hepatic encephalopathy, right upper quadrant pain, ascites and other signs of liver failure are features of hepatoma. Laboratory findings include elevated α-fetoprotein and other lab findings expected in cirrhotic liver.

4. Hepatoma can be focal, multifocal or diffuse. The CT scan in the arterial and portal phase is usually adequate to establish the diagnosis, which is confirmed by ultrasound or CT-guided biopsy. MRI and contrast ultrasound are also useful. Ultrasound shows an expansive tumour in the liver with a hypoechoic rim at the periphery of the tumour is caused by a fibrous capsule or compressed parenchyma. Ill-defined margins are seen in more invasive tumours. On the CT scan, HCC is seen as a hypodense mass, with a hypodense rim of capsule. The tumour is bright if there is superimposed haemorrhage. Large tumours are heterogeneous due

to areas of haemorrhage or necrosis. The characteristic appearance is seen after contrast enhancement. As the tumour is supplied by the hepatic artery, enhances in the arterial phase, but the contrast rapidly washes out and the tumour is seen as a hypodense mass in the portal phase. Invasion of the portal vein and other structures can be seen. MRI also shows similar features. The lesion is dark on a non-contrast scan and shows early arterial enhancement with quick washout in the portal venous images. Angiography shows vascular tumour, with hypertrophied and new vasculature. Cirrhotic patients undergo yearly ultrasound and α-fetoprotein for screening to rule out development of HCC.

5. **Metastasis** is multifocal and does not enhance in the arterial phase, except the vascular metastases such as renal carcinoma, thyroid carcinoma, phaeochromocytoma, neuroendocrine tumours and sarcomas. **Haemangiomas** are the most common benign tumour in liver and might be difficult to differentiate from hepatomas when they are large. They usually show a different pattern of enhancement, which is nodular and slow filling in delayed phases. **Adenomas** and **focal nodular hyperplasia** are also vascular tumours, but they do not show rapid washout and are isodense on the delayed scans. A central stellate scar is seen in **focal nodular hyperplasia** and **fibrolamellar carcinoma.** ^{99m} Tc-sulphur colloid scan shows increased or normal uptake in focal nodular hyperplasia.

6. Surgery is the treatment of choice. Success rate following tumor resection is only 5%. Liver transplant can be performed if there is solitary tumour < 5 cm, or < 3 tumours measuring <3 cm each. Radiology is useful in palliative treatment of hepatocellular carcinoma. Hepatic artery chemoembolisation, percutaneous alcohol ablation, radiofrequency ablation, microwave/laser ablation are all used in treatment. In hepatic artery chemoembolisation, Lipiodol (iodised poppy seed oil), is used along with chemotherapeutic agents, such as Adriamycin and embolic material such as gelfoam. The lipiodol is selectively taken up by the tumour and cleared very slowly and hence the chemotherapeutic agent is selectively delivered to the tumour, without toxic side effects.

Case 3.35: Answers

1. The ERCP shows extensive irregular narrowing and dilatation of the intrahepatic system, with multiple strictures. Irregularity of the common bile duct is also noted.

2. Sclerosing cholangitis. Primary sclerosing cholangitis is obliterative fibrosing inflammation of the biliary tree, with multiple strictures that result from altered bile metabolism and an increase in lithocholic acid caused by bacterial overgrowth.

3. Sclerosing cholangitis has a high association with inflammatory bowel disease (ulcerative colitis in 75% and Crohns disease in 14%). This is called secondary sclerosing cholangitis. Other associations are pancreatitis, cirrhosis, chronic active hepatitis, retroperitoneal fibrosis, Peyronie's diease, orbital pseudotumour, Riedl's thyroiditis, Sjorgren syndrome and liver fluke infestation. The most common location is common bile duct. Intra and extrahepatic ducts are involved in majority. Involvement of cystic duct, only intrahepatic ducts and only extrahepatic ducts are rare presentations.

4. Cholangiography is the mainstay in the diagnosis. This can be done by percutaneous injection of contrast or with ERCP. A non invasive method opacification of biliary tree is MRCP, where the high T2 signal of fluids is used to demonstrate bile ducts in physiological state, without need for invasive procedure. Multifocal strictures are noted, especially at bifurcations, with skip lesions where the bile duct calibre is normal, giving as string of beads appearance with alternating segments of dilatation and stenosis. Small diverticula are seen. Pruned tree appearance is seen due to opacification of central ducts and no visualisation of peripheral ducts. Cobblestone appearance is seen due to nodular mucosal irregularities. Mild ductal dilatation is seen is seen proximal to affected areas. Ultrasound shows echogenic portal triads and biliary casts with wall thickening. CT shows same changes and focal of high density in ducts. MRI shows intermediate intensity in T1 and hyperintesntiy in T2 in periportal areas.

5. The complications are calculi, cholangitis, secondary biliary cirrhosis, portal hypertension and cholangiocarcinoma.

6. Differential diagnoses: **cholangiocarcinoma** (single short segment stricture, irregular, upstream dilatation, mass), **cholangitis** (bile duct thickening, fever), **primary biliary cirrhosis** (limited to intrahepatic ducts, less prominent strictures, crossing of bile ducts) and **AIDS cholangiopathy**.

1. The barium follow-through shows dilated loops of small bowel. In the proximal bowel loops, the spaces between the folds are increased. In the distal small bowel loops, there is dilution of barium, with flocculated clumps of barium.

2. Coeliac disease (coeliac sprue, non tropical sprue, gluten sensitive enteropathy). This is characterised by villous atrophy, cryptic hyperplasia and round cell infiltration. Clinical features are diarrhoea, steatorrhoea, abdominal cramps, fatigue, weight loss, stomatitis, neuropathy, bleeding diathesis, infertility, dermatitis herpetiformis, deficiency of iron, vitamin B_{12} or folate deficiency, decreased levels of cholesterol, calcium, albumin, high alkaline phosphatase (ALP), elevated liver enzymes and increased prothrombin time (PTT). Almost all patients of dermatitis herpetiformis suffer from coeliac disease.

3. Dilated small bowel, decreased peristalsis, decreased folds in jejunum (< 3/inch), increased folds in the ileum (> 5/inch), segmentation of barium (break-up of barium, producing clumps of barium), flocculation (coarse granular clumps of barium), fragmentation, moulage sign (smooth contour with featureless folds) and thick primary mucosal folds are features of malabsorption.

4. Other causes of malabsorption are tropical sprue, disaccharidase deficiency, Whipple's disease, parasites, inflammatory bowel disease, drugs, Zollinger–Ellison syndrome, T-cell lymphoma, abetalipoproteinaemia, lymphangiectasia, agammaglobulinaemia, amyloid, cardiac failure, blind loop syndrome, gastric surgery, pancreatitis, cystic fibrosis and chronic liver disease. Hypoperistalsis is also caused by scleroderma and idiopathic pseudo-obstruction. Nodules are seen in lymphoid hyperplasia, lymphoma, mastocytosis, amyloidosis and eosinophilic enteritis. Bowel wall thickening is caused by infection, irradiation, carcinoid, ischaemia and vasculitis.

5. Complications are – hyposplenism, ulcerative jejunoileitis, cavitatory mesenteric lymph nodes, generalised lymphadenopathy, lymphoma and volvulus. Diagnosis is confirmed by small intestinal biopsy. Treatment is with life long gluten free diet. Lactase free diet should be recommended due to associated lactase deficiency. Vitamin supplements and regular follow-up to rule out lymphoma and carcinoma of GIT is recommended. Relapse occurs due to hidden dietary gluten, diabetes, bacterial overgrowth, intestinal ulceration and lymphoma.

Case 3.37: Answers

1. The first test is a ^{99m}Tc-labelled red blood cell (RBC) scan. This shows an abnormal area of progressively increasing uptake of radionuclide in the right upper side of the abdomen, suggestive of active bleeding in the right colon.

2. This is a superior mesenteric angiography. Late phase of the angiography shows a dense vascular blush in the right side of colon, indicating active bleeding.

3. Colonic bleeding caused by angiodysplasia of colon. Angiodysplasia is a vascular malformation, causing dilatation of the submucosal arteries and veins with thinned mucosa. The aetiology is ischaemic. It is associated with aortic stenosis. The most common location is the antimesenteric border of the caecum and ascending colon. Occasionally it is seen in the descending colon and sigmoid colon. The angiogram shows a cluster of vessels in the antimesenteric border in the arterial phase, with early opacification of a draining ileocolic vein.

4. Gastrointestinal bleeding is classified as upper and lower, depending on location with respect to the ligament of Treitz. Causes of upper gastrointestinal bleeding are oesophageal varices, gastric/duodenal ulcer, gastritis, Mallory–Weiss syndrome, vascular malfomation, aortoenteric fistula and tumours. Lower gastrointestinal bleeding is caused by angiodysplasia, colonic diverticula, inflammatory bowel disease, tumours, vascular malformation and aortoenteric fistula.

5. Gastrointestinal bleeding can be investigated by endoscopy or colonoscopy. If a bleeding source is not identified, radiological procedures are done. Technetium-labelled RBCs or sulphur colloid is used to find the site of bleeding. Angiography can be done in the conventional way or by CT or MRA, which are non-invasive. Digital subtraction angiography is done by introducing catheters into all possible sources of bleeding. Extravastation of contrast in the bowel lumen is noted with bleeding > 1–1.5 ml/min. The labelled RBC scintigraphic technique works on the principle that extravasating labelled RBCs result in an abnormal active focus in the abdomen in a location where normal vascular structures are not visible. Labelled RBCs are prepared in vivo or ex vivo, with technetium-^{99m} as the labelling agent. Scans are taken every few minutes, with delayed images at 24 hours. Unexpected focus of activity and transport along the

gastrointestinal tract indicate the source of gastrointestinal bleeding. This technique is sensitive for detecting bleeding at the rate of 0.1 ml/min and is useful for intermittent bleeding. Technetium-labelled sulphur colloid can detect bleeding as low as 0.05 ml/min, but it is useful in acute bleeding only. Bleeding in the upper abdomen can be masked by uptake in the liver and spleen. Barium studies have very little role in the diagnosis of acute GI bleeding.

6. Gastrointestinal bleeding can be treated by intra-arterial vasopressin infusion or by transcatheter embolisation after superselective catheterisation, using embolic agents such as coils or glue. Complications are bowel infarction and stricture.

Case 3.38: Answers

1. This is a pertechnate scan. There is a focal high activity of the lower abdomen in the left side, of the same intensity as the uptake in the stomach.

2. Meckel's diverticulum.

3. Pertechnate scan is the gold standard in diagnosis of bleeding from Meckel's diverticulum. Since Meckel's diverticulum has ectopic gastric mucosa with its mucoid cells, it takes up Tc^{99m} pertechnate. The patient is prepared for the test, by avoiding any irritative procedure for 48 hours and fasting for 3–6 hours which decreases gastric secretion and intestinal motility. The bowel and bladder are evacuated before the study. 100–300 MBq of Tc^{99m} pertechnate is injected intravenously and scans are acquired for 30–45 minutes. Cimetidine (decreased gastric secretion), pentagastrin (stimulates uptake) and glucagons (decreases intestinal peristalsis) can be used for making the scans better. The scan shows a focal collection of tracer in the lower quadrant of abdomen, appearing at the same time or shortly after the gastric activity and the tracer activity increases in intensity with time parallel to that of the stomach, indicating presence of ectopic gastric mucosa. The Meckel's diverticulum should bleed at rate of atleast 0.1 ml/minute to be picked up by the scan. The sensitivity of this scan is 75–100% and specificity is up to 80%. A false positive scan can be seen if there are other lesions with ectopic gastric musoca such as a duplication cyst with gastric wall, normal small bowel or Barrett esophagus, lesions with increased blood pool – haemangioma, aneurysm,

AVM, hypervascular tumour, duodenal ulcer, appendicitis, ulcerative colitis, Crohn's disease, laxative abuse, intestinal obstruction, intussusception, volvulus, urinary obstruction and meningomyelocele. The test won't be useful after adolescence, since these patients are unlikely to have ectopic gastric mucosa without symptoms. False negative tests are also seen when there is insufficient gastric mucosa or dilution of activity due to peristalsis or hypersecretion. Other tests that would be useful are a contrast study of the small bowel (enteroclysis), where the Meckel's diverticulum would be seen as a smooth, club like intraluminal mass parallel to long axis of distal ileum. Angiogram shows persistent vitelline artery and is useful when the bleeding is more than 1 ml/min.

4. Meckel's diverticulum is the most common congenital abnormality of the gastrointestinal tract. It results from the persistence of the omphalomesenteric duct (which connects the midgut to the yolk sac) and normally obliterates by week 5. It is seen in 2% of the population, located within 0.6 m of the ileocaecal valve in the antimesenteric border, symptomatic before 2 years and is usually 5–6 cm long. It contains ectopic mucosa, which can be gastric (80%), colonic, jejunal or pancreatic. It is supplied by the right vitelline artery. Most patients are asymptomatic and detected incidentally on a barium study. Development of symptoms indicates a complication, the most common being bleeding from peptic ulceration of the gastric mucosa. Definitive treatment of the condition is excision of the diverticulum along with an adjacent ileal segment.

5. This is a barium study of the small bowel. There is a well-defined, smooth filling defect in the distal ileum, parallel to the long axis of the ileum. Complications are acute diverticulitis, acute gastrointestinal bleeding, intussusception, volvulus, bands, internal hernia leading to obstruction and associated malignant tumours (carcinoid, sarcoma, carcinoma).

Case 3.39: Answers

1. The plain film shows a claw (meniscus) sign in the middle of the abdomen at the level of the L2 vertebra, with a soft-tissue opacity protruding into a gas shadow of the colon. Ultrasonography shows a pseudo-kidney sign, with central hyperechogenicity and surrounding hypoechogenicity.

2. Intussusception.

3. Intussusception is a common cause of acute abdomen in infancy, which occurs when a segment of bowel, the intussusceptum, telescopes into the bowel distally, the intussuscipiens. It is usually seen between 6 months and 2 years of age. Most are ileoileal or ileo-ileocolic. Most cases are idiopathic and do not have any lead point other than lymphoid hypertrophy. About 2% have lead points, which include Meckel's diverticulum, duplication cyst, lymphoma, polyps, Henoch–Schönlein purpura and inspissated mucus in cystic fibrosis. Characteristic features include intermittent colicky abdominal pain with drawing up of the legs, vomiting, red-currant jelly stools and palpable abdominal mass. Drowsiness and lethargy can be seen. Mechanical small bowel obstruction and ischaemia are the complications if untreated.

4. A plain X-ray demonstrates a soft-tissue mass in the right upper quadrant, dilated loops or the classic claw sign where the apex of the intussusceptum is outlined by gas in the colon. Bowel obstruction, perforation and a sparse amount of bowel gas are other features. A plain X-ray can be normal. Ultrasonography is a sensitive method in diagnosis. Multiple concentric rings or a pseudo-kidney or doughnut sign can be seen, caused by various appearances of the telescoping bowel loops. Fluid in the intussusceptum indicates vascular compromise.

5. This picture demonstrates air reduction of intussusception. The bowel loops are distended with gas, which has entered the small bowel, indicating successful reduction. The standard treatment is air reduction using oxygen or carbon dioxide. A Foley catheter is inserted into the rectum and a tight seal maintained. Air is delivered inside the bowel, with a maximum pressure of 120 mmHg. Successful reduction is indicated by air entering the small bowel. Three attempts can be made with 3-minute intervals. Reduction is less likely to be successful if the duration of symptoms is > 48 hours, or there is rectal bleeding or small bowel obstruction. Perforation and tension pneumoperitoneum are complications of air reduction. Surgery is performed for failed reductions. Some 5–10% recur after surgical or non-surgical reduction.

1. The barium enema shows absence of haustrations in the colon. There are multiple small ulcers seen, scattered throughout the colon, but more prominent in the descending colon. There are mucosal islands noted in the transverse colon, which is grossly distended. In the second picture, there is an irregular, ulcerative mass in the transverse colon, close to the splenic flexure.

2. Acute exacerbation of ulcerative colitis. Complication seen here is carcinoma in the transverse colon.

3. Ulcerative colitis is an idiopathic inflammatory bowel disease, with symmetrical continuous involvement of the colon. It presents with bloody diarrhoea, fever and cramps. Extracolonic features are iritis, pyoderma gangrenosum, erythema nodosum, pericholangitis, sclerosing cholangitis, chronic active hepatitis, rheumatoid arthritis, spondylitis and thrombotic complications. Usually, ulcerative colitis begins in the rectum and spreads proximally and symmetrically. The rectosigmoid is involved in 95%. When the colitis extends proximal to the splenic flexure it is called universal colitis and when it extends to the terminal ileum it is known as backwash ileitis.

4. The findings on a barium enema depend on the stage. In the acute stage there is fine mucosal granularity and tiny superficial ulcers. Collar-button ulcers, double tracking and thumbprinting are other findings. Pseudopolyps are seen as a result of scattered areas of oedematous mucosa and re-epithelialised granulation tissue within an area of denuded mucosa. The presacral space is widened because of inflammation. Rectal folds are obliterated. In the later stages, the haustra are lost. Inflammatory polyps are seen and the colon is short and rigid. The term 'burnt-out colon' is used when there is distensible colon with no haustral markings and no mucosal pattern. Postinflammatory polyps are small sessile nodules (filiform polyps). Differential diagnoses:

   Familial polyposis: haustrations are seen; no inflammation in polyps

   Cathartic colon: more extensive changes are seen in the right colon

   Crohn's disease is the most important clinical differential diagnosis. It is more common in the small bowel with deep ulcers, a thick ileocaecal valve, eccentric location and transmural skip lesions. Megacolon is uncommon, but fistulas may be seen. There is a slight increase in the risk of carcinoma.

In ulcerative colitis, the colon is involved and the rectum is always involved. There are shallow ulcers with loss of haustrations and a gaping ileocaecal valve. There is symmetrical involvement with no skip lesions. Megacolon is common and there is a high risk of carcinoma.

5. Complications are toxic megacolon (most common cause of death, Transverse colon > 5.5. cm), strictures, obstruction and perforation. There is a 5% risk of malignancy. Risk starts after 10 years of onset. The risk of malignancy is 0.5% per year of colitis. Risk is higher — if the onset < 15 years; pancolitis; when it is in rectosigmoid. The carcinoma is usually annular or polypoid.

6. Treatment is with aminosalicylic acid derivatives, steroids and immunosuppressants. Surgery is done when complications develop.

Case 3.41: Answers

1. The X-ray of the abdomen shows multiple, irregular calcifications in the central portion of the upper abdomen. The CT scan shows an atrophic pancreas. There is a well encapsulated, hypodense fluid collection in the tail and body of the pancreas. There is a peripheral rim of calcification in the wall of the capsule of the cyst.

2. Chronic pancreatitis with pseudocyst formation (probably related to an acute exacerbation).

3. Chronic pancreatitis is a chronic inflammatory disease of the pancreas. It is classified as chronic calcifying and chronic obstructive pancreatitis. It presents with acute exacerbation of epigastric pain, jaundice, steatorrhoea and diabetes mellitus. Alcoholism, congenital/acquired anomalies of the pancreatic duct, sphincter of Oddi dysfunction, trauma, surgical ligation, idiopathic, renal failure and ampullary tumour are common causes of chronic obstructive pancreatitis. Causes of chronic calcifying pancreatitis are hereditary, juvenile tropical pancreatitis, hyperlipidaemia, hypercalcaemia and inborn errors of metabolism.

4. In chronic pancreatitis the X-ray shows irregular calcifications in the pancreatic area. The CT scan shows a small atrophied gland. The duct

is dilated, irregular and beaded. Calcifications are seen in the gland and duct. In an acute attack, the gland is enlarged. Pseudocysts can be seen. Ultrasonography shows similar appearances with an irregular, atrophied gland, and dilated ducts and calculi. MRI shows a low signal in T1 and a high signal in T2. Cholangiography shows a dilated main duct, beading, string-of-pearls appearance caused by multifocal dilatation and stenosis of the duct, side branch ectasia, and intraductal filling defects caused by debris, calculi or protein plugs.

5. Complications are superimposed acute pancreatitis, pseudocyst, pancreatic ascites, thrombosis of splenic/mesenteric/portal vein, pseudoaneurysm of splenic artery and pancreatic carcinoma (2–5%). Occasionally, chronic pancreatitis can involve a focal portion of the pancreas. The most important diagnostic dilemma is differentiating a focal pancreatitis from a pancreatic carcinoma. In focal pancreatitis, there is a mass with irregular margins and upstream ductal dilation. Differentiation might be difficult with CT, MRI or even endoscopic ulrasound. Biopsy is required for diagnosis.

6. If there is biliary obstruction, stenting can be done. Fluid collections are drained percutaneously under radiological guidance. Guided biopsy is required for differentiating from cancer.

Case 3.42: Answers

1. The barium study shows multiple ulcers in the proximal jejunum (marked by arrows). There is considerable mucosal oedema of the duodenum and proximal jejunum. The CT scan shows a heterogeneous, hypodense tumour in the head of the pancreas. A stent is noted in the distal CBD and some contrast in gallbladder from the recent ERCP.

2. Zollinger–Ellison syndrome (ZES).

3. Zollinger–Ellison syndrome is produced by a gastrinoma that stimulates the acid-secreting cells of the stomach to maximal activity, with consequent gastrointestinal mucosal ulceration. It may be sporadic or part of multiple endocrine neoplasia type 1 (MEN-1) syndrome. The characteristic clinical triad is gastric hypersecretion, hypergastrinaemia > 1000 ng/l (increase in serum gastrin by > 200 ng/l after secretin administration) and hyperacidity (basal output > 15 mmol/l). Abdominal

pain, diarrhoea/steatorrhoea, heartburn, nausea, vomiting, weight loss and gastrointestinal bleeding are also seen. Gastrinomas are malignant in 50–75%. The 5-year survival rate is 50%. Prognosis is better for patients with ectopic tumours and no hepatic metastasis.

4. The manifestations of Zollinger–Ellison syndrome are ulcers that are multiple, recurrent and in atypical locations distal to the second part of the duodenum. Other features are: barium dilution caused by hypersecretion of gastric acid in a non-obstructed, non-dilated stomach; thickened folds; prominent area gastricae; and distended proximal small bowel resulting from fluid overload. Unlike pancreatic adenocarcinomas, the islet cell tumours show intense contrast enhancement. Somatostatin receptor scintigraphy is the most sensitive method for detecting ZES. A CT scan is used for localising the tumour and for metastasis. Endoscopic ultrasonography is very accurate in localisation.

5. Complications in a Zollinger–Ellison syndrome ulcer are frequent and include perforation, haemorrhage, reflux oesophagitis and oesophageal stricture. Complications of the islet tumour are malignancy and liver metastases. Treatment is with H_2-receptor antagonists, proton pump inhibitors (omeprazole), gastrectomy and resection of the gastrinoma. Patients with sporadic ZES with no hepatic metastases or surgical contraindications should undergo surgical resection to prevent development of hepatic metastasis.

Case 3.43: Answers

1. The CT scan of the abdomen shows diffuse thickening of the wall of the small bowel. There is also abnormal enhancement of the bowel wall. Three layers can be seen in the bowel wall. The inner and outer layers enhance well and there is a central dark area. Small amount of free fluid is also noted in the left side of the abdomen.

2. Acute graft-versus-host disease (GVHD).

3. GVHD results from reactivity of the allogeneic graft lymphocytes to the recipient. It is a major cause of morbidity in stem cell transplant recipients. The most commonly affected organs are the skin, liver, eye, lung and gastrointestinal tract. It is seen in 30–50% of all bone marrow transplant recipients. The risk is high with mismatched transplants. It develops 10–40

days after transplantation. Clinical features are pruritus and maculopapular rash. Gastric involvement causes nausea and vomiting. Oesophageal involvement causes odynophagia and dysphagia. Small bowel involvement causes fever, abdominal pain and diarrhoea. The bowel wall is injured and replaced by granulation tissue.

4. CT is very useful in evaluating the small bowel and colonic manifestations of GVHD. A CT scan is done with negative oral contrast and positive intravenous contrast, so that the bowel wall can be seen well. It shows dilated fluid-filled bowel loops, bowel wall and fold thickening, separation of bowel loops and mesenteric stranding. The characteristic appearance is the halo sign caused by hyperaemic granulation tissue surrounded by low-density outer wall layers.

5. Differential diagnoses for the appearance of bowel wall thickening and enhancement in a transplant recipient are infection, inflammatory bowel disease and radiation enteritis. The extent of bowel involvement is greater in GVHD than in these diseases. Differentiation from infection might require tissue sample. Treatment of GVHD is with steroids/immunosuppressants/mesenchymal stem cells. However, this treatment makes the patients more prone to infections.

Case 3.44: Answers

1. Barium examination of the small bowel shows dilated duodenum and dilated loops of jejunum and ileum. The folds of the small bowel are very closely placed, like a stack of coins or hidebound. The fold thickness is normal. In addition there are also multiple sacculations, arising from the antimesenteric border (these are the large contrast-filled outpouchings). Stasis of barium in the upper GI tract is indicative of increased transit time.

2. Scleroderma.
   Malabsorption produces diarrhoea, steatorrhoea and deficiencies of fat-soluble vitamins A, D, E and K. Bone pain is produced by hypocalcaemia.

3. Scleroderma is a systemic disease, most obvious in the skin. However, the gastrointestinal tract, respiratory, renal, cardiovascular, genitourinary systems, and vascular structures are also involved. The disease is characterised by obliterative small vessel vasculitis and proliferation of

connective tissue, with fibrosis of multiple organs. It is more common in women and usually seen in those aged 30–40 years. The gastrointestinal abnormalities observed in scleroderma involve oesophageal dysmotility, delayed gastric emptying, intestinal fibrosis and dysmotility, pseudo-diverticula, bacterial overgrowth, pseudo-obstruction, pneumatosis intestinalis, arteritis and colonic dysmotility. The gastrointestinal tract is involved in 80–100% of patients with systemic sclerosis.

4. Small bowel hypomotility is seen in 90% of cases. Barium shows a dilated and atonic duodenum, with reduced peristalsis, proximal to the aorticomesenteric angle and delayed passage of the contrast medium, especially in the recumbent position. The small bowel lumen may also be diffusely dilated with hypomotility and extremely prolonged transit time. In addition there is decreased distance between the valvulae conniventes. This change results from asymmetrical fibrosis involving the circular muscle to a lesser degree than the longitudinal muscle, which produces the stack of coins/hidebound appearance. Sacculation, caused by smooth muscle atrophy, and fibrosis accompanied by small vessel obstruction result in the formation of pseudodiverticula with a broad base

5. Treatment depends on the site of involvement. Good control is achieved when the treatment is commenced before onset of irreversible fibrosis. D-pencillamine has been widely used, with doubtful effectiveness. Anti-inflammatory drugs, anti-fibrotic drugs, immunosuppressive agents and supportive therapies are widely used. Cyclophosphamide, thalidomide and long term prostaglandin infusions are under trial. Pseudoobstruction is managed conservatively with drip and suck technique.

Gastrointestinal Answers

4
GENITOURINARY RADIOLOGY QUESTIONS

Case 4.1

A 44-year-old man presents with abdominal pain, distension and hypertension. On examination, there is no palpable mass.

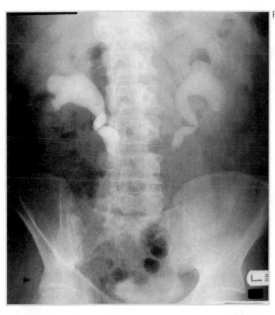
Fig 4.1a

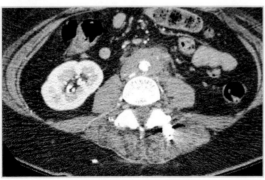
Fig 4.1b

1. What do you find on the intravenous urogram (IVU) and CT scan?
2. What is the diagnosis?
3. What are the mechanism of development, and other causes and associations?
4. What are the characteristic location and the radiological features?
5. What are the differential diagnosis and the treatment?

Answers *on pages 273–293*

Case 4.2

A 76-year-old man presents with sudden onset of difficulty in urination and abdominal distension. Clinical examination showed a large, non-tender mass in the lower abdomen, extending into the pelvis.

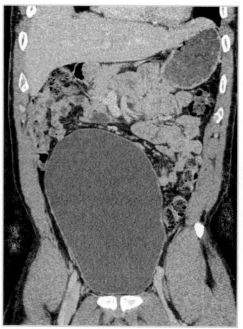

Fig 4.2a

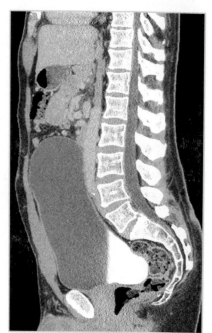

Fig 4.2b

1. What do you observe on the CT scan?
2. What is the diagnosis?
3. What are the causes?
4. What is the role of imaging in this condition?
5. What is the treatment?

Answers on pages 273–293

Case 4.3

A 3-year-old girl presents with recurrent urinary tract infections. Investigations were ordered.

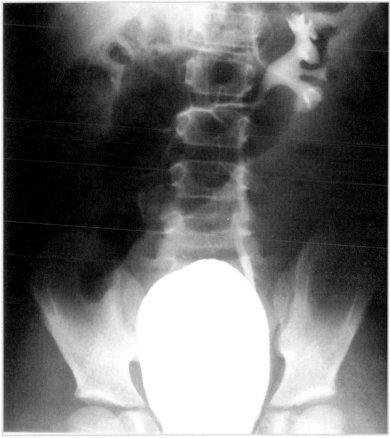

Fig 4.3

1. What is this investigation? How is it done?
2. What are the findings and the diagnosis?
3. What are the causes of this condition and the complications?
4. What other imaging modalities can be used and how is this graded?
5. What is the imaging protocol for recurrent urinary infections?

Answers *on pages 273–293*

Case 4.4

A 40-year-old hypertensive patient presents with fever and bilateral flank pain. On examination, the patient is febrile and tachycardic. There are bilateral masses in the lumbar region, which is tender on the right side.

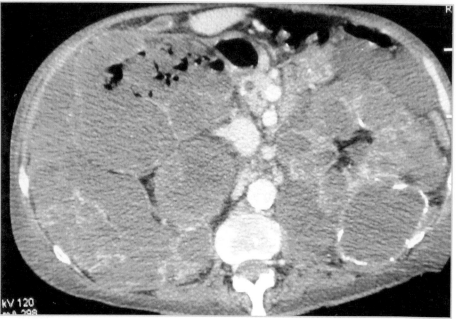

Fig 4.4

1. What are the abnormalities on the CT scan?
2. What is the diagnosis?
3. What are the clinical features of this disease and the associations?
4. What are the radiological features and differential diagnosis?
5. What is the treatment of this disease? How is this disease followed up?

Answers on pages 273–293

Case 4.5

A 9-year-old girl presents with persistent bedwetting and recurrent urinary infections. Clinical examination was unremarkable.

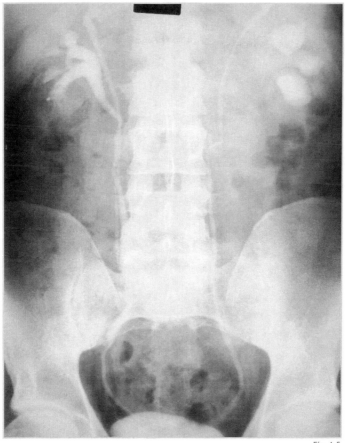

Fig 4.5

1. What do you observe on the IVU?
2. What is the diagnosis and what are the causes of the patient's symptoms?
3. What are the development and clinical features?
4. What is the Weigert–Meyer rule?
5. What are the complications?

Answers *on pages 273–293*

Case 4.6

A 46-year-old woman presents with left loin pain. On examination, there is tenderness in the left costovertebral angle.

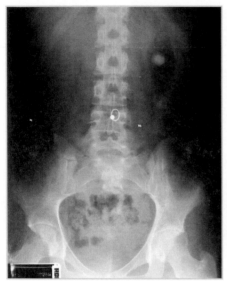
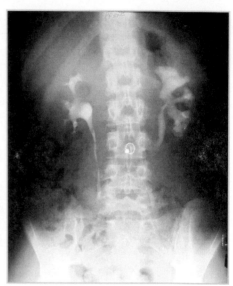

Fig 4.6a   Fig 4.6b

1. What do you see on the X-ray and IVU?
2. What is the diagnosis?
3. What are the types and causes of this disease?
4. What are the clinical and radiological features?
5. What are the complications and treatment?

Answers on pages 273–293

Case 4.7

A 42-year-old man presents with flank pain, fever and chills. On examination, there is tenderness in the right lumbar region, without any palpable mass.

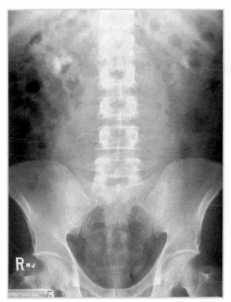

Fig 4.7a

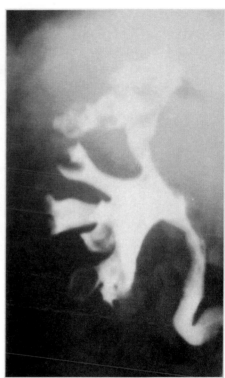

Fig 4.7b

1. What do you see on the plain film and localized view of the right kidney in IVU?
2. What is the diagnosis?
3. What are the pathophysiology and clinical features?
4. What are the radiological features?
5. What are the complications and the differential diagnoses?

Answers *on pages 273–293*

Case 4.8

A 4-year-old girl presents with abdominal pain, fever and pain on micturition. On examination, there is mild, bilateral, renal angle tenderness.

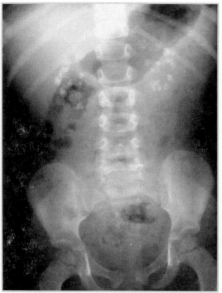

Fig 4.8a

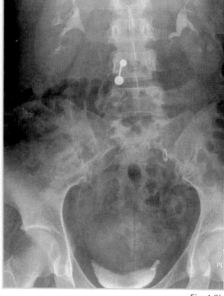

Fig 4.8b

1. What do you see on the plain abdominal X-ray? What do you see in IVU (follow-up IVU done at 13 years of age)?
2. What is the diagnosis?
3. What are the causes of this appearance?
4. What disease does this boy have and what are its clinical features?
5. What are the radiological features?

Answers on pages 273–293

Case 4.9

A 45-year-old man presents with a right-sided abdominal mass. On clinical examination, a non-tender mass is felt in the right lumbar region.

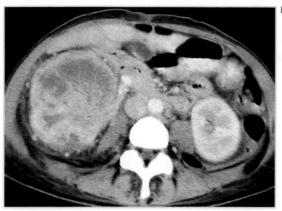

Fig 4.9a

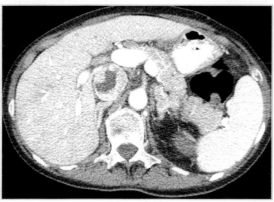

Fig 4.9b

1. What are the findings on the first CT scan?
2. What is the diagnosis? What complication do you see on the second CT scan?
3. What are the important factors to be assessed on the scan?
4. What further investigations are required for confirmation of the diagnosis?
5. What are the various presentations of this disease? What is the cell of origin of this disease?
6. What is the management of this disease?

Answers *on pages 273–293*

Case 4.10

A 40-year-old man presents with haematuria, abdominal pain and malaise. Clinical examination is unremarkable, except for mild tenderness in the left costovertebral angle.

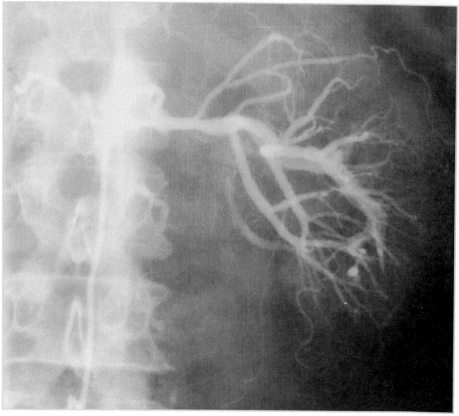

Fig 4.10

1. What is this investigation and what do you find?
2. What is the diagnosis?
3. What is the pathology of this disease?
4. What is it associated with?
5. What are the radiological features?
6. What are the features of involvement of other organs and the treatment?

Answers on pages 273–293

A 12-year-old boy presents with recurrent urinary infections and abdominal pain. On clinical examination, there is no mass or tenderness in the abdomen.

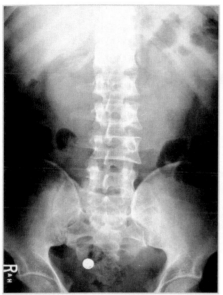

Fig 4.11a

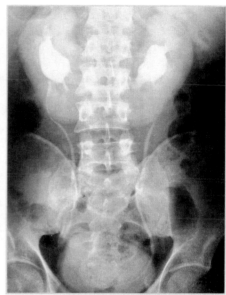

Fig 4.11b

1. What do you observe on the plain X-ray?
2. What do you observe on the IVU and what is the diagnosis?
3. What is the development of this condition?
4. What are the anatomical and radiological features?
5. What other conditions are associated?

Answers on pages 273–293

A 60-year-old woman was investigated for recurrent renal infections. Ultrasonography done as a part of work-up showed a normal right kidney, but the left kidney was not visualised.

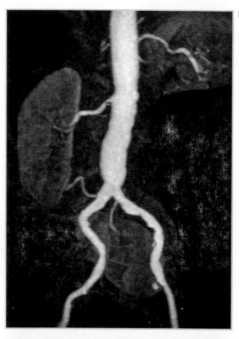

Fig 4.12a

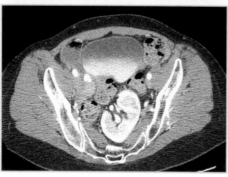

Fig 4.12b

1. What do you observe in these investigations?
2. What is the diagnosis?
3. What is the development of this condition?
4. What are the associated features?
5. What are the complications?

Answers on pages 273–293

Case 4.13

A 55-year-old woman presented with uncontrollable hypertension. On examination, her BP was 180/110 mmHg and there was a bruit in the abdomen.

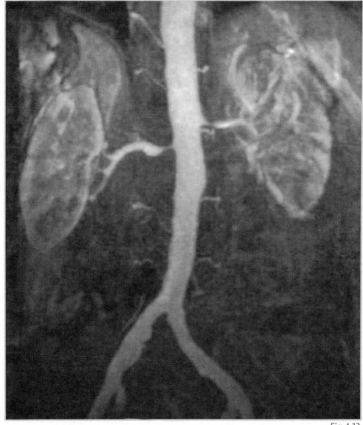

Fig 4.13

1. What is this investigation and what do you observe?
2. What is the diagnosis?
3. What other conditions may cause this disease and what is the pathophysiology related to the hypertension?
4. What are the radiological features on Doppler ultrasonography and MRI?
5. What are the complications and the management?

Answers *on pages 273–293*

Case 4.14

A 32-year-old presents with sudden onset of left loin pain and haematuria. Clinical examination showed tenderness in the left renal fossa.

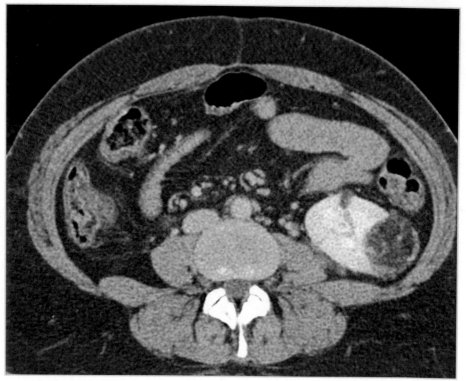

Fig 4.14

1. What do you observe on the abdominal CT scan?
2. What is the diagnosis?
3. What are the types and what is the most important association?
4. What are the radiological features and differential diagnosis?
5. What are the complication and treatment?

Answers on pages 273–293

Case 4.15

A 61-year-old male patient presents with left loin pain and difficulty in urination. On examination, there is a soft mass in the left renal angle. His serum creatinine level was increased.

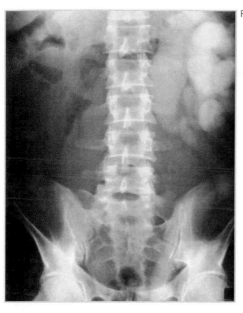

Fig 4.15a

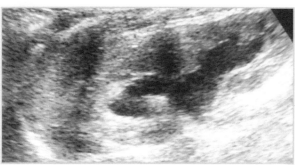

Fig 4.15b

1. What do you see on the delayed IVU film and ultrasound scan?
2. What is the diagnosis? What are the causes?
3. What are the radiological features?
4. What is the differential diagnosis?
5. What is the role of radiology in treatment?

Answers *on pages 273–293*

A 35-year-old woman presented with flank pain and pyuria. On examination, she is febrile and has left renal angle tenderness, without any palpable mass. A urine test demonstrated pyuria.

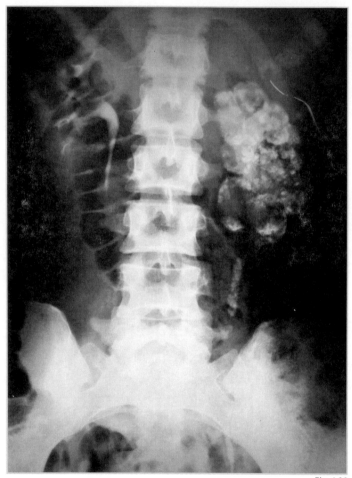

Fig 4.16

1. What do you observe on the IVU?
2. What is the diagnosis?
3. What is the pathophysiology and what are the clinical features?
4. What are the radiological features and differential diagnosis?
5. What are the complications and treatment?

Answers on pages 273–293

A 5-year-old girl presents with severe abdominal pain, vomiting, fever, nausea and burning micturition. On examination, she is febrile and tachypnoeic, and has bilateral renal angle tenderness.

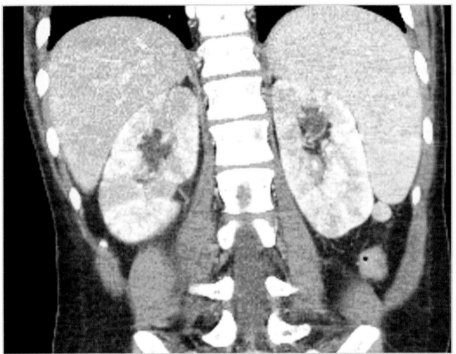

Fig 4.17

1. What do you see on the abdominal CT scan?
2. What is the diagnosis?
3. What are the causative organisms?
4. What are the clinical and radiological features?
5. What are the complications?

Answers on pages 273–293

A 47-year-old woman presents with severe lower abdominal pain, haematuria, dysuria and frequency. Clinical examination revealed mild tenderness in the hypogastric area, but no obvious mass was palpated.

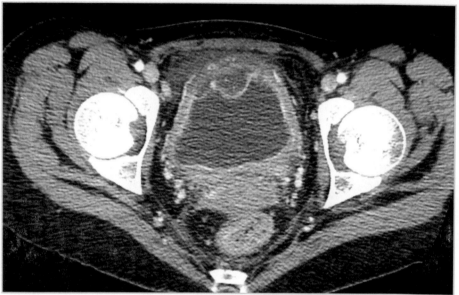

Fig 4.18

1. What do you find on this CT scan?
2. What is the diagnosis?
3. What are the causes and clinical features of this disease?
4. What are the radiological features and differential diagnosis?
5. What are the complications and the treatment?

Answers on pages 273–293

Case 4.1: Answers

1. The IVU shows bilateral dilated ureters, which are medially displaced and taper gradually near the lumbosacral junction. The CT scan shows a hypodense soft-tissue mass in the midline of the retroperitoneum, which is encasing the aorta, with upstream dilatation of the ureters.

2. Idiopathic retroperitoneal fibrosis.

3. Primary retroperitoneal fibrosis is an autoimmune disease that is an immune response to ceroid – a byproduct of aortic plaque that leaks into the retroperitoneum. Malignancy with desmoplastic response (carcinoid, lymphoma, metastases), drugs (methysergide, ergotamine, hydralazine, methyldopa, paracetamol, amphetamines, LSD), fluid collection, aneurysm, radiation and polyarteritis nodosa are other causes of retroperitoneal fibrosis.

4. The characteristic location is the midline of the retroperitoneum around the aortic bifurcation. Proximally it can extend up to the renal hilum. It usually does not extend below the pelvic brim, but occasionally it extends behind the bladder and rectosigmoid. It is associated with other fibrosing conditions such as mediastinal fibrosis, orbital pseudotumour, Riedel's thyroiditis, sclerosing cholangitis and Peyronie's disease. It is seen in men aged 30–60. The IVU shows the classic triad with bilateral hydroureteronephrosis above the level of L4–5, marked medial deviation of the ureters in the middle third and gradual tapering of the ureter. Ultrasonography shows a hypoechoic periaortic mass. A CT scan shows a periaortic hypodense mass, which might show contrast enhancement in the acute stage. MRI shows low-to-medium signal intensity in T1 and T2, the signal depending on the amount of fibrous tissue. Uptake is seen in a gallium scan when there is active inflammation.

5. Differential diagnoses include retroperitoneal lymphadenopathy caused by lymphoma, TB or metastasis, and retroperitoneal sarcomas. Treatment of the causative factor, steroids and the obstruction with nephrostomy or ureteral stents is used in the management of retroperitoneal fibrosis.

Genitourinary Answers

Case 4.2: Answers

1. Coronal image of CT scan shows a massively distended urinary bladder, which is extending out of the pelvis up to the upper abdomen, displacing the bowel loops. Sagittal image shows contrast layering in the dependent portion of the grossly distended urinary bladder. Enlarged prostate is also noted.

2. Bladder outlet obstruction.

3. Causes of bladder outlet obstruction:

   Bladder-neck lesions: transitional cell carcinoma, lymphoma, papilloma, calculus

   Prostate: benign prostatic hyperplasia (BPH), prostatic carcinoma, prostatitis

   Urethra: stricture, calculi, tumour, trauma, TB, congenital, valves, meatal stenosis

   Extrinsic: pelvic lipomatosis, pelvic tumours.

   Bladder obstruction can also be classified as mechanical or neurological/functional obstruction. The most common cause is BPH.

4. Sudden onset of anuria could be a result of renal failure or obstruction. Ultrasonography is vital in differentiating these two. If there is no dilatation of the collecting system and no bladder distension, it implies lack of obstruction and the disease is likely to be prerenal or renal failure, and appropriate medical treatment would be initiated. If there is obstruction, ultrasonography can help to identify the level and cause of obstruction. On an IVU, the bladder trigone is elevated with the fishhook appearance of the lower ureters. The bladder wall is thickened and trabeculated with sacculations. Incomplete bladder emptying, vesicoureteric reflux (VUR), dilated collecting system and postobstructive atrophy of renal parenchyma are also noted.

5. Proximal obstructions can be relieved temporarily by percutaneous nephrostomy. Bladder outlet obstructions require immediate catheter drainage to relieve the obstruction. Definite treatment should be initiated as soon as possible.

Case 4.3: Answers

1. This is a voiding cystourethrogram. The child is catheterised with an 8 French feeding tube or an 5 Fr in a neonate. AP spot films of the bladder and abdomen are obtained. Contrast is introduced by drip infusion with the bottle held 40 cm above the table. The procedure is done under fluoroscopic screening. When the child indicates the urge to urinate or signs of voiding are seen, bilateral oblique views of the bladder are obtained including the catheter. When voiding begins, the catheter is removed. Two pictures of the urethra are obtained during voiding. Fluoroscopy of the renal area is done to observe reflux. After voiding is complete, AP spot views of the bladder and kidneys are carried out.

2. This patient shows reflux of contrast from the bladder into the left ureter and collecting system, which are mildly dilated, indicating a grade III vesicoureteric reflux.

3. **Primary vesicoureteric reflux** results from maldevelopment of the vesicoureteral junction with incompetence of the antireflux flap-valve action. Immaturity is caused by an underdeveloped longitudinal muscle of submucosal ureter. **Secondary** causes of reflux are ureterocele, ureteral duplication, bladder outlet obstruction and periureteral diverticulum. Reflux is seen in 30–50% of children with a urinary tract infection (UTI), and 20% of siblings. Complications of reflux are cystitis, pyelonephritis and renal scarring, hypertension and end-stage renal disease.

4. Vesicoureteric reflux can also be assessed with drect radionuclide cystogram (radioisotope introduced into bladder like conventional VCUG) or indirect radionuclide cystogram (intravenous injection of radioisotope and assessment once the isotope is excreted into bladder). MRI can also be used for this purpose. The international grading system for VUR:

   I: reflux to ureter but not to kidney

   II: reflux into ureter, pelvis and calyces, without dilatation

   III: reflux to calyces with mild dilatation and blunt fornices

   IV: reflux to calyces with moderate dilatation and obliteration of fornices

   V: gross dilatation, tortuous ureters.

5. Imaging protocol for recurrent infections:

Ultrasound – for identifying any structural abnormality that is causing recurrent infections. Ultrasound is poor modality for the diagnosis of acute pyelonephrotis.

Voiding cystoureterography (VCUG) or radionuclide cystography are imaging modalites used for assessment of reflux. All children with infection, < 4 years should undergo a VCUG. Even older children with abnormal ultrasound and repeated infections should get VCUG.

DMSA (^{99m} Tc-labelled dimercaptosuccinic acid) scan is done for diagnosis, assessment of parenchymal scarring in acute and chronic pyelonephritis and for monitoring response to treatment.

Case 4.4: Answers

1. The CT scan shows bilaterally enlarged kidneys the parenchyma of which has been replaced by multiple cysts of varying sizes. Cysts in the posterior aspect of the left kidney show calcified walls. In addition, there are multiple locules of gas seen within the cysts located anteriorly in the right kidney.

2. Autosomal dominant polycystic kidney disease (ADPKD). The presence of gas indicates that some of the cysts have become infected.

3. Adult polycystic kidney disease is an autosomal dominant condition (1/1000). Cysts arise from the nephrons and collecting tubules. Islands of normal parenchymal renal tissue are interspersed between the cysts. Haematuria is one of the presentations and can result from either calculi (in 10%) or associated renal cell carcinoma and warrants ultrasonography or CT. The *ADPKD* gene is located in the short arm of chromosome 16. This has a 100% penetrance and variable expressivity. It is associated with cysts in the liver, pancreas, spleen, lung, thyroid, ovaries, testes, uterus, seminal vesicles, epididymis and bladder. Other associations are berry aneurysms in the circle of Willis, aortic aneurysms, aortic regurgitation, bicuspid aortic valves, aortic coarctation, mitral regurgitation, colonic diverticulosis and mitral valve prolapse. ADPKD presents in the fourth or fifth decade, and in all patients by age 60. Presenting features are hypertension, renal failure, haematuria, proteinuria, pain and renal mass.

4. A plain X-ray can show calcifications or calculi and enlarged renal contours. IVU demonstrates enlarged kidneys with stretching and deformity of collecting system (spider leg deformity). Ultrasonography shows

bilaterally enlarged kidneys, with multiple cysts of varying sizes. The collecting system is distorted or compressed. A CT scan shows the cysts, which might be calcified. Normally they are hypodense. Hyperdense cysts indicate haemorrhage or infection. Swiss-cheese nephrogram refers to the appearance of multiple small cysts with smooth margins. The kidneys become smaller with the onset of renal failure. Associated renal cell carcinoma can be detected. On MRI, the cysts are hypointense in T1 and hyperintense in T2. Differential diagnoses of ADPKD: **multiple simple cysts** (no family history, not diffuse), **von Hippel–Lindau disease** (associated pancreatic cysts, haemangioblastomas, phaeochromocytoma), cysts of renal failure (kidneys small and non-functioning), **infantile PKD** (small cysts, hyperechoic on ultrasonography), **tuberous sclerosis**, **medullary cystic disease**, **multicystic dysplasia**.

5. Complications of cysts: infection, haemorrhage, rupture, calculi and renal cell carcinoma. Death could result from hypertensive disease, uraemia, cerebral haemorrhage caused by aneurysm rupture or hypertension, and cardiac complications. ADPKD is associated with cardiac valvular abnormalities (mitral valve prolapse), berry aneurysms and colonic diverticula. Cysts without complication are followed by ultrasonography to detect renal tumours and other complications. Screening with MRA is done for detecting aneurysms. If MRA is negative, it is repeated every 5 years. If positive, a conventional angiogram is done. If the aneurysm is > 6 mm, it needs endovascular treatment or surgical clipping. If it is < 6 mm, follow-up with angiogram is done after 2 years. Renal failure requires dialysis and transplantation. Patients should be informed of the 50–50 chance of their children being affected by this disease.

Case 4.5: Answers

1. The IVU shows a duplicated collecting system of both kidneys. There is dilation of the collecting system of the lower moiety of the left kidney, which is suggestive of obstruction or vesicoureteric reflux.

2. This is a complete duplex collecting system of the kidneys and ureters. The patient's symptoms result from ectopic ureteric insertion, below the level of the bladder sphincter.

3. Ureteral duplication can be complete or incomplete. Complete duplication is caused by a second ureteral bud arising from the mesonephric duct. Partial duplication is the result of early division of the ureteral bud.

Partial duplication: the ureter may be blind ending if there is no contact with the blastema. There might be a bifid ureter or bifid pelvis. The duplicated ureter enters the main ureter at a distinct angle and there is characteristic ureteroureteral/yo-yo reflux, with the urine moving between the upper and lower pole ureters as a result of peristalsis. It can be associated with pelviureteric junction (PUJ) obstruction of the lower pole.

Complete duplication: there are two ureters draining as per the Weigert–Meyer rule. The upper ureter can insert above or below the bladder sphincter. In males the insertion is always above the sphincter; they may present with urge incontinence or epididymo-orchitis. In females insertion can be below the level of the sphincter, into the urethra or vagina, vestibule, cervix, uterus, fallopian tube or rectum; they present with bedwetting or intermittent dribbling. It is more common in females and is bilateral in 15–40%.

4. The **Weigert–Meyer rule** applies to complete duplication of the ureter. The upper pole moiety inserts ectopically, medially and inferiorly in the lower pole ureter, below the level of trigone, into any of the wolffian duct derivatives. The lower pole ureter inserts orthotopically. An IVU shows a normal appearance of the lower pole. The upper pole can be seen normally or there might be poor visualisation. In this case the upper pole may be obstructed and can have a drooping lily sign (hydronephrotic upper pole causing downward displacement of the lower pole calyces), enlarged kidney, nubbin sign (scarring and decreased function of lower moiety mimicking a mass) and displacement of proximal urine upwards. Ultrasonography shows two separate renal sinuses and absent connection between the upper and lower pole collecting system. An MCUG can detect complications such as reflux in the lower moiety and ureterocele.

5. VUR (common in the lower pole as a result of a shortened ureteral tunnel), obstruction (upper, as a result of ectopic insertion/ureterocele or aberrant artery crossing), ectopic ureteral insertion, ectopic ureterocele (upper), renal dysplasia (upper) and infections (partial duplication) are the complications.

Case 4.6: Answers

1. On the plain X-ray of the abdomen, there is a dense calcific opacity in the left upper quadrant. On the IVU, the opacity is seen within the upper pole calyx of the kidney.

2. Renal calculus.

3. The stones can be composed of calcium, magnesium ammonium phosphate, cystine, uric acid, xanthine and matrix, or be drug induced. Causes of **calcium stones** are hyperparathyroidism, increased gut absorption of calcium, renal calcium leak, renal phosphate leak, hyperuricosuria, hyperoxaluria hypocitraturia and hypomagnesuria. **Struvite stones** are associated with chronic UTIs. **Uric acid stones** are caused by high purine diet and highly cellular malignancies particularly after chemotherapy. **Cystine** stones are seen in cystinuria. **Drugs that cause stones** include indinavir, guaifenesin, triamterene, silicate (overuse of antacids containing magnesium silicate) and sulfa drugs, including sulfasalazine, sulfadiazine, acetyl sulfamethoxazole, acetyl sulfasoxazole and acetyl sulfaguanidine.

4. Loin-to-groin pain caused by ureteric colic is the most common symptom. Flank tenderness and fever are present if there is superimposed infection. 80% of renal stones are radio-opaque. On the IVU, the stones are seen as filling defects in contrast-filled collecting system. They can cause proximal obstruction, with a dilated collecting system. The ureter distal to the calculus is usually small as a result of spasm inflammation/oedema, giving the false impression of a stricture. Stones are bright on ultrasonography, with acoustic shadowing behind them. Ultrasonography can differentiate stones from other filling defects such as clots and tumours. Unenhanced helical CT is increasingly used in the diagnosis of ureteric colic. It can be performed very fast without oral or intravenous contrast. It can demonstrate small calculi and determine other causes of abdominal pain. Obstruction can be detected. Secondary signs of stones are ureteric dilatation, unilateral renal enlargement, unilateral perinephric soft-tissue stranding and symmetrical dilatation of intrarenal collecting system. A rim of oedema around the stones helps differentiation from phleboliths.

5. Haematuria, infection, sepsis and obstruction are the complications. Hydration and analgesics are used in management of acute ureteric colic. 80% of stones which are less than 4 mm, pass spontaneously. Only 20% of stones larger than 8 mm pass spontaneously. Percutaneous nephrostomy is done for emergency relief of obstruction. Percutaneous nephrolithotomy is done through the nephrostomy tract in stones larger than 2.5 cm in diameter, hard or cystine stones, staghorn calculi, lower calyceal stones, stones associated with obstruction, or in cases of ESWL (extracorporeal shock wave lithotripsy) failure or contraindications. ESWL is used in stones that are smaller than 2.5 cm and lodged above the iliac crest. Anaesthesia or sedation is required. ESWL is contraindicated in pregnancy, untreatable bleeding disorders, patients weighing over 300 pounds, tightly impacted or cystine stones, or in cases of ureteral obstruction distal to the stone. Surgical removal of stone may be required for large staghorn calculus.

Case 4.7: Answers

1. Plain film shows small specks of calcification in the upper poles of kidneys on both sides, more on the right side. The IVU shows abnormal, deformed, cup shaped calyces, with contrast extravasation from the papillae in the upper pole. A thin rim of contrast is seen within the medulla of the lower pole of the right kidney (2nd picture), encircling a renal papilla. Lucent filling defects are noted within the upper pole calyx and in the upper ureter.

2. Acute renal papillary necrosis.

3. Renal papillary necrosis is ischaemic necrosis of the renal medulla secondary to interstitial nephritis or vascular obstruction. There are three stages:

   Necrosis *in situ*: the necrotic papilla detach but remain within the bed, unextruded (as noted in the lower pole of the kidney).

   Medullary type (partial papillary slough): single cavity in papilla with the long axis paralleling the long axis of the papilla and communicating with the calyx; it can be bilateral or unilateral.

   Papillary type: total papillary plough. Papillary necrosis presents with flank pain, dysuria, fever, chills, hypertension, proteinuria, pyuria, haematuria and leukoctyosis.

   The causes of renal papillary necrosis are analgesic nephropathy, diabetes mellitus, pyelonephritis, obstruction, sickle cell disease, TB, trauma, renal vein thrombosis, cirrhosis, coagulopathy, dehydration, haemophilia, acute transplant rejection, postpartum state and high-dose urography. Unilateral papillary necrosis indicates obstruction, renal vein thrombosis or acute bacterial nephritis.

4. Abdominal X-ray shows calcified necrotic papilla in the medulla. An IVU shows a normal or small kidney. Occasionally, the kidney is large as a result of obstruction or infection. The earliest sign is a subtle area of contrast extending from the fornix parallel to the long axis of the papilla. Other features are cavitation of the papilla, central or eccentric, widened fornix, club-shaped calyx, rind shadow of papilla, filling defect in calyx, pelvis or ureter (sloughed papilla), decreased density of contrast on the nephrogram and decreased parenchymal thickness. Ultrasonography can show multiple cystic spaces in the renal medulla.

5. Complications are higher incidence of transitional cell carcinoma and squamous cell carcinoma. Differential diagnoses: **hydronephrosis** (does not show necrotic papilla), **congenital megacalicosis** (normal renal function), **postobstructive renal atrophy** and **renal TB.**

Case 4.8: Answers

1. The X-ray shows bilateral, small, punctate calcifications in the distribution of the medulla of both kidneys. The kidneys are not enlarged. The IVU shows a striated nephrogram, with contrast radiating from the collecting system.

2. Nephrocalcinosis caused by medullary sponge kidney.

3. Nephrocalcinosis refers to deposition of calcium salts in the renal parenchyma. Causes of medullary nephrocalcinosis: hyperparathyroidism, renal tubular acidosis, medullary sponge kidney, papillary necrosis, nephrotoxic drug (amphotericin), chronic pyelonephritis, TB, schistosomiasis, hypervitaminosis D, milk alkali syndrome, hyperoxaluria, hypocalcaemia, hypercalcaemia, Bartter syndrome, drugs such as furosemide, ACTH, vitamins E and D, sarcoidosis and hyperuricosuria

    Causes of cortical nephrocalcinosis: chronic glomerulonephritis, renal cortical necrosis (pregnancy, shock, infection, toxins such as methoxyflurane, ethylene glycol), chronic rejection of renal transplant, AIDS nephropathy, chronic hypercalcaemia, oxalosis and Alport syndrome.

4. Hyperparathyroidism, renal tubular acidosis and medullary sponge kidney are the three most common causes of medullary nephrocalcinosis. Medullary sponge kidney is a developmental disease characterised by dysplastic dilatation of the renal collecting tubules, usually seen in young adults. It is asymptomatic and detected incidentally. Occasionally it can produce stones, infections and haematuria with stasis. It can be unilateral, bilateral or segmental. Renal failure is seen in 10%.

5. Medullary nephrocalcinosis is seen as bilateral stippled calcifications of medullary pyramids, which are hyperechoic on ultrasonography and hyperdense on CT. A plain X-ray shows triangular calcifications conforming to the shape of the medullary pyramids. Cortical nephrocalcinosis is seen as a rim-like calcification of the renal cortex. In medullary sponge kidney, the X-ray shows medullary nephrocalcinosis. An IVU shows a striated nephrogram in a

brush-like configuration as a result of contrast radiating to collecting ducts. This should be differentiated from papillary blush, which is an amorphous contrast enhancement and a normal variant. There are cystic tubular dilatations, 1–3 mm, too small for detection with ultrasonography and seen as hyperechoic lesions. It can be associated with hemihypertrophy, hypertrophic pyloric stenosis, Ehler–Danlos syndrome and horseshoe kidneys.

Case 4.9: Answers

Genitourinary Answers

1. The first CT scan of the abdomen shows a normal left kidney. The right kidney is enlarged and there is a large, heterogeneous mass arising from the lower pole, with areas of necrosis in it.

2. Renal cell carcinoma. The second CT scan obtained cranial to the first CT scan shows an expanded IVC, which is filled with tumoural thrombosis, extending from the renal carcinoma.

3. The size of the tumour, spread outside the kidney, involvement of Gerota's fascia and the adrenals, regional lymphadenopathy, extension into renal vein/IVC and liver/lung/bony metastasis are the important factors assessed in the scan.

4. Usually the CT scan is enough to confirm diagnosis and no further investigation such as biopsy is required. In small or indeterminate cases, ultrasonography or CT-guided biopsy is performed. CT scans of the abdomen and chest are done for staging the disease and identifying metastases. MRI is useful in assessing vascular extension into the renal vein, IVC and right atrium.

5. The classic presentation is haematuria, abdominal mass and pain, which are seen in less than 15% of cases. Renal carcinoma can, however, present with a myriad of symptoms, including fever, anaemia, polycythaemia, hypertension, hypercalcaemia, nephrotic syndrome, weight loss, fatigue, cachexia, night sweats, hepatic dysfunction, varicocele, particularly on the left side and polyneuromyopathy. Von Hippel–Lindau syndrome is associated with renal carcinoma. In this syndrome, the tumours are bilateral and multicentric, and occur at a younger age. Renal cell carcinoma originates from the proximal tubular epithelium.

6. Definitive treatment is radical nephrectomy, which can be done by a transperitoneal/retroperitoneal/thoracoabdominal/laparoscopic route. Resection of lymph nodes and thrombus is performed if present. Resection of localised/solitary metastasis gives good results.

Palliative treatments

– nephrectomy – for symptomatic relief

– chemotherapy – renal tumours are refractory; gemcitabine can be tried

– hormonal therapy – megesterol was used, but not much benefit

– immunotherapy – interferons, interleukin 2 (IL-2), lymphokine-activated killer cells, tumour-infiltrated leukocytes, BCG and stem cell transplantation are useful

– radiotherapy – for local symptoms, bone/brain metastasis

– radiofrequency ablation under ultrasonic or CT guidance is performed in small tumours confined to a kidney or tumours in a solitary kidney

– embolisation is useful to reduce vascularity of a large tumour before surgery, if the tumour is in a solitary kidney or as a palliative measure.

Case 4.10: Answers

1. This is a renal angiography of the left kidney. There are multiple small aneurysms in the small- and medium-sized renal arterial branches

2. Polyarteritis nodosa (PAN).

3. Polyarteritis nodosa is a fibrinoid necrotic inflammation of medium- and small-sized muscular arteries and vasculitis in arterioles, capillaries and venules. The organs involved are the kidney, heart, liver, spleen, pancreas, gastrointestional tract, central nervous system (CNS) and skin.

4. PAN is associated with hepatitis B and HIV. Characteristic laboratory finding is elevated pANCAs. Fever, malaise, pain, weight loss, elevated ESR, thrombocytopenia, anaemia and hepatitis B surface antigen positivity are also noted.

5. The characteristic radiological finding in PAN is the presence of multiple (> 10), small (1–5 mm), saccular aneurysms of small- and medium-sized arteries, typically at branching points, as a result of pan-necrosis of the internal elastic lamina. Fusiform aneurysms, stenosis, occlusions and irregularities are also seen. Differential diagnoses for this appearance are SLE, Churg–Strauss syndrome, rheumatoid vasculitis and drug abuse. As a result of vascular disease, kidneys are small and thinned with a lobulated contour.

6. **Chest**: cardiac failure, pleural and pericardial effusion, pulmonary oedema, infarcts. **Liver**: infarcts, gastrointestinal tract – bleeding, infarction, perforation. **Skeletal**: myalgia, ischaemia. **Skin**: purpura, nodules, neuropathy. Complications are hypertension, renal failure, haemorrhage caused by aneurysm rupture, infarction caused by thrombosis and gangrene. Treatment is with corticosteroids and cytotoxic agents.

Case 4.11: Answers

1. The X-ray of the abdomen shows a normal appearance of the bowel. The upper pole of the kidneys appears normal. The lower pole of the kidneys appears more medially placed and overlying the psoas muscles.

2. IVU shows fusion of the lower pole of the kidneys, across the spine, consistent with horseshoe kidney. The calyces of the kidneys are medially placed and the pelvis and ureters are lateral in position, which is a characteristic appearance.

3. Horseshoe kidney is seen in 1/400 children. Kidneys are formed by the union of ureteric buds from the mesonephric ducts, with nephrogenic cords at the level of S1 and S2. Subsequently, they ascend as a result of straightening of the caudal end of the embryo and differential growth of the pelvic structures. Horseshoe kidney occurs as a result of abnormal ventral flexion of the hind end of the embryo or variations in the growth of the pelvic structures, which brings the developing kidneys abnormally close together for a longer period, ending in fusion. The ascent of the fused kidney is limited at the level of the inferior mesenteric artery. Hence, the isthmus is trapped under it, and the horseshoe kidney always lies lower than normal.

4. The kidneys can fuse at the upper or lower pole (90%). The region of fusion is called an isthmus. The isthmus can be fibrous or normal renal tissue and is situated at L4–5 between the aorta and inferior mesenteric artery. Occasionally it might pass between the aorta and IVC or even posterior to these vessels. The long axis of the kidney is oriented medially and the pelvis and ureters are situated more anteriorly. The renal pelvis is usually malrotated and lies anteriorly or laterally, depending on the severity of fusion. There are multiple renal arteries arising from the aorta, including the isthmus artery, which might arise from the renal artery, aorta, or mesenteric or iliac arteries. Males are more commonly affected. IVU, ultrasonography, CT and MRI all detect horsehoe kidneys. Differential diagnosis includes crossed fused ectopia, where the fused kidneys are on the same side of the spine. In pancake kidney, the whole kidney is fused. Occasionally, in marked scoliosis, the axis of the kidneys is altered and it might mimic horseshoe kidney. Malrotated kidneys are another differential diagnosis.

5. Cardiovascular system (CVS), skeletal, CNS and anorectal malformations, hypospadias, undescended testis, bicornuate uterus, ureteral duplication, trisomy 18 and Turner syndrome are associated. Infections are common as a result of urine stasis and associated VUR. The PUJ obstruction is a common complication because of high insertion of the ureter. Recurrent calculi are seen as a result of obstruction or infection. Increased risk of trauma is present, because of the position just anterior to the spine. The morbidity mainly depends on associated infections and stones. Most of them are asymptomatic and there is no reduction in the life span.

Case 4.12: Answers

1. The first picture is MR angiography. The right kidney is normal and supplied by a right renal artery arising from the aorta. There is no kidney in the left renal fossa. The left kidney is located in the pelvis and is supplied by a branch from the left common iliac artery. CT scan shows the presence of left kidney deep inside the pelvis cavity.

2. This is an ectopic pelvic kidney. The appearances of an ectopic kidney are the same as the normal kidney, except that it is in an abnormal place. There might be non-rotation of the collecting system and hence the renal pelvis can be situated anteriorly.

3. Pelvic kidney is the most common type of renal ectopia. During development the ureteral bud separates from the wolffian duct around week 4 and ascends towards the urogenital ridge. The metanephric blastema develops above the ureteric bud by week 5. A period of rapid caudal growth in the embryo assists in migration of this structure out of the pelvis and into its eventual retroperitoneal location in the renal fossa. This migration and rotation are complete by week 8. In the pelvic kidney ascent is prevented, probably by the interior mesenteric artery. The pelvic kidney is supplied by aberrant arteries, depending on the level of arrest. Usually, it is supplied by branches from the aorta or iliac arteries.

4. An ectopic kidney is associated with a lot of other conditions such as renal agenesis, uterine abnormalities (unicornuate/bicornuate/aplastic uterus, duplicate/rudimentary vagina, undescended testis, hypospadias, duplicate urethra), adrenal cardiac and skeletal anomalies.

5. Hydronephrosis can occur as a result of alterations in the course of the ureter and there is increased risk of trauma, because of the pelvic location. Complications result from associated anomalies. VUR is also a feature.

Case 4.13: Answers

1. The first picture is MR angiography of the renal arteries. There is bilateral, high-grade narrowing of both renal arteries, involving their origins from the aorta and proximal 2 cm on each side. Atheromatous narrowing of the aorta is also noted.

2. Bilateral renal arterial stenosis (due to atherosclerosis).

3. Causes of renal arterial stenosis are: Atherosclerosis 60–90%, (ostia and prox 2 cm), fibromusclar dysplasia, dissection, thromboembolism, aneurysm, AV fistula, vasculitis, polyarteris nodosa, radiation, neurofibromatosis and retroperitoneal fibrosis. Due to stenosis, there is decreased flow which leads to decreased perfusion pressure of glomeruli, which produces renin in juxtaglomuerlar apparatus. Renin converts angiotensinogen to angiotensin I. which is converted by ACE (angiotensin converting enzyme) in vascular endothelium to angiotensin II, which releases aldosterone, which increases salt and water retention and vasoconstriction. Haemodynamically significant lesions are – elevated

renin >1.5:1, collateral vessels, > 70% stenosis, transtenotic pressure gradient > 40mmHg and decrease in renal size. Patients present with abdominal pain, flank pain, haematuria, hypertenion, oliguria/anuria and low urine sodium.

4. Screening is indicated for those with hypertension and bruit, accelerated/ malignant hypertension, severe hypertension < 25 or > 50 years, unilateral small kidney, diastolic pressure > 105 mmHg, sudden worsening, and refractory and impaired renal function after an ACE inhibitor. Investigations used for diagnosis are IVU, ultrasonography of the abdomen with Doppler, CT/MRA and captopril scintigraphy. The IVU shows delayed appearance of contrast with increased density and delayed washout, with notching of ureter as a result of the collaterals. Doppler ultrasonography may visualise the stenotic areas but it is technically challenging because of bowel gas, collaterals and multiple renal arteries. Peak systolic velocity in renal artery > 150 cm/s, ratio of peak renal artery velocity to peak aortic centre stream velocity > 3.5, poststenotic spectral broadening and absent flow during diastole. CT and MRA show good visualisation of renal arteries and preclude the need for conventional angiography unless intervention is contemplated.

5. Complications are renal failure, hypertension, cardiac failure and stroke. Antihypertensive therapy with ACE inhibitors or angiotensin II receptor antagonists is used for mild cases. Renal angioplasty is indicated for high-grade stenosis with stent placement. There is a high success rate for non-ostial lesions (80%). Surgical revascularisation is done if angioplasty fails. Poor results are seen in middle and old age group patients after revascularization.

Case 4.14: Answers

1. The CT scan shows a well-defined mass in the lateral aspect of the lower pole of the left kidney, which is very dark and shows attenuation values of fat. (Fat has a very low density, lower than soft tissue and fluids.) Few areas of enhancement are seen within this mass, due to blood vessels.

2. Renal angiomyolipoma.

3. Angiomyolipoma is a benign renal choristoma, which is composed of vascular, muscular and fatty elements. There is no true capsule.

Haemorrhage is common. Angiomyolipoma is associated with tuberous sclerosis in 20% and seen in 80% of patients with tuberous sclerosis. There is also an association with neurofibromatosis and von Hippel–Lindau syndrome. Isolated angiomyolipoma is solitary, unilateral, more on the right site, common in females and has no features of tuberous sclerosis. In angiomyolipoma associated with tuberous sclerosis, the tumour is equal in males and females, bilateral, multifocal and larger. Small angiomyolipomas are asymptomatic. Large ones present with haemorrhage and abdominal pain.

4. Angiomyolipomas are diagnosed by the characteristic presence of fat. Ultrasonography shows a well-defined, echogenic (bright) lesion, with increased vascularity. There is posterior sound transmission. A CT scan shows a mass with attenuation values of fat. High density is seen if there is haemorrhage. MRI shows a high signal in T1 and T2 and suppresses on STIR sequences. There is a chemical artefact at the junction of the tumour and renal tissue (chemical shift artefact is a common artefact in MRI – seen at the junction of fat and water). Angiography shows a tumour with a spoke-wheel pattern of vascularity. Usually the tumours are small and asymptomatic. Differential diagnoses for fat-containing tumour: lipoma, fat in renal cell carcinoma, liposarcoma, Wilms' tumour.

5. Complications are haematoma, haemoperitoneum and rupture. Wunderlich syndrome is haemorrhagic shock caused by massive bleeding into an angiomyolipoma or the retroperitoneum. Small lesions are followed up annually with ultrasonography. Larger lesions are followed up every 6 months. Larger tumours presenting with pain or bleeding are treated with emergency laparotomy with resection/nephrectomy or embolisation.

Case 4.15: Answers

1. This is a delayed film in IVU. There is no contrast in the right kidney. The left kidney is enlarged and there is massive dilatation of the left pelvicalyceal system and the ureter

2. Left hydroureteronephrosis caused by obstruction. Hydronephrosis is aseptic dilatation of the collecting system. Obstruction can be caused by intrinsic, intramural or extrinsic pathologies. The common cause of acute obstruction is passage of calculus/blood clot, instrumentation, inadvertent surgical suture, sulphonamides or pregnancy. Chronic obstruction is a

result of PUJ obstruction, tumours (ureteric and extrinsic), retroperitoneal fibrosis and pelvic mass, bladder outlet masses (BPH, prostate carcinoma), urethral polyps/neoplasms/strictures, posterior urethral valve and ureterocele.

3. In acute obstruction, the kidney is of normal size, with an increasingly dense nephrogram, delayed opacification of the collecting system, dilated collecting system and a ureter with blunting of the calyceal angle. Delayed films show the level of obstruction. In chronic obstruction, the kidney is large, with wasted parenchyma, poor density nephrogram, a thin band of dense contrast surrounding calyces, delayed opacification of the collecting system and a dilated collecting system. Ultrasonography shows separation of the renal sinuses and dilated collecting system. Hydronephrosis is graded into three types:

Grade 1 – mild separation of central sinuses, ovoid

Grade II – rounded separation of collecting system

Grade 3 – severe.

The amount of dilatation depends on the duration of obstruction, renal output and presence of decompression. Doppler ultrasonography shows a high resistive index of > 0.77, which helps in differentiation from false-positive cases. In the bladder the ureteral jet is not seen. Complications of hydronephrosis are pyonephrosis, contrast extravasation and papillary necrosis.

4. Differential diagnoses for dilated collecting system without obstruction: full bladder, overhydration, medications, diabetes inspidus, after an IVU, reflux, pregnancy, postobstructive, postinfective, postsurgical, megaureter, megacalycoses, extrarenal pelvis, parapelvic cysts and sinus vessels. Occasionally false-negative appearances are seen, in hyperacute obstruction, dehydration, spontaneous decompression or staghorn calculus filling the pelvis. Hydronephrosis is seen in 80% of pregnant women because of the effect of progesterone on smooth muscle relaxation and compression of the ureter at the pelvic brim by an enlarged uterus. This dilatation is physiological, common in the right side and seen up to the pelvic brim, and resolves within a few weeks after delivery.

5. Percutaneous nephrostomy is done to relieve obstruction. Under ultrasonic and fluoroscopic guidance a needle is advanced into a lower pole calyx and a drainage tube introduced.

Case 4.16: Answers

1. IVU shows normal excretion of right kidney. The left kidney is small, scarred and shows extensive dystrophic calcification, extending to the left ureter.

2. Renal tuberculous.

3. Renal TB is caused by *Mycobacterium tuberculosis.* The urogenital tract is the second most common site for TB involvement after the lungs. Infection spreads via a haematogenous route. During initial seeding, the *Mycobacterium tuberculosis* lodges in the periglomerular capillaries, with resulting immune reaction that produces caseating granulomas in the cortex. The organisms spill from the nephrons and are trapped in the narrow segment of the loop of Henle, which results in ulcerous lesions of the papilla that erode into the calyces. The collecting system is affected by contiguous spread from the renal parenchyma to the urothelium. Haematogenous spread directly to the collecting system is unusual. Clinically the salient features are sterile pyuria, dysuria, urgency, frequency, haematuria and a past history of TB.

4. The X-ray might show features of pulmonary TB (pulmonary findings are seen in < 50% of patients with renal TB). Renal TB is usually bilateral, but asymmetrical on X-rays and 75% of cases are unilateral. An X-ray is useful only in the later stages, when the kidney goes into the autonephrectomy phase where it is small, scarred and non-functioning with extensive dystrophic calcifications. Parenchymal calcifications are seen. The earliest change in IVU is an irregular feathery appearance of papilla as a result of erosion. Small cavities are subsequently seen from the calyx into the papilla. Strictures of the infundibula and pelvis are seen as dilated calyces. A phantom calyx indicates incomplete visualisation of calyx as a result of stenosis. Kinking of the renal pelvis and thick collecting system is another feature. The kidneys are scarred in the later stages and small, with distortion of the collecting system, although they are large in the early stages. Tuberculomas are seen that displace the collecting system. Ultrasonography and CT show cavities, granulomas, distorted collection system, scars, strictures and calcifications. Differential diagnoses are renal abscess, renal tumours, pyelonephritis and xanthogranulomatous pyelonephritis. The extensive calcification in a small kidney is, however, fairly specific for renal TB.

5. Complications are autonephrectomy with loss of renal function, extension to adjacent pararenal space and psoas, and extension to adjacent organs. Antituberculous therapy is used for treatment.

Case 4.17: Answers

1. The CT scan shows enlargement of both kidneys. There are multiple, large, wedge-shaped poorly perfused areas in both kidneys. There is no stone or hydronephrosis. No contrast is seen in collecting system. Scarring is seen in the upper pole of the left kidney.

2. Acute pyelonephritis, with upper pole scarring of left kidney from prior infection.

3. Acute pyelonephritis is inflammation of the upper urinary tract. It usually involves the pyelocalyceal lining and extends centrifugally along the medullary rays. Common organisms are *E. coli, Proteus* and *Klebsiella* spp. *Enterobacter* and *Pseudomonas* spp. are other organisms. It is more common in females. VUR is a predisposing factor. Stasis and obstruction are also predisposing factors.

4. Acute pyelonephritis presents with fever, chills, nausea, vomiting, flank pain and tenderness. Leukocytosis, pyuria, bacteriuria, microscopic hematuria, bacteremia and positive urine culture are also seen. Imaging can be done, but it is not sensitive or specific. Radiological features are:

IVU: normal in 75%. Kidneys can be enlarged/immediately dense nephrogram/non-visualised kidneys/mucosal striations/compressed collecting system/delayed opacification of collecting system

Ultrasonography: normal/enlarged kidney/oedematous and hypoechoic/ loss of central sinus complex/wedge-shaped hypoechoic areas, loss of corticomedullary differentiation/thick wall of renal pelvis

CT: enlarged kidneys/hypodense wedge-shaped areas from papilla to capsule, which enhance in delayed scans/striated nephrogram/loss of corticomedullary differentiation/effaced calyces.

MRI: wedge-shaped increased signal intensity in T2

Scintigraphy: focal areas of decreased uptake in DMSA scan. This is a sensitive and specific examination.

5. Complications of acute pyelonephritis are renal abscess, perinephric abscess, pyonephrosis and scarring with recurrent infections. Prompt treatment with antibiotics results in resolution without scars. Delayed treatment can result in chronic pyelonephritis with scarring, decreased renal function, hypertension and renal failure.

Case 4.18: Answers

1. The CT scan shows extensive thickening of the wall of the bladder. There is abnormal enhancement of the wall and a layer of oedema seen in between intensely enhancing layers of the bladder wall.

2. Acute cystitis.

3. Cystitis is infection of the bladder. Causes of cystitis are: infections – bacterial/non-bacterial (viral, TB, *Chlamydia* spp., schistosomiasis, fungal) – radiation, chemical, autoimmune, hypersensitivity, haemorrhagic and interstitial cystitis. The route of infection is usually ascending from urethra, but descending infection from kidney, particularly TB, haematogenous and lymphogenous routes are also possible. Clinical features are dysuria, urgency, frequency, suprapubic pain, haematuria, dyspareunia, abdominal cramps and incontinence. Acute haemorrhagic cystitis is an unusual and severe form of cystitis with haematuria and dilated urethra. Cyclophosphamide cystitis is seen following chemotherapy. Tumoral cystitis is focal and mimics a tumour. Eosinophilic cystitis is secondary to an allergic process. Emphysematous cystitis is seen in diabetics and immunocompromised individuals. It is caused by fermentation of urinary glucose to carbon dioxide, usually by *E. coli* species.

4. Diagnosis is established with urinary cultures. Severe cases require cystoscopy. Imaging does not play an important role in cystitis. It is used for confirming diagnosis and evaluating complications. Ultrasonography shows diffuse wall thickening and irregularity. Gas in the wall is seen in emphysematous cystitis. CT also demonstrates wall thickening and irregularity. Intense wall enhancement with oedema and layering is noted. Soft tissue stranding may be seen in the perivesical space in severe inflammation. Gas is seen in the lumen and wall, if there is infection with gas-forming organisms. Haemorrhagic cystitis shows high-density clots in the wall. In severe cystitis, necrosis of the bladder wall and perforation will be seen. Differential diagnoses include frequency-dysuria syndrome, interstitial cystitis and carcinoma in situ.

5. Antibiotics are used for treatment of cystitis, based on the urine culture and sensitivity. Complications are chronic/recurrent urinary infection, such as bladder haemorrhage, necrosis, pyelonephritis and acute renal failure.

5
ENDOCRINOLOGY AND HAEMATOLOGY
QUESTIONS

Case 5.1

A 28-year-old woman presents with a neck swelling and difficulty in swallowing. On clinical examination, there is a firm, non-tender swelling in the right side of the neck, that is mobile with deglutition.

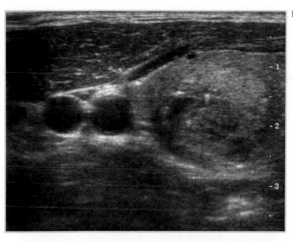

Fig 5.1a

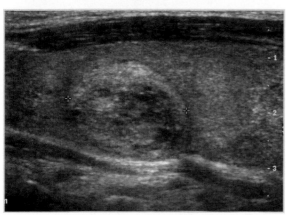

Fig 5.1b

1. What do you see on ultrasonography of the thyroid?
2. What is the diagnosis?
3. What are the causes of this appearance?
4. What are the radiological features?
5. What is the role of imaging and what is the management protocol?

Answers *on pages 315–333*

Case 5.2

A 34-year-old woman presents with severe headache, abdominal pain and palpitations. She is known to have hypertension that does not respond to medication.

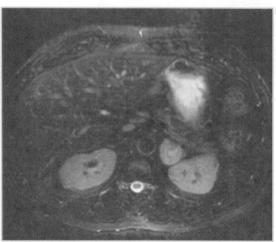
Fig 5.2a

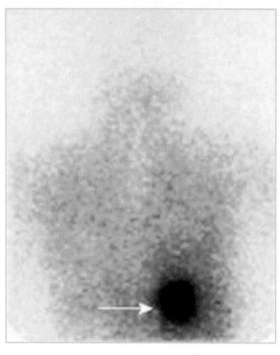
Fig 5.2b

1. What do you observe on the MR scan?
2. What is the investigation shown on the second picture?
3. What is the diagnosis? What are the common presentations of this condition?
4. What are the radiological features?
5. What is the radiological differential diagnosis? How will you manage this patient?

Answers *on pages 315–333*

Case 5.3

A 37-year-old woman presented with headache, weight gain and visual difficulties. Clinical examination showed bitemporal hemianopia with normal power and reflexes. MRI was done for diagnosis. There was a sudden deterioration in her consciousness level on the second day of admission and a second MRI was done.

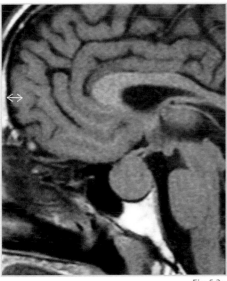

Fig 5.3a

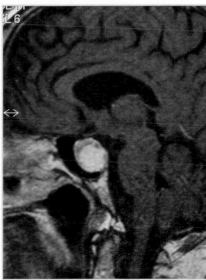

Fig 5.3b

1. What are the findings in this MRI?
2. What is the diagnosis? What complication do you see on the second MRI?
3. What are the types of this disease?
4. What are the radiological findings? What are the important factors to be obtained from MRI?
5. What are the complications and differential diagnosis?

Answers on pages 315–333

Case 5.4

A 31-year-old woman presents with neck pain, worse on swallowing, increased sweating and some loss of weight. Laboratory investigations were unremarkable.

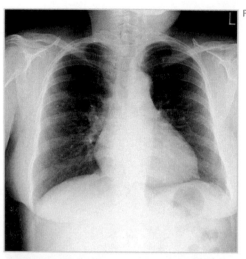

Fig 5.4a

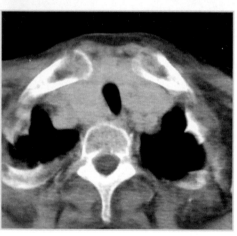

Fig 5.4b

1. What do you find on the X-ray and CT scan?
2. What is the diagnosis?
3. What are the types of this disease?
4. What is the role of imaging in this disorder?
5. What is the differential diagnosis?

Answers on pages 315–333

Case 5.5

A 5-year-old boy presents with headache, growth retardation and visual disturbances. On examination he has no focal neurological deficit, but has bitemporal hemianopia.

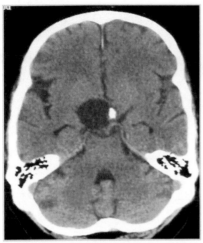

Fig 5.5a

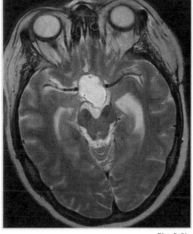

Fig 5.5b

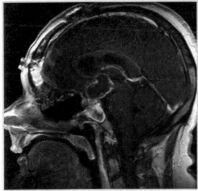

Fig 5.5c

1. What are the findings on the CT scan?
2. What do you observe on the MR scan?
3. What is the diagnosis? What is the differential diagnosis?
4. What are the clinical presentations?
5. What are the radiological features?

Answers *on pages 315–333*

Case 5.6

A 37-year-old man presents with bone pain, abdominal pain and constipation. Clinical examination shows diffuse, generalised bony tenderness.

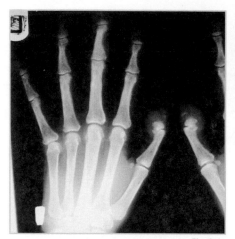
Fig 5.6a

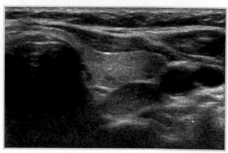
Fig 5.6b

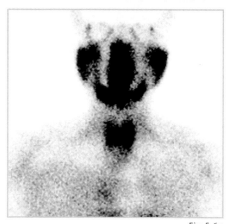
Fig 5.6c

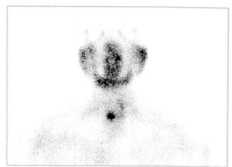
Fig 5.6d

1. What do you observe on the plain X-ray and ultrasonography?
2. What is the investigation in the third and fourth pictures? What is the diagnosis?
3. What are the causes of this condition?
4. What are the clinical features?
5. What are the other radiological features?

Answers on pages 315–333

Case 5.7

A 23-year-old woman presents with intermittent pain in her hands, grittiness in her eyes and excessive sweating. Clinical examination revealed midline neck swelling with prominent bruit, proptosis and swelling of the hand and leg. An X-ray of the hand was done as part of the clinical work-up.

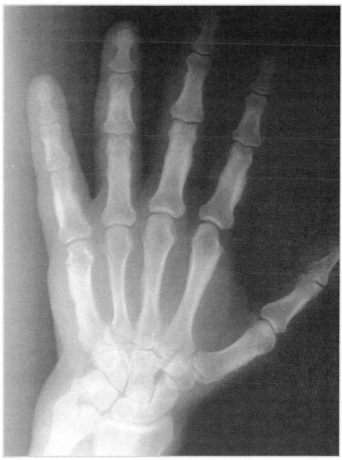

Fig 5.7

1. What are the findings on the X-ray of the hand?
2. What is the diagnosis?
3. What are the pathology and clinical features?
4. What are the radiological features?
5. What is the differential diagnosis?

Answers *on pages 315–333*

A 13-year-old girl presents with tetany, diffuse body pain and dental caries.

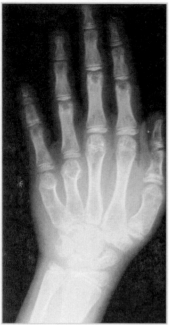

Fig 5.8a

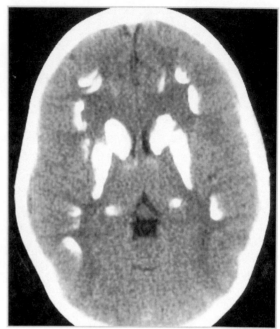

Fig 5.8b

1. What are the findings on the X-ray of the hand and the brain CT scan?
2. What is the diagnosis?
3. What is the pathophysiology?
4. What are the radiological features?
5. What is the differential diagnosis?

Answers on pages 315–333

Case 5.9

A 1-year-old boy presents with persistent abdominal pain. He was born after a difficult and prolonged labour and needed intensive care after birth. Clinical examination did not show any focal areas of rebound tenderness and vital signs were normal.

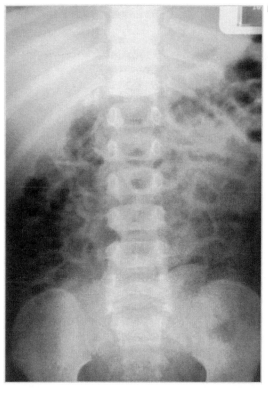

Fig 5.9a

1. What do you see on abdominal X-ray?
2. What is the diagnosis?
3. What are the causes of these findings?
4. What are the clinical and radiological features?
5. What is the differential diagnosis?
6. What is the management of this condition?

Endocrinology Questions

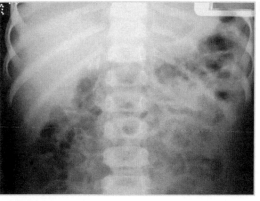

Fig 5.9b

Answers on pages 315–333

Case 5.10

A 67-year-old man presents with back pain and fatigue. He has a chronic medical condition. On examination, he has restriction of movements and tenderness in the spine.

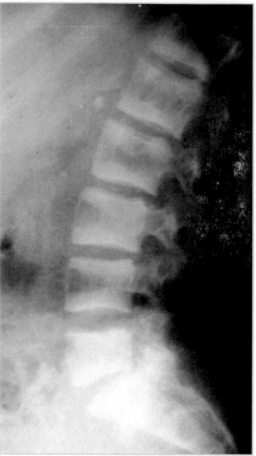

Fig 5.10

1. What do you find on the X-ray of the spine?
2. What is the diagnosis?
3. What is the pathophysiology of this disease and what are the components of the disease?
4. What are the radiological features?
5. What is the differential diagnosis?

Answers on pages 315–333

Case 5.11

A 14-year-old boy with a chronic medical history presents with abdominal and back pain. Clinical examination revealed tenderness in the left upper quadrant, without any palpable mass.

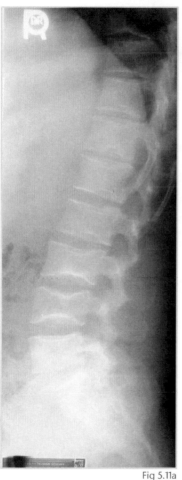

Fig 5.11a

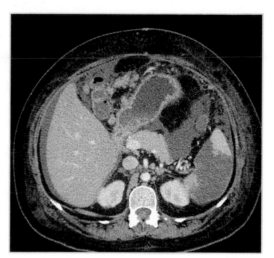

Fig 5.11b

1. What do you find on the X-ray and CT scan of the abdomen?
2. What is the diagnosis?
3. What are the causes of this disease?
4. What are the radiological features?
5. What are the other features of this disease?

Answers *on pages 315–333*

A 9-year-old boy presented with severe pain in her knees and hips. On examination the hip and knee joints are tender and there is limitation of movements.

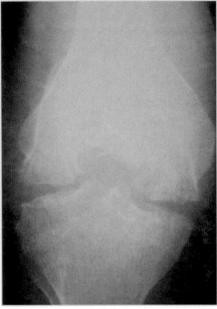

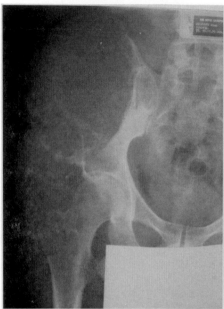

Fig 5.12a   Fig 5.12b

1. What do you observe on the plain X-rays of the right knee and pelvis?
2. What is the diagnosis?
3. What is the differential diagnosis for this radiological appearance?
4. What are the clinical and radiological features of this disease?
5. What are the differential diagnoses?

Answers on pages 315–333

Case 5.13

A 61-year-old woman presents with backache and headache. Clinical examination showed severe tenderness in the spine and other bones.

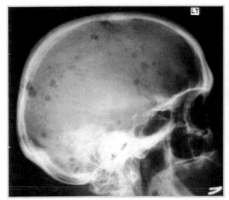

Fig 5.13a

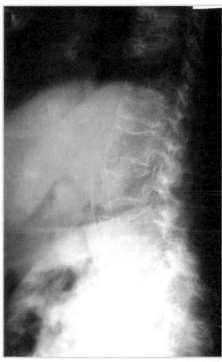

Fig 5.13b

1. What do you see on the X-rays of the skull and spine?
2. What is the diagnosis?
3. What is the origin of this lesion? What are the types of presentation?
4. What are the clinical and radiological features?
5. What is the differential diagnosis?

Answers *on pages 315–333*

Case 5.14

A 27-year-old man presents with abdominal pain and jaundice. Clinical examination shows an enlarged, non-tender liver. No other abdominal mass is palpated.

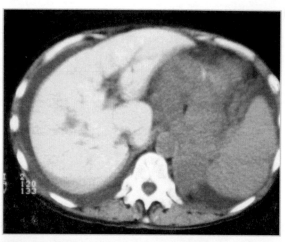

Fig 5.14a

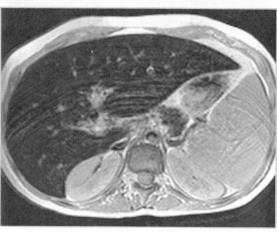

Fig 5.14b

1. What do you observe on the CT scan of abdomen? What does MRI show?
2. What is the diagnosis?
3. What other conditions produce a similar appearance on the CT scan?
4. What are the clinical and radiological features of this condition?
5. What are the complications and treatment of this condition?

Answers on pages 315–333

Case 5.15

A 6-year-old girl presented with failure to thrive, recurrent infections and headache.

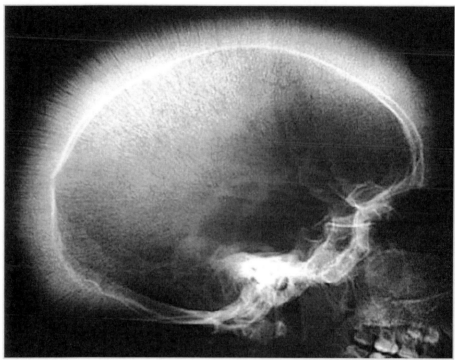

Fig 5.15

1. What do you observe on the plain X-ray?
2. What is the diagnosis?
3. What is the differential diagnosis for this radiological appearance?
4. What are the clinical features of this disease?
5. What are the radiological features?

Answers on pages 315–333

Case 5.16

A12-year-old boy presents with low backache, which is severe on bending. Clinical examination elicted point tenderness of the L3 vertebra. There is a restriction of spinal movement.

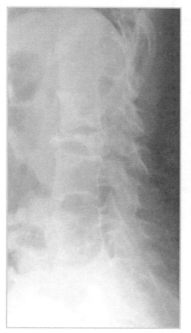

Fig 5.16a

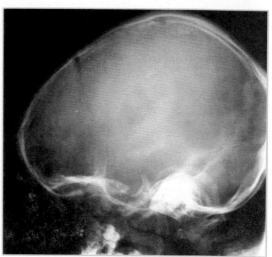

Fig 5.16b

1. What can you observe on the plain film of the spine and the X-ray of the skull?
2. What is the diagnosis?
3. What are the other causes for the radiological appearance of the spine?
4. What are the clinical and radiological features?
5. What is the management of this disease?

Answers on pages 315–333

Case 5.17

A 63-year-old woman presents with fatigue, weight loss, dyspnoea and chest pain.

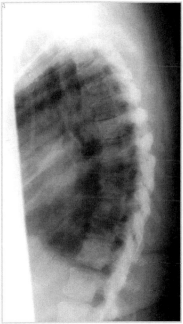

Fig 5.17a

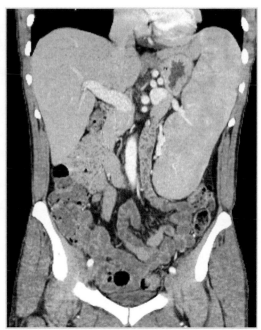

Fig 5.17b

1. What do you find on the X-ray and CT scan?
2. What is the diagnosis?
3. What is the pathology?
4. What are the associations?
5. What are the radiological features and differential diagnosis?

Answers *on pages 315–333*

Case 5.18

A 24-year-old man presents with swellings in the groin, abdominal pain and weight loss. Clinical examination revealed firm, rubbery lumps in the groin and axilla.

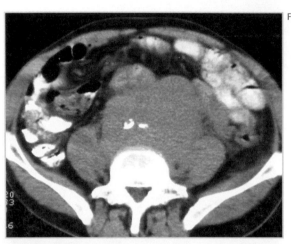

Fig 5.18a

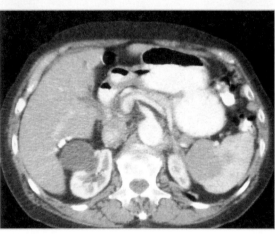

Fig 5.18b

1. What do you observe on the CT scan?
2. What is the diagnosis?
3. What are the types of disease?
4. What are the radiological features?
5. What is the differential diagnosis?

Answers on pages 315–333

Case 5.1: Answers

1. Ultrasonography shows a large nodule in the right lobe of the thyroid which has a heterogeneous echo pattern with tiny specks of calcification.

2. Thyroid nodule

3. Nodules in the thyroid are caused by adenomas (adenomatous nodule, follicular adenoma, ectopic parathyroid adenoma), inflammation, haematoma, abscess, carcinoma (papillary, follicular, medullar, anaplastic, lymphoma, metastasis). Nodules suggesting malignancy are in the following circumstances: < 20 years, > 70 years, male, dysphagia/ dysphonia, history of neck irradiation, clinically firm/hard/immobile and cervical lymphadenopathy.

4. In thyroid scintigraphy, a nodule can be hot, warm or cold, depending on the relativeuptake of the isotope. Hot nodules indicate autonomously functioning nodules (adenomatous hyperplasia or autonomous adenoma), warm nodules suggest normal thyroid function and cold nodules indicate hypofunctional or non functional thyroid tissue. Cold nodules are due to non functioning adenoma, cyst, thyroiditis, granuloma, abscess, carcinoma, metastasis or lymphoma. 5–8% of warm or cold nodules are malignant. Ultrasound is very sensitive in the diagnosis of nodules. Normal thyroid is homogeneously isoechoic to muscle tissue. Normal thyroid measures 2 cm in anteroposterior direction. Thyroid enlargement can be diffuse or there can be multiple, small nodules Thyroid nodules are usually hypoeehcoic, but they can be anechoic or hyperechoic.

5. Imaging cannot reliably differentiate benign and malignant nodules. A nuclear thyroid scan can detect only whether or not the nodule is functioning. To exclude malignancy, a fine-needle aspiration (FNA) biopsy should be performed under ultrasonic guidance. If the lesion is well defined and appears purely cystic, no further biopsy is required. FNA is indicated in the following situations: solid nodule with microcalcifications – if measuring > 1 cm; solid nodule with coarse calcifications > 1.5 cm; or mixed solid and cystic nodule or cystic with mural nodules > 2.0 cm. Other nodules can be followed up with regular ultrasonography, every 6 months. FNA of thyroid nodules can be used to categorise tissue into the following diagnostic categories: malignant, benign, thyroiditis, follicular neoplasm, suspicious or non-diagnostic.

Case 5.2: Answers

1. MRI shows a left adrenal mass of high signal intensity (anterior to the left kidney). There is no calcification or invasion of adjacent structures.

2. This is an MIBG (*meta*-iodobenzylguanine) scan, which is very sensitive for detection of phaeochromocytomas. It is taken up by chromaffin tissue.

3. Phaeochromocytoma. This is a vascular tumour of chromaffin tissue origin. It commonly arises from the adrenal medulla, and 10% are bilateral, extra-adrenal/seen in children/malignant. It can be seen in the organ of Zuckerkandl, carotid body or urinary bladder. Hypertension, cardiac arrhythmias, dilated cardiomyopathy, MI, pulmonary oedema and hypertensive crisis are complications. It is seen equally in men and women and is common between the third and fifth decades. Increased production and urinary excretion of urinary catecholamines are seen. It is associated with MEN-2a and -2b syndromes, von Hippel–Lindau syndrome, neurofibromatosis, tuberous sclerosis and Sturge–Weber syndrome. Headache, sweating, palpitations, tremor, nausea, weakness, anxiety, epigastric pain, flank pain, constipation and weight loss are the presenting features.

4. In phaeochromocytoma, there is an elevation of plasma metanephrine, urine metanephrine, catecholamines and vanillylmandelic acid. Ultrasonography and CT show a vascular adrenal mass, which enhances intensely with contrast administration. Extra-adrenal phaeochromocytoma can be seen anywhere from the skull base to the bladder, along the sympathetic chain. The common sites are the organ of Zuckerkandl (close to the inferior mesenteric artery origin), bladder wall, heart, mediastinum, carotid and glomus jugulare bodies. MRI is very sensitive in detection of adrenal and extra-adrenal tumours. The lesion is typically bright on T2-weighted images, more than any other adrenal tumour. An MIBG scan is useful in those cases that have positive lab findings, with normal CT/MRI. ¹¹¹In-labelled pentatreotide is also useful. A PET (positron emission tomography) scan is very sensitive. Venous sampling is seldom required nowadays because of the high sensitivity of CT, MRI, MIBG and PET.

5. Radiological differential diagnoses include other tumours of the adrenal such as adenomas, carcinomas and metastasis. Adenomas can be differentiated by CT and MRI. In MRI, fat-containing adenomas show loss of signal in oppose phased images. Contrast-enhanced CT

can also differentiate adrenal adenoma from metastasis. An adrenal tumour in the presence of elevated catecholamines is more likely to be a phaeochromocytoma than an adenoma. Surgical resection is required for the control of hypertension. The patient is prepared for surgery with α blockers followed by β blockers and volume expansion with isotonic sodium chloride, to reduce the effect of high circulating catecholamines during surgery.

Case 5.3: Answers

1. Sagittal view of MRI shows a homogeneous mass in the sellar region extending into the suprasellar region, which is elevating the optic chiasma.

2. Pituitary macroadenoma. In the second film, high signal is seen within the enlarged pituitary, indicating development of haemorrhage into the macroadenoma.

3. Pituitary adenoma is a benign tumour arising from the anterior lobe of the pituitary gland. It can be a macroadenoma, which is > 10 mm, or a microadenoma, which is < 10 mm. Pituitary adenomas are classified based on the hormones that they secrete. Prolactinoma, corticotrophic adenoma, somatotrophic adenoma, gonadotroph cell adenoma, thyrotroph cell adenoma, plurihormonal adenoma, non-functioning null cell adenoma and oncocytoma are the various types. Prolactinoma is the most common type and is large and presents with infertility, amenorrhoea, galactorrhoea, elevated prolactin levels, headache and impotence.

4. Macroadenomas are larger than 10 mm, seen in the sella and extends into the suprasellar region. CT/MRI shows a isodense/intense tumour, which enhances homogeneously on contrast. Microadenomas are small (<10 mm) and may be seen as a small dark lesion in the bright signal of the pituitary gland in MRI. After contrast, the normal pituitary gland enhances and the adenoma is seen as an area of low signal intensity. Subtle signs of small microadenoma are: height of the gland > 10 mm, convexity of the gland, depression of floor, erosion of sella, deviation of pituitary stalk and asymmetry of the gland. When there is haemorrhage in the tumour, high signal is seen in T1 and T2. Calcification may be seen, as an area of signal void. Important factors to be assessed in macroadenoma are – extension to the supraesllar region, parasellar region, compression of the optic chiasm, ventricles and carotid artery.

5. Necrosis, obstructive hydrocephalus, pituitary apoplexy and encasement of carotid artery are the complications. Differential diagnoses are meningioma, metastasis, aneurysm, craniopharyngioma, Rathke's cleft cyst, epidermoid and histiocytosis.

Case 5.4: Answers

1. The X-ray shows widening of the upper part of the superior mediastinum. The soft-tissue density in the mediastinum is seen in contiguity with the soft tissue of the neck, which is also enlarged. The CT scan shows a large thyroid gland, with multiple areas of high and low signal density, extending into the superior mediastinum, with side to side compression of the trachea.

2. Retrosternal goitre. A goitre is retrosternal if most of it is below the level of the thoracic inlet.

3. Goitre is enlargement of the thyroid gland. This may be diffuse or nodular and functionally toxic, non-toxic, or hypofunctioning. Most retrosternal goitres are an extension of the cervical goitre through the fascial planes into the mediastinum. In 1% a purely intrathoracic goitre can be seen. Retrosternal goitre is prone to compress adjacent structures such as the trachea, larynx, superior and inferior laryngeal nerves, oesophagus and SVC.

4. AP and lateral views of the neck confirm the presence of a mass in the thyroid region and potential extension to the mediastinum. Ultrasonography is useful for characterising the internal architecture of the gland and identifying nodules that may then be biopsied by fine needle aspiration or Truecut biopsy to exclude malignancy. Benign and malignant nodules cannot be differentiated on the basis of scintigraphy ultrasonography. CT and MRI of the neck and the superior mediastinum are used to assess the extension into the mediastinum and compression of adjacent structures. Most of the retrosternal goitres are seen in the anterior mediastinum, anterior to the subclavian and innominate arteries. In 10–15% the goitre can be seen posteriorly. Radionuclide thyroid scan is used to assess the activity and function of the nodule and for diagnosis of ectopic mediastinal thyroid.

5. Differential diagnosis for retrosternal goiters are other anterior mediastinal masses such as lymphoma, germ cell tumours, aneurysms and lymphadenopathy. Treatment depends on the functional status of the thyroid. Hyper or hypo functioning thyroid should be corrected medically. Surgical treatment is undertaken when medical treatment fails, when there are symptoms of tracheal compression and in proven malignancy.

Case 5.5: Answers

1. The axial view on a CT scan shows a cystic lesion with circumferential calcification in the sellar and suprasellar regions. The adjacent structures are normal.

2. An axial MR scan shows a cystic lesion with a high signal intensity in the suprasellar region. The sagittal view shows peripheral contrast enhancement. There is superior displacement of the optic chiasma.

3. Craniopharyngioma. A suprasellar mass in a child is considered a craniopharyngioma unless proven otherwise. Differential diagnoses of a cystic lesion in the suprasellar region include necrotic pituitary adenoma (no calcification), dermoid cyst (fatty component seen), epidermoid cyst (high signal in diffusion images, minimal enhancement), arachnoid cyst (angular margins, no solid component/enhancement), Rathke's cleft cyst (no solid component, calcification rare), cystic optic chiasmal hypothalamic glioma (solid with necrotic areas, calcification rare, enhancement seen) and thrombosed aneurysm.

4. Craniopharyngioma is a benign tumour that arises from squamous epithelial remnants along Rathke's duct/pouch. Pathologically the tumour has a cyst with a solid component. The cyst has fluid similar to motor oil, containing blood products, protein products and cholesterol. It is lined by stratified squamous epithelium. This is the most common tumour of the suprasellar cistern. It is commonly seen between 5 and 10 years of age. There is a second peak at 40–50 years. Most of them are a combined sellar and suprasellar mass. Clinical findings are variable. Growth retardation (compression of the hypothalamus), diabetes insipidus (pituitary compression), bitemporal hemianopsia (optic chiasma compression), headaches, nausea, vomiting, seizures, cranial nerve palsies (cavernous sinus involvement), growth delay, obesity and hydrocephalus are some of the clinical features. In children, growth delay is a common manifestation.

Endocrinology Answers

Diabetes insipidus is more commonly seen with eosinophilic granuloma of the stalk and precocious puberty is more common with a hypothalamic hamartoma.

5. CT and MRI are useful in the diagnosis. The three characteristic features are cyst, calcification and contrast enhancement. CT shows a hypodense cyst, with mural nodule. Calcification is seen in 90%. The solid component shows rim enhancement and there is no enhancement of the cystic component. The MRI signal is variable depending on the content of the cyst, which can be protein, blood or cholesterol. It can be hypointense in T1 and hyperintense in T2 or it can be hyperintense in T1 if the contents are proteinaceous or cholesterol. The solid component is isointense and enhances on contrast. A cystic component extends anteriorly or laterally and typically wraps around the solid component. MRI also demonstrates compression of adjacent structures. Hydrocephalus is seen as a result of compression of the foramen of Monro.

Case 5.6: Answers

1. The X-ray of the hand shows subperiosteal resorption of the lateral aspect of the proximal phalanges of the second to fourth digits. There is also resorption of the terminal phalanx of the fifth digit. Ultrasonography of the neck shows a hypoechoic mass behind the left lobe of the thyroid.

2. This is a technetium thallium subtraction imaging. Initially Thallium chloride is injected intravenously and images are recorded over neck for 15 minutes. Thallium concentrates in normal thyroid and enlarged parathyroid glands, proportional to regional blood flow and cellularity. Subsequently, ^{99m}Tc pertechnate is injected and images are acquired at 1 minute interval for 20 minutes. Pertechnate concentrates only in thyroid. The images of pertechnate scan are subtracted from the thallium scan, by the computer and if there is persistent uptake in the lower neck, it indicates the site of the parathyroid adenoma. In this patient, in the fourth image, there is increased focal uptake in the lower part of the neck, but no uptake is seen in the thyroid. This patient has parathyroid adenoma and hyperparathyroidism.

3. Primary hyperparathyroidism is caused by a parathyroid adenoma in 80–85%, hyperplasia in 10–15% and a carcinoma in 2–3%.

4. The clinical features are a result of increased bone resorption and hypercalcaemia. Stones, bone pain, arthralgias, muscular aches, peptic ulcer, pancreatitis, fatigue, depression are also seen. It is more common in women.

5. Technetium ^{99m} sestamibi can also be used for localising parathyroid adenomas. It localises in myocardium and mitochondria rich tumours proportional to regional blood flow and cellularity. It washouts of thyroid quickly, but retained in abnormal parathyroid glands. Ultrasound, CT scan and MRI are also useful in diagnosing small adenomas. In ultrasound, normal parathyroids are not usually seen, but parathyroid adenomas are seen as hypoechoic areas posterior to the thyroid gland. In 10%, parathyroid adenomas can be ectopic and situated in anterior mediastinum. CT scan is obtained from hyoid bone upto tracheal bifurcation, with contrast administration. Adenomas are seen as enhancing soft tissue masses. MRI also shows adenomas as contrast enhancing soft tissue masses. The most recent radipharmaceutial is ^{99m} Tc tetrofosmin, which is taken in parathyroid adenomas, like sestamibi. Surgical treatment includes removal of adenoma and preoperative biopsy of another normal parathyroid. If there is evidence of hyperplasia in the normal parathyroid, then removal of all parathyroids and autotransplantation is undertaken. Radiological interventions include ethanol ablation of the parathyroid adenoma.

Case 5.7: Answers

1. The X-ray of the left hand shows formation of lacy subperiosteal new bone in the ulnar aspect of the diaphysis of the metacarpal and proximal phalanx of the fifth digit.

2. Thyroid acropachy.

3. Thyroid acropachy is a rare condition occurring in 1% of patients with Graves' disease. It is common in females and can post-date thyrotoxicosis, ophthalmopathy and dermopathy; it can occur occasionally in euthyroid and hypothyroid patients.

4. The characteristic triad is finger clubbing (not toes), swelling of digits and periosteal reaction in long bones. The characteristic appearance is lacy subperiosteal new bone in the diaphyses of short tubular bones of the hands and feet and less commonly in the long bones of the forearms and legs. The new bone formation is shaggy, spiculated and perpendicular to the shaft. The most commonly involved bones are the metacarpals, and proximal and middle phalanges of the first, second and fifth digits. The periosteal reaction is asymptomatic, but may present with bone or joint pain. The clinical course is benign and resolution occurs after treatment of the thyroid disease. Serum thyroid-stimulating immunoglobulin is markedly elevated.

5. Differential diagnosis includes cause of **hypertrophic pulmonary osteoarthropathy**. This can be primary or secondary to pulmonary and cardiovascular disorders. A lamellar/single, regular/irregular periosteal reaction is seen in the diaphysis and metaphysis. Onion-skin periosteal reaction can be seen. **Pachydermoperiostitis** is a rare hereditary disorder, characterised by digital clubbing, pachydermia (thickening of the facial skin and/or scalp) and periostosis. Subperiosteal new bone formation is seen in the distal tibia, fibula, radius, ulna, metacarpals, phalanges and metatarsals. The periosteal reaction is shaggy, with irregular excrescences and diaphyseal expansion, starting at the epiphyseal region. Acro-osteolysis and ossification of the ligaments and interosseus membranes are seen. Cortical thickening and narrowing of the medullary cavity are seen. **Hypervitaminosis A, Caffey's disease, diaphyseal dysplasia** and **venous stasis** are the other causes.

Case 5.8: Answers

1. The X-ray of the hand shows short fourth and fifth metacarpals. The CT scan of the brain shows diffuse, dense calcification in the basal ganglia and in the cortex.

2. Pseudohypoparathyroidism.

3. Pseudohypoparathyroidism is a congenital, X-linked dominant, inherited disease that is characterised by renal and skeletal resistance to parathyroid hormone (PTH) as a result of end-organ resistance, anti-enzymes or defective hormone. It is often associated with hyperparthyoidism caused by hypocalcaemia. There is hypocalcaemia, hyperphosphataemia and normal serum levels of PTH.

4. The radiological features are short metacarpal/metatarsal bones in the first, fourth and fifth digits (the epiphysis of which appear the last), accelerated epiphyseal maturation, dwarfism, multiple exostosis, calcification of the dura mater/basal ganglia,/dentate nucleus and soft-tissue ossification/calcification. Metacarpal sign refers to shortening of the fourth and fifth metacarpals and is assessed by drawing a tangential line along the heads of the fourth and fifth metacarpals, which intersects the third metacarpal. In a normal individual the line passes over the head of the 3rd metacarpal.

5. Differential diagnoses of short metacarpals producing a short metacarpal sign are pseudohypoparathyroidism, pseudo-pseudohypoparathyroidism, multiple epiphyseal dysplasia, juvenile chronic arthritis, Turner syndrome, Klinefelter syndrome, hereditary multiple exostosis, idiopathic, basal cell naevus syndrome, sickle cell anaemia, Beckwith–Weidemann syndrome and melorheostosis. Differential diagnoses for basal ganglia calcification are idiopathic, hyperparathyroidism, pseudohypoparathyroidism, pseudo-pseudohypoparathyroidism, TORCH infection, tuberous sclerosis, Fahr syndrome, Cockayne syndrome and lipoid proteinosis.

Case 5.9: Answers

1. The plain X-ray shows bilateral, dense areas of calcification in the retroperitoneum, above the level of the renal shadows.

2. Bilateral adrenal calcification, following adrenal haemorrhage.

3. Adrenal haemorrhage is caused by physiological stress, trauma or hypercoagulopathy. It is more common in neonates. In neonates, the adrenal glands are large, well-vascularised organs; they are also prone to hypotension and/or asphyxia. Any condition leading to hypoxia may lead to shunting of blood flow to vital organs and damages the endothelial cells, making them more prone to haemorrhage. The complexity of the adrenal vasculature may make it disproportionately susceptible to massive intraglandular haemorrhage. In times of physiological stress or shock, endogenous adrenocorticotrophic hormone (ACTH) release increases blood inflow rates to critical organs severalfold. As many patients with adrenal haemorrhage also have coexisting renal vein thrombosis, one theory is that the eccentric musculature of the adrenal vein encourages turbulence and local stasis, which, in turn, contribute to adrenal vein thrombosis.

4. In neonates, adrerenal haemorrhage is usually preceded by a palpable mass. Other clinical features are jaundice, hypotension and anemia. Plain X-rays may show mass effect with anteromedial displacement of bowel loops and caudal displacement of kidneys. Calcifications are seen after resolution and can be seen as early as 1–2 weeks and are peripheral or egg shell shaped. Ultrasound shows hyperechoic lesion. CT scan shows adrenal enlargement with hyperdense haemorrhage. MRI can accurately characterise the stage. In acute stage, the haemorrhage is iso – low signal in T1 and low signal in T2. In subacute stage, there is initially a high signal rim, followed by complete high signal in T1. Fluid levels can be seen. High signal in T2 can be seen due to lysis and clots. Ultrasound- the adrenals are detected as large, hyperechoic masses.later they reduce and become cystic and eventually completely not visualized with resolution of haematoma.

5. Differential diagnoses for plain film appearances include hydronephrosis, multicystic dysplastic kidney, neuroblastoma and other retroperitoneal masses. There might be adjacent soft-tissue stranding. Bilateral adrenal calcification is seen in Wolman's disease, which is a lysososomal storage disease. In Waterhouse–Frederichen syndrome massive bilateral adrenal haemorrhage occurs in cases of meningococcal septicaemia.

6. If there is a suspicion of haemorrhage on ultrasonography, CT or MRI, the best course of action is to follow up with serial imaging, to exclude an underlying malignancy. Haemorrhage undergoes change in density, becomes cystic in 3–4 weeks and shows eventual resolution with or without residual calcification. Complications include adrenal insufficiency with volume loss and shock, adrenal pseudocysts and calcifications. Unilateral haemorrhage is rarely significant. It is more common on the right side. An abscess is a complication of a haemorrhage. Underlying malignancy has to be excluded. Deaths result from massive blood loss in neonates and adrenal insufficiency in adults.

Case 5.10: Answers

1. The X-ray of the spine shows abnormal vertebrae, which have normal density in the middle, but increased density at the upper and lower aspects of the vertebrae giving them a 'rugger jersey' appearance.

2. Renal osteodystrophy.

3. Renal osteodystrophy is a skeletal manifestation of chronic renal failure. Renal insufficiency causes decreased conversion of 25-hydroxy 1, 25 hydroxy vitamin D to active vitamin D, resulting in vitamin D deficiency, which causes reduced intestinal calcium absorption. Low calcium levels lead to osteomalacia (calcium phosphate product remains normal as a result of hyperphosphatasia). Another mechanism is phosphate retention caused by renal insufficiency. Maintained calcium × phosphate product lowers serum calcium, which increases PTH production; this is associated with vitamin D resistance and leads to an increase in calcium × phosphate product with soft-tissue calcification. The combination of the above two mechanisms also produces increased serum phosphate, which inhibits vitamin D activation via feedback regulation. The pathological features are osteopenia, rickets, secondary hyperparathyroidism, osteosclerosis and soft-tissue calcifications.

4. Rugger jersey spine is produced as a result of osteosclerosis. This might be the sole manifestation of renal osteodystrophy. It commonly affects the dorsolumbar spine. Other bones such as pelvic bones, ribs, long bones, facial bones and skull bones may be affected. The appearance might increase or regress after renal transplantation.

5. Differential diagnoses of osteosclerosis are diffuse metastasis, Paget's disease, myelofibrosis, fluorosis, osteopetrosis, mastocytosis, melorheostosis, hypothyroidism, phosphorous poisoning, hypervitaminosis D, sickle cell disease, tuberous sclerosis and pyknodysostosis.

Case 5.11: Answers

1. Lateral X-ray of the spine demonstrates demineralization of vertebral bodies and thinning and central compression, causing biconcave H-shaped vertebrae. Multiple H-shaped lumbar and lower dorsal vertebra. CT scan of the upper abdomen shows a large, wedge shaped, hypodense, unperfused area in the spleen. There is trace free fluid in the peritoneal cavity.

2. Sickle cell anaemia with splenic infarct and biconcave deformity of vertebral bodies caused by the pressure of nucleus pulposus on softer vertebral bodies.

3. Sickle cell disease is a haemolytic anaemia, characterised by abnormally shaped, sickled, red blood cells, which are removed from the circulation

and destroyed, leading to anaemia. The term 'sickle cell disease' applies to all patients with at least one HbS chain and one other abnormal β-globin chain. The term 'sickle cell anaemia' is used when the patient has homozygous HbSS. Sickle cell trait is heterozygous HbSA, with one normal haemoglobin, and is benign. The abnormal shape of the cells impairs the ability to pass through small vascular channels, resulting in sludging and congestion of vascular beds. This results in infarct throughout the body. Acute pain crisis is the result of bone marrow infarction.

4. Sickle cell disease is characterised by infarcts in different parts of the body. In the skeleton, the skull is expanded with hair on end appearance. One of the common appearances of sickle cell patients is an H-shaped vetebra, which is due to infarction of the endplates in the vertebra. This is a central square shaped endplate depression due to microvascular end plate occlusion and subsequent overgrowth of surrounding portions of endplate. This is pathognomonic of sickle and is called Lincoln log of H shaped vertebra. Other bone manifestations are infarcts in long bones and aseptic necrosis of heads of humerus and femurs. Osteomyelitis (salmonella infection common), is usually superimposed on areas of infractions. Medullary infarcts show typical calcification. In hands and feet, expansion of medulla and thinning of cortex produces typical appearance of sickle cell dactylitis.

5. **Spleen**: infarction, leading to autosplenectomy; calcified, small, dense spleen; sequestration syndrome. By 5 years, 94% are asplenic, making them prone to infection with capsulated bacteria.

Kidneys: renomegaly, glomerulosclerosis, nephritic syndrome, renal failure.

Brain: stroke, atrophy, cognitive impairment

Lungs: pneumonia, acute lung syndrome, pulmonary fibrosis. Respiratory complications leading to death.

Miscellaneous: hepatitis, infarction, gallstones, iron overload, cardiac infarction, priapism, retinal artery occlusion, skull infarction, subperiosteal haematoma, sensorineural hearing loss. Treatment consists of transfusion and specific therapy of the complication.

Case 5.12: Answers

1. The X-ray of the right knee shows expansion of the epiphysis and metaphysis, with coarse trabeculations and widening of the intercondylar notch. The X-ray of the pelvis shows a large, expansile, lucent lesion in the right iliac bone, with no periosteal reaction or fracture.

2. Haemophilic right knee and joint haemophilic pseudotumour involving the right innominate bone.

3. Haemophilia is an X-linked disorder with deficiency in coagulation factor VIII. Haemophilic arthropathy is caused by repeated bleeding into joints, which results in a reactive pannus formation that erodes bone. It is seen in the first and second decades.

4. Haemophilic arthropathy is common in knee joints. Ankle, elbow and shoulder joints are also affected. The changes are bilateral. There is haemarthrosis, enlarged epiphysis (synovial hyperaemia), juxta-articular osteoporosis and widening of the intercondylar notch. Erosions, joint space narrowing, subchondral cysts and osteophytes are seen. In the knee, bulbous femoral condyles, widening of the intercondylar notch, flattening of the condylar surfaces, genu valgum, slanted tibial plateaus, squared patella and contracted hamstrings are noted. MRI shows hypertrophied synovium, haemorrhage and erosions. Haemophilic pseudotumour is seen in the hip. It is a haemorrhagic cystic swelling in bone or muscle, and produces multiloculated, expansile lesions in flat bones, with bony destruction and soft-tissue extension and pathological fracture. MRI shows haemorrhage in varying stages. CT shows mass with high density and destruction. Bleeding in urinary tract and retroperitoneum can cause obstructive uropathy. IVU can show papillary necrosis. Submucosal bleeding in GIT causes thumbprinting in barium enema.

5. Widening of the intercondylar notch is also caused by haemophilia B (Factor IX deficiency) juvenile rheumatoid arthritis (JRA), haemophilia, gout, TB, synovial osteochondromatosis and synovial haemangioma. The combination of intercondylar notch widening and widened epiphysis is seen only in haemophilia and JRA. Expansile lesions such as the pseudotumour can also be caused by giant cell tumours, aneurysmal bone cysts, plasmacytomas, hydatid cysts and brown tumours of hyperparathyroidism.

Endocrinology Answers

Case 5.13: Answers

1. The X-ray shows multiple, punched-out, lytic lesions of varying sizes in the skull. The spine has low density (osteopenia) with mild wedge compression fractures of multiple vertebrae.

2. Multiple myeloma.

3. Multiple myeloma is the most common primary malignant neoplasm of bone in adults, which is characterised by monoclonal proliferation of myeloma cells. It is seen in the fifth to eighth decades and is common in men. Myeloma can be disseminated or focal (< 2%). The disseminated form can be seen anywhere in the axial skeleton – anywhere where is there red marrow – although it is more common in the vertebrae, ribs and skull. Solitary plasmacytoma is seen in the vertebrae, pelvis, skull, sternum and ribs.

4. Clinical features are bone pain, renal insufficiency, proteinuria, hypercalcemia, Bences jones proteinuria, normochronic normocytic anaemia and increased globulin production. Radiological features are diffuse low density of bones with coarse trabecular pattern (15%). Punched out lesions with endosteal scalloping and uniform size is a pathognomonic finding. Expansile osteolytic lesions, soft tissue mass adjacent to bone lesion and involvement of mandible are other features. Nephrocalcinosis may be seen due to hypercalcemia. Spine lesions – interspersed on background of osteopenia, soft tissue mass, doesn't involve pedicles first (metasis involves pedicles first). Sclerosis – may be seen after chemo or radiotherapy, and may the main presentation (3%). Can be locally sclerotic or diffusely sclerotic. Often a skeletal survey is done to identify myelomatous foci in bones. On bone scintigraphy, the lesions do not show increased uptake, except in sclerotic myeloma and in healing fracture in myeloma which responded to treatment. MRI can be done to scan all the bones of the axial and appendicular skeleton for myelomatous involvement in the bone marrow. MRI is also used to evaluate cord compression. POEMS syndrome – polyneuropathy, organomegaly, endocrine anomalies, myeloma and skin changes may be ecountered. 10% develop amyloidosis of GIT, kidneys and joints.

5. Differential diagnosis:

    Diffuse osteopenic form: postmenopausal osteoporosis and (it is difficult to exclude myeloma in a patient with diffuse osteoporosis), hyperparathyroidism, particularly with compression fracture of vertebrae

Lytic lesions: metastasis (not punched out, spares mandible), amyloidosis, myeloid metaplasia

Expansile lytic lesion similar to solitary plasmacytoma: renal cell carcinoma metastasis, giant cell tumour, hydatid cyst

Sclerotic lesion: lymphoma, osteopoikilosis, mastocytosis, myelosclerosis, osteoblastic metastasis, renal osteodystrophy

Spinal tumour: metastasis (involves posterior elements, large paraspinal mass).

Case 5.14: Answers

1. This is a non-contrast CT scan of the abdomen. (Note the lack of contrast in aorta and blood vessels.) The liver is very bright and spleen is of normal density. In MRI, the liver appears very dark. Pancreas is also dark.

2. Haemochromatosis. This is excess iron deposition in various parenchymal organs, particularly in the liver, pancreas and the heart.

3. High density in the liver is seen in CT as a result of deposition of iron (haemochromatosis, haemosiderosis), copper (Wilson's disease), iodine (amiodarone toxicity), gold (gold therapy for rheumatoid arthritis), thorotrast, thallium and glycogen storage disease.

4. Primary haemochromatosis is caused by excessive absorption and retention of dietary iron, which accumulates in parenchymal cells of the liver, pancreas, heart and pituitary gland. It is an autosomal recessive disorder. The excess iron is bound to transferrin and stored in periportal hepatocytes. The reticuloendothelial cells are not affected (unlike haemosiderosis). Clinical features are hyperpigmentation, hepatomegaly, arthralgia, diabetes mellitus, cardiac failure and infertility. Diagnosis can be confirmed by liver biopsy. High density is seen on a liver CT scan. MRI shows a diffusely low signal in T2-weighted images as a result of the presence of iron. The spleen signal is normal, because there is no accumulation here. The pancreas may show low signal intensity when it is affected. Secondary haemochromatosis (haemosiderosis) is increased iron deposition without organ damage and is seen in transfusional iron overload, excessive dietary iron (Bantu siderosis) or erythroid hyperplasia (thalassaemia). The iron is deposited in reticuloendothelial cells, with sparing of parenchymal cells. In MRI, there is signal loss in liver, but less

than for the primary form and the signal is more than background noise. The signal is low in spleen and bone marrow, but normal in the pancreas, because it does not have reticuloendothelial cells.

5. Complications are cirrhosis, hepatocellular carcinoma (15–30%), type 1 diabetes mellitus and congestive cardiomyopathy. Treatment is with phlebotomies before for reduction of iron load in the body at the rate of one or two times a week for up to 1–4 years, before development of cirrhosis. Normal life expectancy is seen with early diagnosis and treatment.

Case 5.15: Answers

1. The X-ray of the skull shows dense bone with expansion of diploic space with hair-on-end appearance

2. Thalassaemia.

3. Differential diagnoses for hair-on-end appearance: thalassaemia, sickle cell disease, hereditary spherocytosis, glucose-6-phosphate dehydrogenase deficiency, iron deficiency anaemia, haemangioma, neuroblastoma and osteosarcoma.

4. Thalassaemia major is an inherited disorder of haemoglobin synthesis. Normal adult haemoglobin has two α and two β chains. In α-thalassaemia there is a deficiency of α chains and in β-thalassaemia of β chains. Thalassaemia major is the severe form and it is homozygous. Clinical presentation is retarded growth, retarded secondary sexual characters, pigmented skin, high bilirubin, high uric acid, hypochromic/microcytic anaemia, thrombocytopenia and leukopenia.

5. The following are the radiological features of thalassaemia.

   Skull: the diploic spaces are widened with thinned cortex, coarse trabeculations, hair-on-end appearance in frontal bones, frontal bossing, opacified maxillary sinuses caused by marrow hyperplasia, narrow nasal cavity

   Appendicular skeleton: expansion of marrow, cortical thinning, osteopenia and premature epiphyseal fusion; bone lesions are less with systemic blood transfusion (secondary haemosiderosis is a complication); pathological fracture may be encountered

Chest: cardiomegaly, posterior mediastinal mass as a result of extramedullary haematopoiesis

Ribs: widening of ribs, rib-within-rib appearance

Abdomen: hepatosplenomegaly, gallstones.

Case 5.16: Answers

1. The lateral view of the lumbar spine shows complete flattening of L3 vertebral body (vertebral plana) with preservation of the adjacent disc spaces. X-ray of the skull shows a well-defined, geographical, lucent defect in the parietal bone, close to the vertex.

2. Eosinophilic granuloma.

3. The causes of vertebra plana are eosinophilic granuloma, neuroblastoma metastases, Ewing's sarcoma, aneurysmal bone cyst, leukaemia, lymphoma, infection and trauma. Causes of multilevel platyspondyly are osteogenesis imperfecta, Morquio syndrome, Cushing syndrome, lymphoma, leukaemia, Gaucher's disease and metastasis.

4. Eosinophilic granuloma is characterised by expanding erosive accumulations of histiocytes, usually within the medullary cavity. It can be a single or multiple skeletal lesions, and it predominantly affects children, adolescents and young adults. Solitary lesions are more common. Any bone can be involved, but the most common sites include the skull, mandible, spine, ribs and long bones. In the skull, it produces a well-defined, geographical, lytic lesion. In the spine, it is most commonly seen at at the thoracic level and it may present with progressive bone pain. The highest frequency is seen at between 5 and 10 years of age. Scoliosis can be seen, and pathological fracture can occur. Eosinophilic granuloma can produce expansile lytic lesions of the vertebral bodies and the posterior vertebral elements. A paraspinal soft-tissue mass may occasionally occur. Involvement of the second cervical vertebra is an extremely rare occurrence, but it may cause atlantoaxial instability. MRI shows low signal intensity in T1 and high intensity in T2, and can show extradural soft-tissue space exquisitely. Contrast enhancement may be seen. Bone scan appearance is variable. It can be hot, cold or cold with ring of reparative activity. If diagnosis is uncertain, biopsy is required.

5. The bone lesion is usually self-limiting and at least 50% reconstitution of vertebral height may be expected. Lesions with no neurological deficit or mild non-myelopathic signs are followed up or treated with bracing, which prevents progressive kyphosis. Chemotherapy is used for the systemic form of the disease. Surgical decompression is done in severe lesions. Low-dose radiotherapy is used if surgery is not possible.

Case 5.17: Answers

1. The X-ray of the spine shows dense vertebral bodies. The CT scan of the abdomen shows a massively enlarged spleen on the left side.

2. Myelofibrosis.

3. Myelofibrosis is a haematological disorder, where the bone marrow elements are replaced by fibrous tissue, which is associated with extramedullary haematopoiesis, splenomegaly, anaemia and changes in platelets, and polycythaemia.

4. It is associated with metastatic carcinoma, chronic infection, poisoning, acute myeloid leukaemia, polycythaemia, McCune–Albright syndrome and histiocytosis. The characteristic locations are red marrow-containing bones such as in the spine, pelvis, femora, humeral shafts, skull and peripheral bones.

5. The radiological features are generalised increased density in all bones, spine and skull, small lucent lesions and obliterated diploic space. Other findings are splenomegaly, rugger jersey spine and jail bar ribs. MRI shows hypointense marrow in T1-weighted image as a result of fibrosis. Normal bone marrow is bright because of fat. Differential diagnoses for **dense bones with splenomegaly** are chronic leukaemia, lymphoma and mastocytosis. Differential diagnoses for **dense bones without splenomegaly** are osteoblastic metastases, fluorosis, osteopetrosis and chronic renal disease.

Case 5.18: Answers

1. The CT scan shows a large, hypodense mass in the retroperitoneum at the level of pelvic brim, which is encasing the calcified iliac arteries. In the second picture at a higher level, there is splenomegaly with a lobular, hypodense mass adjacent to the hilum.

2. Lymphoma.

3. Lymphoma is divided into Hodgkin's and non-Hodgkin's types. There are four types of Hodgkin's lymphoma: lymphocyte predominant, lymphocyte depleted, mixed and nodular sclerosing. Non-Hodgkin's lymphoma is classified as low, intermediate and high grade, based on the Working group classification. Retroperitoneal nodes are involved in 20–30% of Hodgkin's lymphoma and 50–55% of non-Hodgkin's lymphoma patients.

4. In the abdomen lymphoma usually affects the paraaortic and paracaval lymph nodes. Abdominal lymph nodes are considered enlarged when they measure > 10 mm in the short axis. The lymph nodes are homogeneously hypodense and can show contrast enhancement. Necrosis and calcification can be seen after treatment. Occasionally lymphoma presents as a conglomerate, lobulated mass, encircling the aorta and causing anterior displacement. The spleen is considered to be enlarged when it measures > 13 cm in the craniocaudal dimension. Focal lesions can be seen in the liver, spleen and kidney. When a diagnosis of lymphoma is suspected, a CT scan of the chest, abdomen and pelvis is performed for staging the disease. Staging of Hodgkin's lymphoma depends on the lymph node groups involved and whether nodes on either side of diaphragm are involved.

5. Differential diagnoses for diffuse lymphadenopathy in the abdomen are metastasis, TB (more extensive areas of necrosis), HIV and granulomatous disease. Other causes of retroperitoneal masses are sarcomas, lymphangiomas and extension of tumours from adjacent organs.

6
NEURORADIOLOGY
QUESTIONS

Case 6.1

A 34-year-old woman presents at hospital with sudden onset of severe headache.

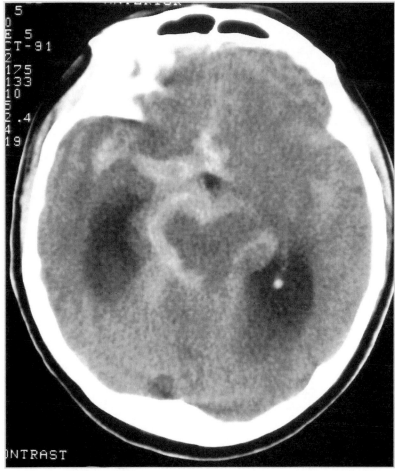

Fig 6.1

1. What does the CT scan show?
2. What is the diagnosis and what are the common complications of this condition?
3. Are further radiological investigations required with this CT appearance?
4. What is the classic presentation of this condition?
5. What conditions are associated with this abnormality?
6. How is this condition managed and what is the role of radiology?

Answers *on pages 367–398*

Case 6.2

A 4-year-old girl presented with nystagmus, syncopal episodes and weakness of the upper limbs. On examination, there was decreased power in the upper extremities. Reflexes were exaggerated.

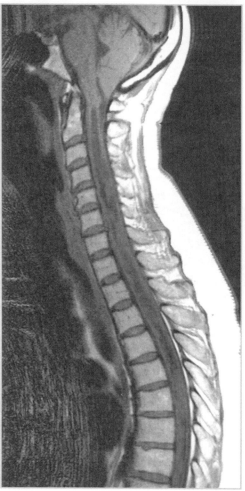

Fig 6.2

1. What are the findings on MRI?
2. What is the diagnosis?
3. What are the types of the disease?
4. What are the radiological features?
5. What are the clinical features and associations of this condition?

Answers on pages 367–398

Case 6.3

A 7-year-old girl with developmental delay presents with sudden-onset diffuse headache and seizures. An urgent CT scan of the head was done before and after intravenous contrast administration.

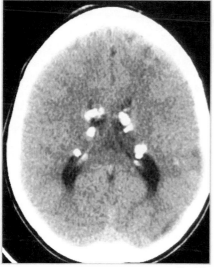

Fig 6.3a

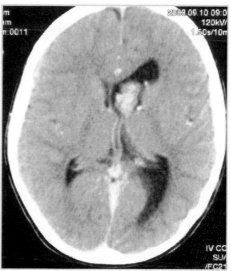

Fig 6.3b

1. What do you observe on the CT scans of the brain?
2. What is the cause for the developmental delay and seizures?
3. What are the clinical features?
4. What is the cause of the sudden-onset headache? What are the other complications?
5. What are the radiological features and treatment of this condition?

Answers *on pages 367–398*

Case 6.4

A 31-year-old man presents with sudden onset of weakness in both legs. Clinical examination showed power of 1/5 and exaggerated reflexes in both lower limbs.

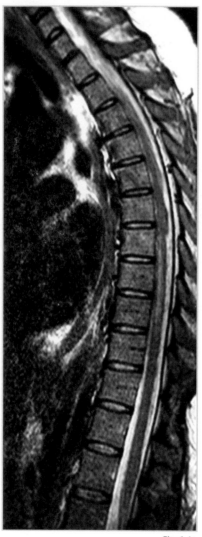

Fig 6.4a

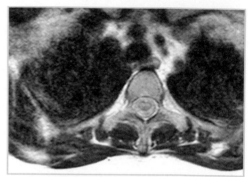

Fig 6.4b

1. What do you observe on MRI of the spine?
2. What is the diagnosis?
3. What are the pathophysiology and clinical features of this condition?
4. What are the radiological findings?
5. What are the differential diagnosis and treatment?

Answers on pages 367–398

Case 6.5

A 13-year-old girl presents with pain in the neck and both arms. Clinical examination showed increased reflexes, loss of power and sensation in all four limbs.

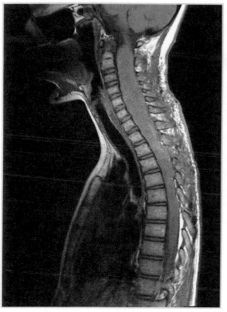

Fig 6.5a

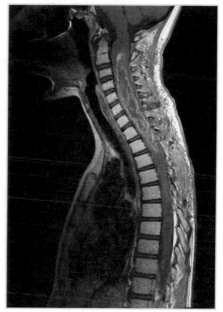

Fig 6.5b

1. What do you see on MRI of the spine?
2. What is the diagnosis?
3. What are the different types of this disease?
4. What are the radiological features?
5. What is the differential diagnosis?

Answers on pages 367–398

Case 6.6

A 85-year-old man patient presents with altered level of consciousness, loss of memory and headache. On examination there is weakness on the left side.

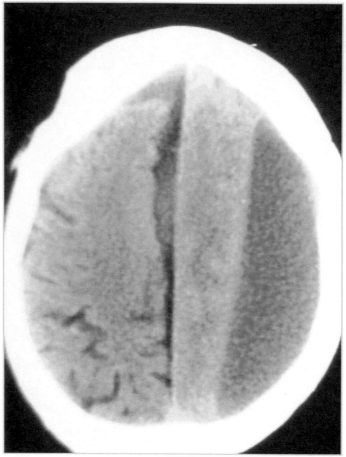

Fig 6.6

1. What are the findings on the CT scan?
2. What is the diagnosis?
3. What is the mechanism?
4. What are the radiological features?
5. What is the prognosis?

Answers on pages 367–398

Case 6.7

A 31-year-old man presents with weakness in his arms and legs and reduced vision. On examination the power and tone on his limbs are decreased and there are exaggerated reflexes. The visual acuity is reduced.

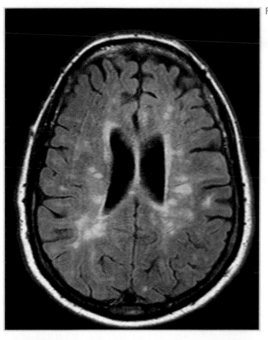

Fig 6.7a

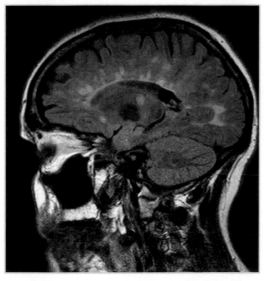

Fig 6.7b

1. What are the findings on MRI of the brain?
2. What is the diagnosis?
3. What are the clinical features?
4. What are the radiological features? What other investigations are required?
5. What is the radiological differential diagnosis? What is the management?

Answers *on pages 367–398*

Case 6.8

A 39-year-old woman presents with severe headache, weakness of the right arm, fever and vomiting. On examination she is febrile, and has neck stiffness and right hemiparesis.

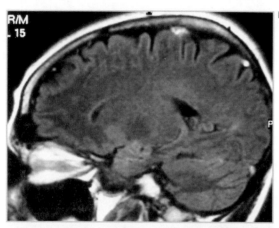
Fig 6.8a

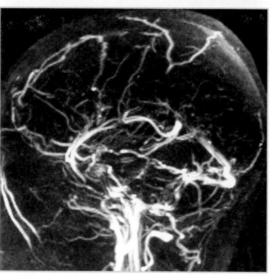
Fig 6.8b

1. What do you observe in these investigations?

2. What is the diagnosis?

3. What are the predisposing factors?

4. What are the clinical features and treatment?

5. What are the imaging features?

Answers on pages 367–398

Case 6.9

A 31-year-old man with C3 HIV presents with headache and right hemiparesis.

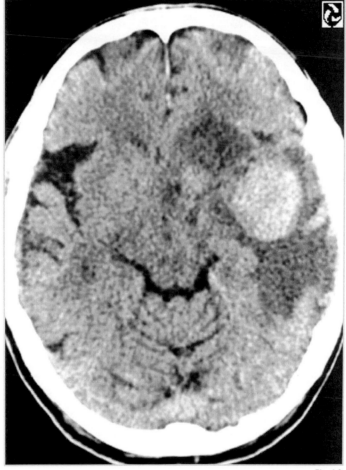

Fig 6.9

1. What do you find on the CT scan?
2. What is the diagnosis?
3. What are the clinical features and pathology of this disease?
4. What are the radiological features?
5. What is the most common differential diagnosis?
6. What is the treatment?

Answers *on pages 367–398*

A 56-year-old woman develops left-sided weakness, speech disturbance and altered consciousness. A CT scan was done with and without contrast.

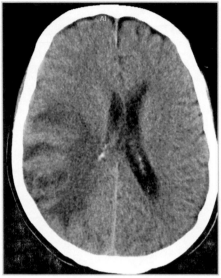
Fig 6.10a

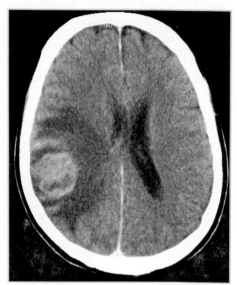
Fig 6.10b

1. What are the abnormalities seen on the brain CT scan?
2. What is the diagnosis?
3. What are the other organs which may be involved when these lesions are present in the brain and what other investigations should be done?
4. What are the radiological features and what is the most sensitive investigation in diagnosis? What conditions cause haemorrhage in this scenario?
5. What is the treatment?

Answers on pages 367–398

Case 6.11

A 13-year-old boy, who had a recent bone marrow transplantation, presents with severe headache, nausea, vomiting, fever and seizures. On examination, he is febrile. There is a left hemiparesis.

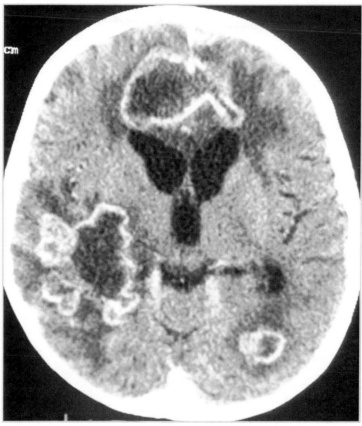

Fig 6.11

Neuroradiology Questions

1. What are the findings on the CT scan?
2. What is the diagnosis?
3. What are the causative agents and how is the brain affected?
4. What are the clinical features?
5. What are the radiological findings?
6. What is the differential diagnosis?

Answers *on pages 367–398*

Case 6.12

A 21 year old presents after a road traffic accident with loss of consciousness, headache and vomiting. On examination, there is weakness in the left arm and leg.

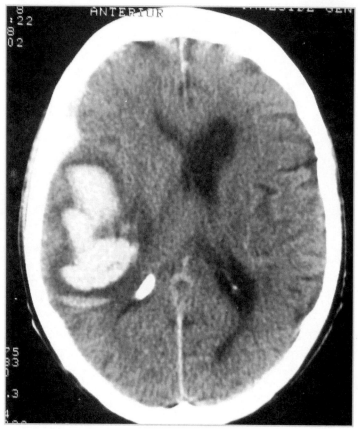

Fig 6.12

1. What are the findings on the CT scan?
2. What is the diagnosis?
3. What is the mechanism? What is the usual location?
4. What are the radiological features?
5. What are the other non-traumatic causes of this appearance? What are the complications and treatment?

Answers on pages 367–398

Case 6.13

A 2-year-old boy presents with recurrent generalised tonic–clonic seizures and delayed milestones.

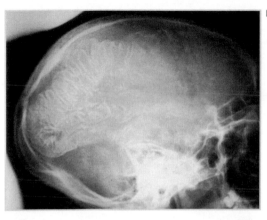

Fig 6.13a

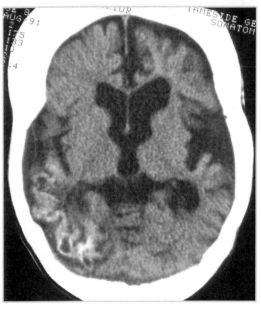

Fig 6.13b

1. What do you see on the skull X-ray?
2. What do you note on the CT scan of the brain?
3. What is the diagnosis?
4. What is the development of this condition?
5. What are the radiological features and differential diagnosis?

Answers *on pages 367–398*

Case 6.14

A 33-year-old man with HIV presents with headache and seizures.

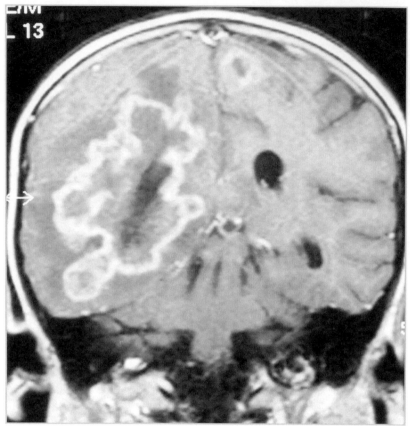

Fig 6.14

1. What do you observe on MRI?
2. What is the diagnosis?
3. What is the pathology of this disease?
4. What are the radiological features of this disease?
5. What is the most common differential diagnosis in this clinical setting?
6. What are the complications?

Answers on pages 367–398

Case 6.15

A 36-year-old woman presents with sudden onset of seizures and headache. Clinical examination did not detect any neurological deficit.

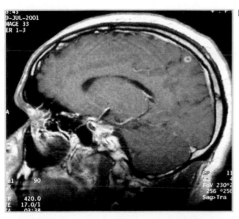

Fig 6.15a

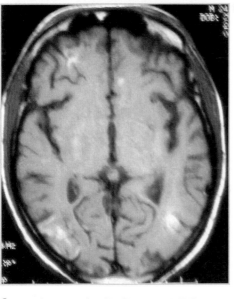

Fig 6.15b

1. What are the findings on MRI?
2. What is the diagnosis?
3. What are the characteristic location and pathology?
4. What are the radiological features?
5. What are the differential diagnoses?

Answers *on pages 367–398*

A 29-year-old man presents with headache and loss of consciousness. On clinical examination, there is decreased power in the right arm and leg.

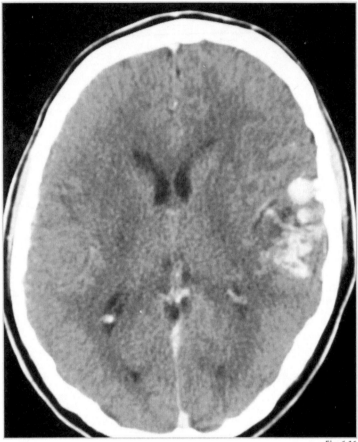

Fig 6.16

1. What do you see on the CT scan?
2. What is the diagnosis?
3. What are the causes, types and vascular supply? What are the common locations?
4. What are the imaging findings and what is the role of radiology in treatment?
5. What are the complications and prognosis?

Answers *on pages 367–398*

Case 6.17

A 28-year-old man who was involved in a road traffic accident presents with headache, drowsiness and history of loss of consciousness. On examination he is disoriented and does not respond to verbal stimuli.

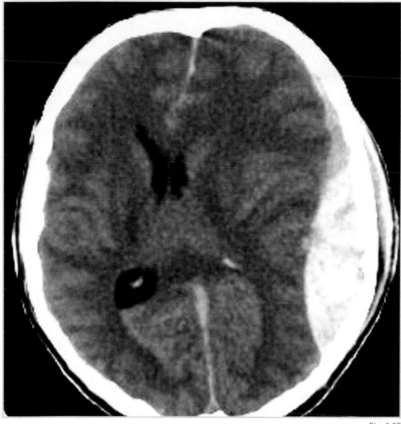

Fig 6.17

1. What are the findings on the CT scan?
2. What is the diagnosis?
3. What is the mechanism?
4. What are the clinical and radiological features?
5. What is the treatment of this condition?

Answers *on pages 367–398*

A 11-year-old girl presents with loss of pain and temperature sensation in the upper limbs and muscle weakness.

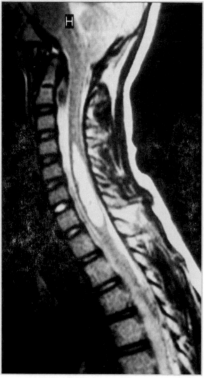

Fig 6.18a

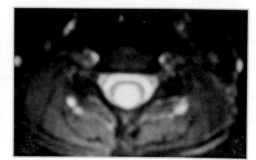

Fig 6.18b

1. What are the findings on MRI?
2. What is the diagnosis?
3. What are the types of disease?
4. What are the clinical presentations and treatment?
5. What are the radiological features?

Answers on pages 367–398

Case 6.19

A 14-year-old boy presents with headache and focal seizures. On examination he does not have any neurological deficit.

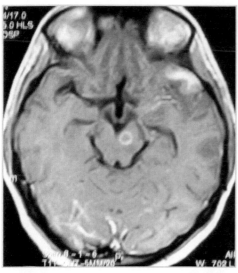

Fig 6.19a

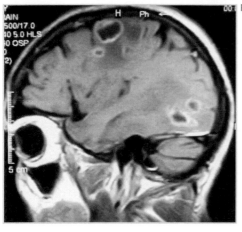

Fig 6.19b

1. What are the findings on the MR scan?
2. What is the diagnosis?
3. What is the mode of spread to the brain?
4. What are the clinical features?
5. What are the radiological findings?
6. What is the differential diagnosis?

Answers *on pages 367–398*

A 27-year-old patient was brought to A&E unconscious after he was found collapsed by the road side. On examination, his GCS (Glasgow Coma Score) was 4.

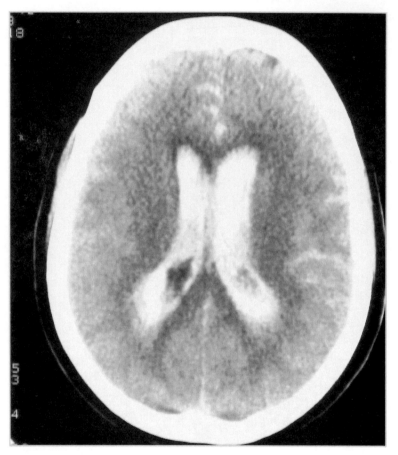

Fig 6.20

1. What are the findings on the CT scan?
2. What is the diagnosis?
3. What are the causes?
4. What are the radiological findings?
5. What are the complications and treatment?

Answers on pages 367–398

Case 6.21

A 47-year-old woman presents with left-sided sensorineural deafness and tinnitus.

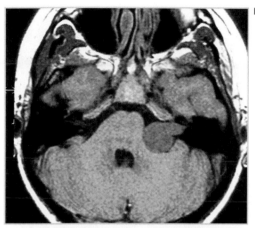

Fig 6.21a

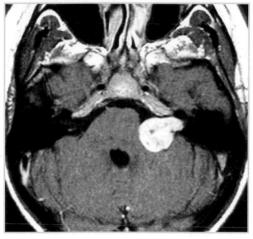

Fig 6.21b

1. What are the findings on MRI?
2. What is the diagnosis?
3. What is the origin of this lesion? What are the pathological and clinical features?
4. What are the radiological features and the associations?
5. What is the differential diagnosis?

Answers *on pages 367–398*

Case 6.22

A 65 year old presents with headache, seizures and right-sided hemiparesis. Clinical examination showed dense hemiplegia on the left side.

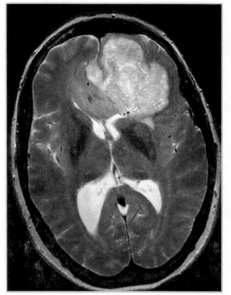

Fig 6.22a

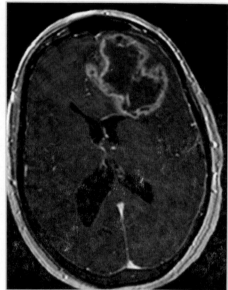

Fig 6.22b

1. What are the findings on the MRI scan of the brain?
2. What is the diagnosis?
3. What is the pathology and what are the common locations?
4. What are the associations, other types and mode of spread?
5. What are the radiological features?
6. What is the differential diagnosis?

Answers on pages 367–398

Case 6.23

A 45-year-old woman presents with headache, seizures and amnesia. She also has chronic cough and dyspnoea. Clinical examination showed mild decrease in power in all four limbs.

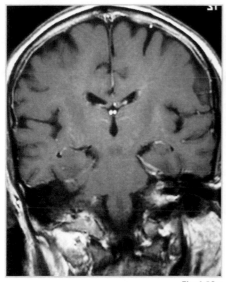

Fig 6.23a

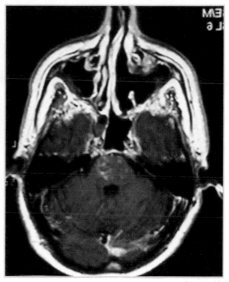

Fig 6.23b

1. What do you find on MRI?
2. What are the causes of this appearance?
3. What is the most likely diagnosis in this patient?
4. What are the radiological features?
5. What are the other areas of the nervous system brain affected by this disease and what is the treatment?

Answers on pages 367–398

Neuroradiology Questions

Case 6.24

A 49-year-old man, hospitalised for bowel obstruction, develops sudden onset of quadriparesis and confusion.

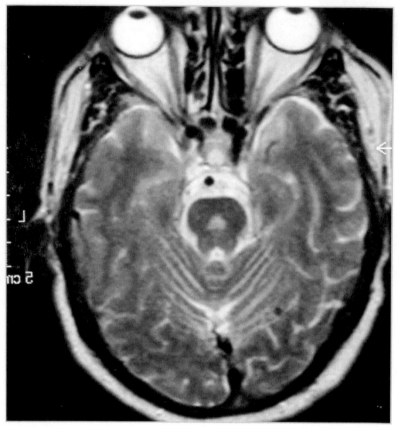

Fig 6.24

1. What are the findings on MRI?
2. What is the diagnosis?
3. What are the causes of this appearance?
4. What are the typical locations?
5. What are the radiological features and differential diagnosis?

Answers on pages 367–398

Case 6.25

A 38-year-old woman presents with headache and seizures. On clinical examination, there are no remarkable neurological findings.

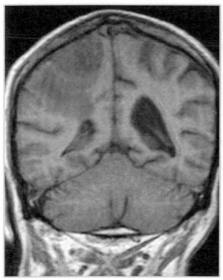
Fig 6.25a

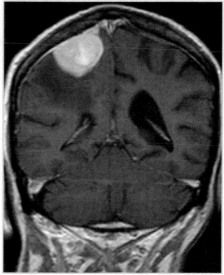
Fig 6.25b

1. What are the findings on MRI?
2. What is the diagnosis?
3. What are the cell of origin, common locations and associations?
4. What are the types and radiological appearances?
5. What are the differential diagnoses and treatment?

Answers on pages 367–398

Case 6.26

A 23-year-old woman presents with headache, gait disturbance and nystagmus. On examination cerebellar signs are positive.

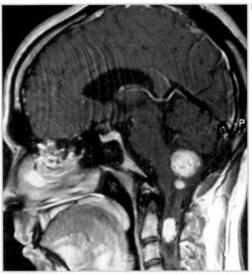
Fig 6.26a

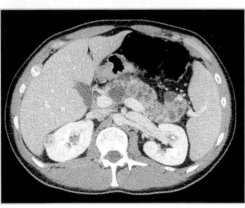
Fig 6.26b

1. What do you observe on MRI?
2. What is the diagnosis?
3. What is the underlying associated condition?
4. What do you observe on the CT scan of the abdomen?
5. What are the radiological findings?
6. What is the differential diagnosis?

Answers *on pages 367–398*

Case 6.27

A 35-year-old woman presented with severe headache and photophobia.

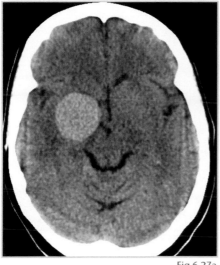

Fig 6.27a

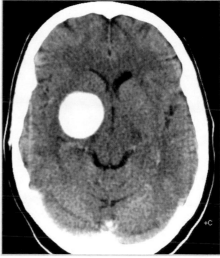

Fig 6.27b

1. What do you see on this CT scan?
2. What is the diagnosis?
3. What are the causes, risk factors and common locations?
4. What are the radiological findings?
5. What is the recent role of radiology in the treatment of this condition?

Answers *on pages 367–398*

Case 6.28

A 56-year-old woman presents with sudden onset of weakness in the left arm and leg. On examination, she is fully conscious, but she has power of 0/5 in her left arm and leg with exaggerated deep tendon reflexes and brisk plantar response.

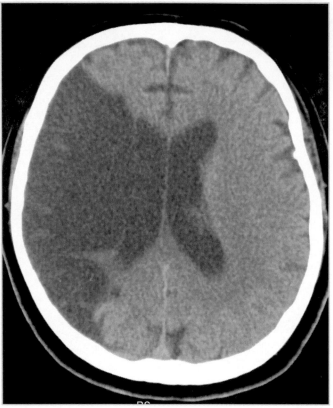

Fig 6.28

1. What do you observe on the CT scan of the brain?
2. What is the diagnosis?
3. What are the causes of this disease? What is the common location?
4. What are the tests that are used for early diagnosis? What are the radiological features?
5. What are the contraindications for thrombolysis?

Answers *on pages 367–398*

Case 6.29

A 52-year-old woman presents with weakness in her right arm. On examination, the power is 3/5 in the right arm with exaggeration of the deep reflexes.

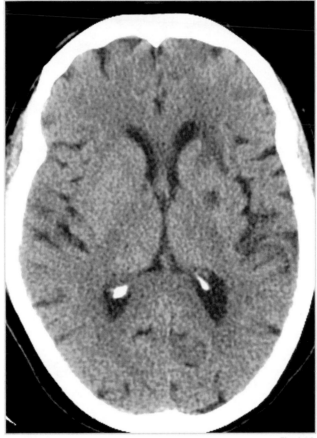

Fig 6.29

1. What do you see on the CT scan?
2. What is the diagnosis?
3. What are the causes? What is the most common location?
4. What are the clinical syndromes?
5. What are the findings on CT and MRI?

Answers *on pages 367–398*

Neuroradiology Questions

A 14-year-old boy presents to the hospital with intractable seizures over the past year. His seizures begin with a feeling of déjà vu followed by motionless stare and fumbling. Clinically no neurological deficit was observed.

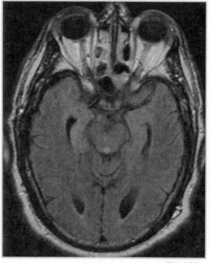

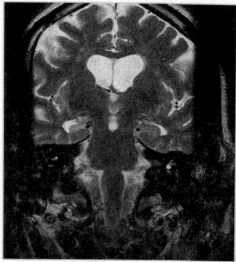

Fig 6.30a

Fig 6.30b

1. What is this investigation and what do you observe?

2. What is the diagnosis?

3. What are the causes of epilepsy?

4. What is the relationship of this lesion to epilepsy?

5. What is the role of MRI in the diagnosis of epilepsy?

Answers on pages 367–398

Case 6.1: Answers

1. This is a CT scan examination without contrast. The bright density consistent with fresh blood is seen in the sulci and basal cisterns. In addition, the laterial ventricles appear marginally dilated.

2. The patient has subarachnoid haemorrhage. The most common cause is rupture of aneurysm. Other causes are arteriovenous malformations, hypertension and cryptogenic causes. The patient has developed acute hydrocephalus, which is caused by decreased drainage of cerebrospinal fluid.
   Complications of subararachnoid haemorrhage are rebleeding, vasospasm (seen in 70–90%) leading to stroke in 50%) and mortality (10% die before reaching hospital). Other medical complications which may develop are – electrolyte disturbances, arrhythmias, neurogenic pulmonary oedema and hypoxia.

3. If CT scan demonstrates subarachnoid haemorrhage, a conventional angiography is required to determine the presence of aneurysm. This is being replaced by CT/MR angiography, which identifies the aneurysm and determines if it is appropriate for intervention. On the other hand, if CT is normal, a lumbar puncture is done, to exclude subarachnoid haemorrhage. Presence of blood and xanthochromia confirms the diagnosis.

4. Headache of sudden onset is the classic presentation. Other presentations are meningism (photophobia, vomiting, neck stiffness), nerve III palsy, seizures, altered consciousness and focal neurological deficits.

5. Marfan syndrome, Ehler–Danlos syndrome, polycystic kidney disease, coarctation of the aorta and arteriovenous malformation (AVM) are associated.

6. Calcium channel blockers are used to reduce vasospasm. Aneuryms are managed by surgical clipping or endovascular coiling. AVMs are managed by embolisation with coils. Cerebral oedema is managed by steroids. Hydrocephalus requires shunting. Risk of rebleeding is 10–20% in the first 2 weeks and 50% in the first 6 months. The mortality rate from rebleeding is 70–90%. Radiology not only is used in diagnosis, but also plays a major role in treatment. GDC (Gugielmi detachable coils) are employed to embolise the aneuryms using selective catheterisation of the involved arteries.

Case 6.2: Answers

1. The sagittal views of the brain stem and upper cervical spine show herniation of the cerebral tonsil below the level of the foramen magnum. There is also an abnormal, long segment of low signal intensity in the cervical and thoracic spinal cord.

2. Arnold–Chiari I malformation associated with syringohydromyelia of the upper cervical cord.

3. Arnold–Chiari malformation is a congenital malformation resulting from defective neural tube closure. There are four types:

    I: downward herniation of the cerebellar tonsils below the level of foramen magnum

    II: caudal herniation of tonsils and vermis, small posterior fossa, towering cerebellum, beaked tectum

    III: Chiari II findings + encephalocele

    IV: severe cerebellar hypoplasia.

4. In the normal sagittal pictures of the craniocervical junction, the cerebellar tonsils are above the level of the foramen magnum. If they extend below the foramen magnum, they do not extend > 5 mm. Any descent > 5 mm is considered to be tonsillar herniation and is a feature of Arnold–Chiari I malformation. The fourth ventricle can be elongated, but remains in the normal position. It is associated with syringomyelia in 50% of cases. Syringomyelia is seen as a low signal intensity lesion in T1- and high signal intensity in T2-weighted images.

5. Arnold–Chiari I malformation is associated with intermittent compression of the brain stem, which manifests as nerve palsies, atypical facial pain, respiratory depression and long tract signs. Associated features are syringomyelia (50%), hydrocephalus (25%), basilar invagination (30%), Klippel–Feil anomaly (10%) and atlanto-occipital fusion (5%).

Case 6.3: Answers

1. The pre-contrast scan shows dense calcified nodules in the subependymal region of the ventricles on both sides. The post-contrast scan shows a densely enhancing mass in the region of the foramen of Monro, which is expanding the frontal horn of the left lateral ventricle.

2. The patient suffers from tuberous sclerosis. Calcified subependymal nodules are characteristic of tuberous sclerosis. Developmental delay and seizures are common features of this condition.

3. Tuberous sclerosis is an autosomal dominant disease with multisystem involvement including neurological, cutaneous, ocular, renal, cardiac, pulmonary and other organs. Deletions in chromosomes 9 and 11 are identified. Classic clinical triad is seizures, learning disability and adenoma sebaceum, which are found in less than 50% of patients. Diagnosis is made on finding one of the following: adenoma sebaceum, ungual or subungal fibromas, cortical or subependymal harmatomas, or giant cell tumours. Hypopigmented macule, shagreen patches, infantile spasm, retinal hamartomas, renal hamartomas, cysts, cardiac rhabdomyomas or first–degree relative sufferer favours a presumptive diagnosis. Ninety per cent have skin and brain lesions. Seizures start before age 2 years.

4. The child has developed subependymal giant cell astrocytoma within the left lateral ventrical (seen in 2nd CT scan). This is a recognised complication of tuberous sclerosis. This is the cause of the headache. Renal angiomyolipomas, cysts, cardiac rhabdomyomas, pulmonary lymphangioleiomyomatosis and cutaneous changes are the other complications.

5. In the CNS, the characteristic features are cortical tubers, white matter abnormalities, subependymal nodules and subependymal giant cell astrocytomas, which are caused by a migration abnormality of dysgenetic neurons. Subependymal nodules are the hallmark of this lesion and are seen as dense calcified nodules along the ventricular margins. Cortical tubers are hypointense in T1 and hyperintense in T2. White matter lesions are seen as straight or curvilinear bands extending from the ventricles towards the cortex. Subependymal astrocytomas occur near the foramen of Monro and cause obstructive hydrocephalus. Regular follow-up is done with MRI of the brain and ultrasonography of the kidneys and heart. Neurosurgical intervention is necessary for complications such as development of astrocytoma and hydrocephalus.

1. This is T2-weighted MRI of the thoracic spine. The mid-thoracic cord shows an abnormal area of high signal intensity within it from levels T4 to T7. There is also some diffuse swelling of the spinal cord.

2. Transverse myelitis. This is inflammation across both sides of one level or segment of the spinal cord.

3. Transverse myelitis is an acute inflammation of the spinal cord, caused by a rapidly developing lesion that affects both halves of the cord, occurring in the absence of any known disease compressing the spinal cord, and resulting in bilateral motor, sensory and autonomic dysfunction. Pathologically, it is characterised by perivenular inflammation and demyelination. It can occur as an isolated incident (idiopathic, as a result of abnormal activation of the immune system against the spinal cord). Secondary causes are viral (herpes simplex, herpes zoster, cytomegalovirus, Epstein–Barr virus, polio, human T-cell leukaemia virus, echovirus, HIV, influenza, rabies, *Mycoplasma pneumoniae*, Lyme disease, borreliosis, syphilis, TB), vaccination (rabies, cowpox), autoimmune diseases (SLE, Sjögren syndrome, sarcoidosis), multiple sclerosis (MS), paraneoplastic syndrome and vascular (spinal artery thrombosis, vasculitis). Most patients have a viral illness close to the onset of radiological findings. Clinical features are limb weakness, sensory disturbance, bowel and bladder dysfunction, back pain and radicular pain.

4. MRI is used mainly to exclude a mass, which might be in the cord or outside the cord. MRI shows high signal in the affected segment in T2-weighted images and low signal in T1-weighted images. The cord is expanded. There is contrast enhancement, which can be patchy, mostly occurring in the periphery of a centrally located lesion. These changes extend to three or four vertebral segments of the cord. Other lesions such as herniated discs, tumours, stenosis and abscesses are excluded with MRI.

5. Differential diagnosis – **Multiple sclerosis** (other multiple lesions in brain, never extends more than 2 vertebral segments in the cord. In transverse myelitis, enhancement is in the periphery of a centrally located area of high T2 weighted images. In multiple sclerosis, the lesions show enhancement in the central zone of peripherally located high signal intensity on T2 weighted images), **Acute disseminated encephalomyelitis**, **Sarcoidosis**, **Infarct** (thoracic level, single

Neuroradiology Answers

lesion, contrast enhancement not common, acute onset, vascular history), **Vasculitis** (clinical history of SLE and vaculitis), **Radiation** (> 4000 cGY, 1–3 year latency, peripheral enhancement may be seen), **Spinal cord tumours** (solid or cystic mass with enhancement) and **AV fistula** (> 50 years, long history, serpigionous flow voids, dorsolumbar level). Steroids are used in the treatment of transverse myelitis. Recovery may be absent, partial or complete and is seen in 1–3 months. Many patients show good recovery.

Case 6.5: Answers

1. Sagittal views of the MRI of the cervical spine show a large hypointense mass in the cervical spinal cord, which has expanded the cord. The lesion enhances after contrast administration.

2. Spinal cord tumour – astrocytoma.

3. Spinal tumours can be divided into intramedullary (within the cord), intradural extramedullary (within the thecal sac, outside the cord) and extradural (outside the thecal sac):

    Intramedullary: astrocytoma, ependymoma, haemangioblastoma, metastasis

    Intradural extramedullary: neurofibroma, meningioma, lipoma, dermoid, drop metastasis

    Extradural: metastasis, lymphoma, myeloma, sarcoma, chordoma, disc prolapse, haematoma, abscess, neurofibroma, osteochondroma, vertebral body tumours.

4. Spinal cord tumours are diagnosed with MRI. Most of the tumours are gliomas. Ependymomas are common in the filum terminale, especially in children. Astrocytomas are seen in the cervical cord. Haemangioblastomas are seen in the posterior columns and can be associated with other haemangioblastomas in the brain, especially in von Hippel–Lindau syndrome. Astrocytomas are usually associated with cysts. The cyst can be intratumoral or peritumoral and syringomyelic, extending the whole length of the cord. In MRI the tumour can be of same signal intensity as the cord or have a lower signal in T1 and a brighter one in T2. Cysts are low signal in T1 and higher in T2. Good contrast enhancement is seen.

5. Differential diagnoses for intramedullary tumours are syringomyelia, intramedullary abscess, myelitis and haematomyelia.

Case 6.6: Answers

1. The CT scan shows a large crescenteric hypodense collection in the right parietal area. There is mass effect, with obliteration of the sulci in the right grey–white matter interface.

2. Chronic subdural haematoma.

3. Chronic subdural haematoma is usually more than 3 weeks old. This might occur as a result of trivial head trauma. It is more common in old age, those with alcohol abuse, epilepsy, coagulopathy and ventricular shunts. It is believed to occur as a result of minor injuries that tear fragile capillary bed, which results in repeated episodes of rebleeding. It is more common in elderly people, because the brain is atrophic and the bridging veins connecting the surface of brain to the diploic veins are stretched, fragile and easily damaged. The bleeding is surrounded by thick and vascular neomembrane.

4. Usually, a history of trauma is absent. The haematoma is in the subdural space, so it is crescenteric with a medial concavity. It can, however, also be biconvex similar to an extradural haematoma, as a result of compartmentalisation caused by fibrous septa. Unlike acute subdural haematoma, the density of the haematoma is very low, in the range 0–25 HU, which is lower than for brain but higher than for CSF. In long-standing cases, the density might be even lower than for CSF. High-density components are seen if there is acute bleeding within the chronic haematoma. Fluid sedimentation levels are seen as a result of sedimented fresh blood with proteinaceous fluid layered above. There is displacement/effacement of sulci, with displacement of ventricles. When the haematomas are bilateral, no midline shift is seen. If contrast is administered, the surrounding neomembrane will enhance and cortical veins are seen in the periphery of the haematoma rather than passing through it. MRI is useful in isodense subdural haematomas.

5. Usually chronic subdural haematomas present with ill-defined neurological signs and symptoms, with cognitive deficit, behavioural abnormality and non-specific headache. Liquefied chronic subdural haematomas commonly can be treated with drainage through one to two burr holes. Burr holes are placed so that conversion to a craniotomy is possible if needed. A closed drainage system is sometimes left in the subdural space for 24–72 hours postoperatively. Small catheter drainage via a twist drill craniotomy at the bedside has also been described as adequate treatment. A non-liquefied, chronic, subdural haematoma cannot be decompressed adequately by burr holes and must be removed by craniotomy. Bilateral chronic haematomas must be drained from both sides, usually during the same operation, through burr holes placed on each side of the head. Outcome after drainage of chronic subdural haematoma correlates with the preoperative neurological state. Early diagnosis before significant neurological deterioration correlates with a favourable prognosis. Of patients 80% regain normal function, especially if they are younger.

Case 6.7: Answers

1. MRI of the brain (FLAIR sequence – Fluid attenuated inversion recovery) shows elongated, oval hyperintense lesions extending perpendicularly from the corpus callosum\in the sagittal view. The second axial image shows multiple hyperintense, bright lesions in the white matter surrounding the ventricles.

2. Multiple scelerosis (MS).

3. MS is the most widespread acquired demyelinating disease. The aetiology is uncertain and is probably an autoimmune response against myelin, triggered by a previous virus infection or exogenous agent acting on inherited susceptibility. There are many types, including the **classic Charcot's, neuromyelitis optica (Devic syndrome), Balo concentric sclerosis** and **Schilder's diffuse sclerosis**. The classic form has four subtypes: **relapsing–remitting, chronic progressive, secondary progressive** and **benign.** Most patients present in the third or fourth decade. Fifteen per cent are seen before age 20 years and 10% after age 50 years. Females are more commonly affected. Clinical symptoms are double vision (optic neuritis), weakness, numbness, tingling and gait disturbance, loss of sphincter control, blindness, paralysis and dementia.

4. MR has the highest sensitivity in the diagnosis of MS (85%), even better than evoked potentials and CSF oligoclonal bands. Sagittal FLAIR (fluid attenuation inversion recovery) sequences are the most sensitive. This sequence suppresses the fluid signal from the CSF, which appears as dark, and any subtle high signal in the subcallosal region will be seen as a bright lesion. Most plaques are iso- or hypointense in T1-weighted images and hyperintense in T2-weighted images. They are typically ovoid, from medial to lateral, and are mainly close to the periventricular white matter. They extend perpendicularly from the surface of the corpus callosum (**Dawson's fingers** – as a result of perivenular demyelination). Other appearances are small subcortical punctuate lesions, tumour-like plaques involving a large part of centrum semiovale, and confluent periventricular and peritrigonal plaques. Plaques can enhance in the acute stage. CSF analysis for oligoclonal bands is the other test that could be performed to confirm the diagnosis.

5. Other diseases that produce white matter hyperintensities are degeneration, vasculitis, metastases, infection and haemorrhage. Oval hyperintensities in the periventricular white matter, resulting from perivenous demyelination, are specific for MS and not seen in any of the above conditions. Immunomodulators such as interferon-β1a and -1b, glatiramer acetate and nalalizumab, corticosteroids and immunosuppressants such as cyclophosphamide, methotrexate, mitoxantrone and azathioprine are used for disease pharmacotherapy. Supportive methods include medication to relieve spasticity, pain, trigeminal neuralgia and depression.

Case 6.8: Answers

1. The first picture, which is a T1 weighted MRI acquired in the sagittal plane shows an abnormal high signal deep to the inner table of skull vault, which indicates clot. The second test is MR venography, which shows irregular obliteration of the superior sagittal sinus.

2. Superior sagittal sinus thrombosis.

3. The causes of cerebral venous thrombosis are idiopathic, infections, tumour, trauma, dehydration, shock, cardiac failure, hypercoagulable states (antiphospholipid syndrome, protein C and S disease, polycythaemia vera, thrombocytopenia, thrombocytosis, sickle cell, DIC), HIV, SLE, nephritic syndrome, chemotherapy (asparaginase) and Behçet's disease.

4. The clinical features are headache, nausea, vomiting, visual blurring, drowsiness, lethargy, seizures, stroke and fever. Systemic anticoagulation is used for treatment of sinus thrombosis. Thrombolysis/surgical thrombectomy is reserved for extensive, occlusive thrombus.

5. A CT scan shows a dense clot in the sinuses in non-contrast (**cord/dense triangle sign**). On contrast scans, the clot does not enhance and is seen as filling defects. One of the signs of sinus thrombosis is an empty **delta sign**, in which the walls of the dural sinus enhance and the clot does not enhance and is seen as a filling defect. Focal haemorrhage in the brain and infarct can be seen. There is gyriform enhancement of the periphery of the infarct. MRI shows a high signal intensity thrombus within the sinuses, which is isointense in T1 and hypointense in T2. In the subacute phase, it is initially bright in T1 and dark on T2, and later bright in both T1 and T2. Chronic thrombus is isointense in T1 and hyperintense in T2. MR or CT venography exquisitely demonstrates the venous anatomy and the exact location of the thrombosis is identified. In thrombus, there is partial or total non-visualisation of dural sinus, with collateral vessels.

Case 6.9: Answers

1. The non-contrast CT scan shows a large dense lesion with surrounding oedema in the left parietal cortex.

2. Primary intracerebral lymphoma.

3. Primary cerebral lymphoma is seen in 6% of AIDS patients and is the AIDS-defining illness in a third of these cases. It is usually a high-grade, B-cell, non-Hodgkin's lymphoma, with a doubling time of only 14 days. The tumour expresses Epstein–Barr virus, which can be detected in the CSF and DNA.

4. It is commonly seen in the periventricular white matter, subependymal region, basal ganglia, thalamus and corpus callosum; 40–75% are in contact with ependyma or leptomeninges. It is multifocal in 50% and usually large − > 4 cm. As a result of its high cellularity, the tumour is hyperdense in non-contrast CT and iso- to hypointense in T1- and T2-weighted sequences. There is mass effect and oedema. Contrast enhancement can be homogeneous, heterogeneous or ring like.

Haemorrhage, calcification and necrosis are uncommon features. Leptomeningeal involvement is seen in metastatic spread from lymphoma and is usually associated with parenchymal disease.

5. These lymphomas in HIV patients have some differences from those in a non-HIV patient. They occur in younger populations, are more often multiple, and show more prominent oedema and ring enhancement. The most common differential diagnosis is toxoplasmosis.

6. Primary cerebral lymphoma is practically unresectable. On average 2–3 years survival is now achieved with multi drug chemotherapy and radiotherapy. High-dose steroids and radiation are used for palliation.

Case 6.10: Answers

1. The pre-contrast scan shows a rounded mass approximately 4 cm in diameter in the right parietal cortex which is surrounded by low-density vasogenic cerebral oedema. The scan on the right, done after contrast administration, shows contrast enhancement and the mass becomes brighter than the previous scan. A hypodense area noted within the mass probably represents area of necrosis.

2. Cerebral metastasis.

3. Headache, focal neurological weakness and altered consciousness are the common symptoms. Other causes of enhancing mass in the brain are primary tumour, lymphoma and infections. The lung, breast and colon are the sites of common primaries. Any primary tumour can metastasise to the brain. If a primary tumour is not already known, it can be searched for by doing a chest X-ray, mammogram and staging CT of the chest, abdomen and pelvis. A bone scan can be done to assess skeletal metastasis.

4. Contrast-enhanced MRI is the most sensitive method and is the most cost-effective method for screening cerebral metastasis in a patient with a known primary. On CT, the metastasis is seen as a nodular or isodense mass, which enhances on contrast administration. Ring-enhancing metastasis can be seen. On MRI, the lesion is hypointense in

T1, hyperintense in T2, and can show homogeneous, heterogeneous and ring enhancement in contrast scans. Melanoma, choriocarcinoma, kidney, thyroid, germ cell tumours, breast and lung are tumours that cause haemorrhagic brain metastasis. They are seen as bright and hyperdense on a non-contrast CT scan. A follow-up CT scan should be done after the haemorrhage resolves, to assess the underlying tumour.

5. High intracranial pressure can be reduced by using intravenous dexamethasone. The survival is poor and ranges from 18 months to 24 months. A solitary lesion can be treated with surgery or stereotactic radiosurgery. Radio- and chemotherapy are palliative treatment options.

Case 6.11: Answers

1. The CT scan shows multiple ring-enhancing lesions. The larger lesions are seen in the midline frontal region and right parietal region and a small lesion is seen in the left occipital region. The lesions are surrounded by vasogenic oedema.

2. Cerebral abscesses caused by *Aspergillus*.

3. Streptococci, anaerobic organisms, *Bacteroides* spp., staphylococci and fungi are common causative organisms. The infection can extend from adjacent sinuses/middle ear/mastoid or by penetrating trauma, surgery, septicaemia, or may be cyptogenic. Predisposing factors are immunosuppressive drugs, HIV, steroid use, trauma, lung infections (bronchiectasis, empyema, bronchopleural fistula, pneumonia) and cardiac lesions (endocarditis, right-to-left shunt).

4. Headache, drowsiness, confusion, seizures, focal neurological deficit, fever and leukocytosis are the clinical features. Complications are daughter abscesses and rupture into the ventricular system.

5. The most common location of abscess is the corticomedullary junction. It is more common in the frontal and temporal lobes. A CT scan shows a hypodense area with mass effect, which shows rim enhancement. The wall is thin, smooth with relative thinning of the medial wall. Gas can be seen within the lesion. There is extensive perilesional oedema, which can

produce mass effect and compression of the ventricles. Satellite nodules can be seen. MRI shows a hypointense lesion in T1 and hyperintense in T2, with the rim appearing hypointense in T2. Contrast enhancement of the rim is seen. There is high signal perilesional oedema.

6. Differential diagnoses: cystic glioma, metastasis, ganglioma, pilocytic astrocytoma, haemangioblastoma, infarct, cyst and cavitating haematoma.

Case 6.12: Answers

1. The CT scan shows a very dense lesion seen in the right parietal lobe, with compression of the right lateral ventricle and a midline shift to the left side. There is a subfalcine herniation and is minimal vasogenic oedema surrounding the lesion, which is seen as a low-density area.

2. Acute cerebral intraparenchymal haematoma.

3. Intraparenchymal haematomas are caused by shear strain injury by a blunt or penetrating trauma, with blood separating the neurons. The most common location for a traumatic intracerebral haematoma is low frontal and anterior temporal white matter or basal ganglia. Hypertensive haematomas are common in basal ganglia, external capsule, thalamus, brain stem and cerebellum, and cerebral hemispheres.

4. In a non-contrast CT scan, haematoma is seen as a high-density lesion (50–70 HU), surrounded by a hypodense oedema. The density of the haematoma increases in the first few days as a result of haemoglobin and clot retraction. Layering may be seen. The density of the haematoma increases in the first week, after which the density decreases starting from the periphery to the centre, and becomes isodense haematoma. Contrast is not advisable because it might increase intracerebal pressure. There might be rim enhancement in the second week as a result of a break in the blood–brain barrier. The MRI appearance of haematoma depends on the stage of haematoma and the type of haemoglobin.

Stage	Time (days)	Haemoglobin	T1	T2
Hyperacute	< 24 hours	Oxyhaemoglobin	Iso-	Hyper-
Acute	1–3	Deoxyhaemoglobin	Hypo-	Hypo-
Subacute early	4–7	Methaemoglobin intracellular	Hyper-	Hypo-
Subacute chronic	8–14	Methaemoglobin extracellular	Hyper-	Hyper-
Chronic	> 14	Haemosiderin	Hypo-	Hypo-

5. Common causes of haematoma are chronic hypertension, trauma, rupture of aneurysm, rupture of AV malformation, hemorrhagic infarction, amyloid angiopathy, coagulopathy, haemorraghic tumour (metastasis from choriocarcinoma, melanoma, renal cancer, thyroid cancer), glioblastoma multiforme, ependymoma, venous infarction, ecclampsia, septic embolism and vasculitis. Complications are herniation (transtentorial, subfalcine, etc), extension to ventricles, porencephaly, gliosis and atrophy. Large intracranial haematomas with rising intracranial pressure require urgent surgical evacuation.

Case 6.13: Answers

1. The skull X-ray shows extensive tram-track calcifications on the surface of the brain, involving the parieto-occipital region.

2. The CT scan shows an area of calcification along the gyrus in the right parieto-occipital lobe, and there is generalised brain atrophy, with some associated prominence of the ventricular system of the brain.

3. Sturge–Weber syndrome.

4. Sturge–Weber syndrome is a vascular malformation that is caused by persistence of the primordial sinusoidal plexus stage of brain development. Clinically there is port wine stain on the face in the trigeminal nerve distribution, seizures/hemiatrophy opposite to the side of the naevus, learning disability and homonymous hemianopia. In the brain, leptomeningeal vascular malformation is seen. Glaucoma, choroidal haemangioma and buphthalmos are also seen. An angiomatous malformation can be seen in the viscera, such as the kidneys, spleen, ovaries, thyroid, pancreas, lungs and intestines.

5. X-ray shows characteristic tram track cortical calcification of the gyri underlying the pial angioma, most commonly in the pariteooccipital region. CT scan shows the calcification and contrast enhancement of the angioma, with atrophy of the underlying brain. There is enlargement of the choroid plexus and thickening of the skull. MRI shows areas of gliosis with hypointensity in T1 and hyperintesnsity in T2. Angiography shows capillary blush, deep medullary draining veins and large subependymal veins. Differential diagnosis include Klippel Trenauny syndrome, Wyburn Mason syndrome and thrombosed cavernous angioma of brain.

Case 6.14: Answers

1. MRI shows a large rim-enhancing lesion in the right cerebral hemisphere with compression of the right lateral ventricle. A smaller similar lesion is also noted in the left cerebral hemisphere.

2. Cerebral toxoplasmosis.

3. Toxoplasmosis is an opportunistic infection caused by reactivation of an obligatory intracellular parasite *Toxoplasma gondii*. It is the most common CNS infection in the AIDS population. It is the most common cause of a focal mass in the HIV population and is seen in 5–30% of these patients. It is commonly seen in the grey–white matter junction and basal ganglia. Multiple lesions are quite common and a solitary lesion is seen in only 14% of cases. The lesions are usually small, < 4 cm. Pathology shows necrotising encephalitis. Abscesses have a thin capsule.

4. A CT scan shows an isodense or hypodense lesion. MRI is isointense to hypointense in both T1 and T2, with a mild hyperintense rim of oedema in T2 and ring or solid contrast enhancement. Occasionally T2-weighted images show a hyperintense centre with enhancing isointense rim. Haemorrhage and necrosis are seen. A rare variant is diffuse toxoplasmosis, which shows patchy areas of high signal in T2 in the grey–white matter junction, which show enhancement. When the immunity is very low, the capsule formation can be subtle or absent.

5. The most common differential diagnosis is lymphoma.

	Toxoplasmosis	Lymphoma
Number	Multiple	Solitary/few
Size	Small (< 4 cm)	Large (> 4 cm)
Location	Grey–white junction, BG	Periventricular, subependymal
Corpus callosum/ subependyma	Not involved	Involved
Mass effect/oedema	Pronounced	Slight
Enhancement	Ring, thin walled	Homo-/heterogeneous, thick walled
Haemorrhage	May be seen	May be seen
Meningeal enhancement	Not seen	Seen occasionally
CT	Hypo-/isodense	Hyperdense
PET	Low or normal metabolism	High metabolism
Thallium-201 SPECT	No uptake	High uptake
Gallium	High uptake	No increase in uptake
Spectroscopy		
Choline	Relative elevation	Low
N-Acetylaspartate	Low	Low
Lipid/lactate	High	low
CSF	*Toxoplasma* spp.	Epstein–Barr virus
Clinical outcome	Good prognosis	Bad prognosis.

6. A reasonable protocol in suspicious cases is to start a trial of anti-toxoplasmosis drugs (clindamycin, pyrimethamine) and do a repeat MRI after 2–3 weeks. If there is a good response, anti-toxoplasmosis therapy is continued for life. If there is no response or an increase in the size of the lesion, a brain biopsy is indicated.

Case 6.15: Answers

1. Contrast-enhanced, sagittal view of MRI shows a small area of ring enhancement in the parietal cortex. The axial images show multiple enhancing areas in other areas of the brain.

2. Neurocysticercosis.

3. Neurocysticercosis is produced by the larval stage of *Taenia solium*. It is the most common CNS parasite infection. The infection is acquired by ingestion of food/water contaminated by ova of the adult tapeworm. The embryophore is dissolved by gastric acid and enzymes, the oncosphere is liberated, embryos invade the intestinal wall and disseminate to different parts of body, where they develop into the larval stage, cysticercus. Common locations in the brain are the meninges, basal cisterns, parenchyma and ventricles. It can involve the spinal cord or it could be a mixed lesion. It is usually asymptomatic and can produce symptoms after 5–7 years.

4. There are four stages of cysticercosis: **vesicular, colloidal vesicular, nodular granular** and **granular calcified stage.** In the early stages a clear fluid-containing cyst is seen, which is hypodense in CT, low signal in T1 MRI and high signal in T2, with surrounding oedema. In the colloidal vesicular stage, the appearances are similar, but a central hypointense mural nodule is seen in T2, which shows homogeneous enhancement. In the nodular granular stage, the cyst becomes smaller, isointense with brain in T1, hypointense in T2. CT shows enhancement of the nodular ring. In the calcified stage, there is a speck of calcification.

5. Differential diagnoses for rim-/nodular-enhancing lesions are TB, fungal infection, toxoplasmosis, metastasis, pilocytic glioma, ganglioma, haematoma, infarct and demyelination. Antihelmintics such as praziquantel and albendozole are used in treatment. Symptomatic treatment involves use of antiepileptics, analgesics (for headache), corticosteroids/glycerol/mannitol for cerebral oedema.

Case 6.16: Answers

1. The CT scan shows tortuous, serpiginous, enhancing lesions in the left temporal lobe.

2. Cerebral AV malformation.

3. AVM is a malformation that consists of a nidus of abnormal, dilated, tortuous arteries and veins with no intervening normal brain parenchyma. The affected arteries have thin walls with gliotic parenchyma in vessels. AVMs are a congenital malformation. They may be associated with other syndromes such as Wyburn–Mason syndrome and Sturge–Weber syndrome. AVMs can be pial or dural. Other malformations are cavernous angiomas, capillary telangiectasia and cortical venous anomaly. Most AVMs are supplied by pial branches of the internal carotid artery. Occasionally dural branches of the external carotid artery supply them. Most are located in a supratentorial location. The most common locations are in parietal and frontal lobes. Infratentorial location is seen in 10%.

4. Non-contrast CT scan shows an irregular hyperdense lesion with large feeding arteries and draining veins. Calcifications can be present. Haemorrhage can be occasionally seen. Usually there is no oedema or mass effect, but when there is haemorrhage, there will be mass effect. On contrast CT scans, there is serpigeneous dense enhancement due to tortuous vessels. If the AVM is thrombosed there is no contrast enhancement. MR shows a flow void with serpigeneous contrast enhancement. Angiogram shows dilated efferent and afferent vessels with AV shunting. Transcatheter embolisation is done by imaging guided catheterisation. Embolisation alone is successful in 40–50%. Surgery and targeted radiation therapy is often necessary after transcatheter embolisation.

5. Complications are haemorrhage, infarction and atrophy. AVMs are seen by the end of the fourth decade and they present with headaches, seizures, mental deterioration and neurological deficit. Risk of rebleeding is 2–3% per year. Mortality rate is 10%.

Neuroradiology Answers

Case 6.17: Answers

1. The CT scan shows a well-defined, lentiform, bright haematoma in the left parieto-occipital region. There is oedema in the underlying brain and compression of the left lateral ventricle with subfalcine herniation to the right side.

2. Acute extradural haematoma.

3. Extradural haematoma is an accumulation of haematoma between the dura mater and the inner table of the skull. Direct trauma results in laceration of arteries, usually the middle meningeal artery. Occasionally meningeal veins, dural venous sinuses or diploic veins are lacerated. It is more common in younger children.

4. Patients present early after injury, with loss of consciousness. There might be a lucid interval, where the patient is normal and then deteriorates. Focal neurological signs, such as hemipariesis and seizures, might develop. Venous bleed is slow and presents late. CT is the main test used for diagnosis. Acute haematoma is hyperdense, subacute is isodense and chronic is hypodense. If there is a hypodense swirl within the haematoma, it indicates active bleeding. The most common location is the temporoparietal region. It is usually associated with skull fractures in 85%. The haematoma is in the extradural compartment and appears lentiform in shape (subdural haematoma is crescenteric). The venous sinuses are separated from the skull. The haematoma produces a mass effect with effacement of underlying gyri and sulci, and displacement of ventricles and herniation. MRI shows signal intensity depending on the stage of haematoma. It shows displacement of venous sinuses away from the inner table.

5. Emergency surgical decompression is indicated and the haematoma is evacuated. Following evacuation, patient should be ventilated, sedated and monitored in ICU. Monitoring of intracranial pressure (ICP) and cerebral perfusion pressure (CPP) is done by placement of ICP monitor. (Ideally – ICP < 25 mmHg and CPP > 70 mmHg). Diuretics are used to reduce brain oedema. Lumbar/ventricular puncture for drainage of CSF or partial lobectomy are done occasionally, if ICP cannot be controlled. Follow-up CT scan is performed if there is poor response to surgery.

Case 6.18: Answers

1. The sagittal view of MRI shows a long cavity within the spinal cord. The cavity has high signal intensity in T2-weighted images, extending through the cervical and upper thoracic levels. The axial T2-weighted image shows a bright fluid-containing space in the centre of the cervical spinal cord

2. Syringomyelia.

3. Syringomyelia is a cavity in the spinal cord that may communicate with the central canal, but not lined by ependymal tissue. Hydromyelia is dilatation of central canal of spinal cord. Although many mechanisms for syrinx formation exist, the exact pathogenesis is not yet known. It is caused by interrupted flow of CSF through the perivascular space of cord between subarachnoid space and central canal. The causes are trauma, post inflammatory, tumours, vascular insufficiency and idiopathic. Syringomyelia is associated with Chiari malformation, Dandy Walker syndrome, spinal dysraphism, myelocele, scoliosis, diastomatomyelia, Klippel Feil syndrome, segmentation defects and tethered cord.

4. Loss of pain and temperature, trophic changes in the skin, muscle weakness, spasticity, hyperreflexia and abnormal plantar reflexes are seen. It is usually seen in the cervical cord, and can extend into the thoracic level or the brain stem. Treatment options are suboccipital/cervical decompression, laminectomy with syringotomy, insertion of syringopleural or syringoperitoneal/lumboperitoneal/syringoperitoneal shunt, fourth ventriculostomy, terminal ventriculostomy, percutaneous needling and neuroendoscopic surgery.

5. MRI is the imaging procedure of choice. It shows a longitudinal CSF-filled cavity, low signal in T1 and high signal in T2. Usually the wall is smooth, but it may be beaded with metameric haustrations in syringomyelia secondary to tumour. Traumatic syringomyelia has septations, irregular borders and arachnoid loculations. Serial examinations are required for evaluating changes in cavity size over time. Phase contrast MRI can be used to analyse CSF flow dynamics. CT shows low-density areas, with no contrast enhancement. The cord is enlarged. A CT myelogram will demonstrate delayed filling of the cysts. In hydromyelia, the central canal is dilated with CSF. Differential diagnoses for syringomyelia include other intramedullary lesions such as tumours, infarcts, demyelination, infections, and vascular malformations.

Case 6.19: Answers

1. MRI shows multiple, small, ring-enhancing lesions in the brain. In the first scan, it is seen in the midbrain. In the second, there are multiple lesions in the cerebral and cerebellar hemispheres.

2. Tuberculoma of the brain.

3. TB spreads by haematogenous dissemination to the subependymal or subpial focus (**Rich** focus) and subsequent seeding of the brain parenchyma

4. Tuberculoma is granuloma formation within the brain parenchyma. It is common in the cerebellar hemispheres and may be associated with tuberculous meningitis. It is common in children and young adults. It is solitary in 70%. Clinical features are headache, seizures and focal neurological deficits.

5. The imaging findings of tuberculoma are variable, because it is an evolving granuloma. In the acute phase, a CT scan may be normal or hypodense focus. After the inflammation is established, it is usually isodense or hypodense with ill-defined margins as a result of minimal surrounding oedema, and shows marked contrast enhancement. When the granuloma caseates, it is hypo-/iso-/hyperdense, with occasional calcifications. Contrast enhancement can be homogeneous or nodular or rim enhancement (target sign – central calcification in isodense lesion with rim enhancement). Calcification can be seen. In early stages, MRI shows a hypointense lesion in T1, hyperintense in T2 and homogeneous nodular enhancement. After a granuloma is formed, the lesion is iso- to hyperintense on T2 with rim enhancement. The core is hypointense in T1 and hyperintense in T2.

6. Differential diagnoses: cysticercosis, toxoplasmosis, bacterial abscess, fungal infections, lymphoma, glioma, metastasis, vasculitis.

Case 6.20: Answers

1. There is high-density blood in the subarachnoid space and all the ventricles.

2. Intraventricular haemorrhage.

3. Intraventricular haemorrhage usually extends from a subarachnoid bleed. The causes are rupture of an aneurysm, rupture of an AVM, spontaneous intracerebral haemorrhage, ventricular angiomas, bleeding tumours, blunt head trauma and ventriculitis.

4. A CT scan shows high-density blood in the ventricles. MRI shows signal changes depending on the age of the haemorrhage.

5. If the patient responds to treatment, hydrocephalus is the main complication. The ventricles are dilated and there may be periventricular hypodensity due to transependymal edema. Intraventricular haemorrhage as such is not a bad prognostic indicator. It usually resolves on its own. The primary condition such as an aneurysm or AVM should be treated. If hydrocephalus develops, external ventricular drainage is done with intraventricular catheter. Drainage is done even when there is haemorrhage near the outlet orifices and hydrocephalus is imminent. The drainage should be slow when there is an unruptured aneurysm. The sudden lowering of CSF pressure might cause a big difference in transmural pressure, which results in rupture of aneurysm. Thrombolytics can be introduced through the catheter to relieve obstruction.

Case 6.21: Answers

1. MRI shows a well-defined, rounded lobular mass arising in the left cerebellopontine angle. The mass is seen extending into the internal acoustic meatus. The mass is isointense on a non-contrast scan and shows intense contrast enhancement.

2. Acoustic neuroma.

3. Acoustic neuroma arises from the vestibular division of the eighth nerve. In 15% it arises from the cochlea; 85% of these lesions arise from inside the internal auditory canal and extend to the cerebellopontine angle. The tumour is a schwannoma with cellular dense regions (Antoni A) and loose areas with widely separated cells in reticulated matrix (Antoni B). Clinically it presents with sensorineural deafness that is slowly progressive, tinnitus, pain, diminished corneal reflex, unsteadiness, vertigo, ataxia and dizziness.

4. A CT scan shows a round, isodense mass arising from the internal auditory canal and extending into the cerebellopontine angle. There is a funnel-shaped component extending into the internal auditory canal. The cerebellopontine angle cistern is widened. Hydrocephalus can be seen. The mass is isodense in non-contrast with areas of cyst formation and necrosis and no calcification. There is homogeneous enhancement. MRI shows iso- or hypointense signal in T1, hyperintense signal in T2 and an intense enhancing homogeneous mass on contrast. Acoustic neuroma is usually diagnosed by high-resolution axial MRI. Images are acquired in axial and coronal planes, without contrast. Normally there is high signal around the roots of nerve VIII. Absence of this high signal indicates a neuroma. Large tumours do not require further evaluation. If there is small lesion that is suspicious, contrast is administered for evaluating tumours. **Intracanalicular neuroma**: this type of acoustic neuroma is confined to the internal auditory canal, and is best diagnosed by contrast-enhanced MRI. Bilateral acoustic neuroma are associated with type 2 neurofibromatosis, which are rare, familial and result from deletion of gene chromosome 22.

5. Differential diagnoses: **meningiomas** (broad based, no intracanalicular extension, dural tail), **aneurysm, epidermoid cyst** (high signal in T1, increased diffusion signal), **arachnoid cyst** (same signal as CSF in all sequences), ependymoma, **trigeminal neuroma** and **metastasis**.

Case 6.22: Answers

1. The MRI scan shows a large heterogeneously enhancing mass in the left frontal cortex, with central areas of necrosis and peripheral enhancement, with compression of the frontal horn of the left lateral ventricle.

2. Glioblastoma multiforme.

3. Glioblastoma multiforme is the most malignant form of all gliomas and is the most common primary brain tumour. The peak age is 65–75 years. The common locations are in the cerebral hemisphere – white matter of centrum semiovale – in the frontal and temporal lobes. Other locations are corpus callosum (butterfly glioma), posterior fossa and extra-axial sites.

4. It is associated with neurofibromatosis 1, Turcot syndrome and Fraumeni syndrome. Multifocal glioblastoma multiforme is caused by spread of primary glioblastoma multiforme or malignant degeneration in a diffuse low-grade glioma of the brain known as gliomatosis cerebri, or as an inherited abnormality. The tumour spreads by direct extension along the white matter, through the subependymal route, via CSF or by haematogenous spread.

5. A CT scan shows a heterogeneous mass with areas of haemorrhage, necrosis and cyst formation. The margins are not well defined and there is a significant mass effect with oedema, compression of ventricles and midline shift to the contralateral side. Usually there is diffuse heterogeneous enhancement and occasionally it may show a rim enhancement such as an abscess. MRI shows an ill-defined lesion, hypointense in T1 and heterogeneously hyperintense in T2, with surrounding oedema. There is significant contrast enhancement of the solid portions. Increased uptake is seen on the PET scan.

6. Differential diagnoses for rim-enhancing lesions: abscess, lymphoma, metastasis, haematoma, resolving infarct and tumefactive demyelination

Case 6.23: Answers

1. MRI of the brain shows contrast enhancement of the meninges, surrounding the brain (note the bright areas surrounding the brain; in normal brain, no enhancement is seen around the brain parenchyma).

2. Causes of leptomeningeal enhancement are sarcoidosis, histiocytosis, Wegener's granulomatosis, meningitis (bacterial, fungal, viral, neurosyphilis, chemical), tumours (meningioma, gliomatosis cerebri, glioblastomatosis, melanoma, sarcoma, lymphoma, CSF spread from primary tumours such as medulloblastoma, germinoma, pineoblastoma).

3. Neurosarcoidosis. Sarcoidosis is a multisystemic disease process, characterised by presence of inflammatory granulomas. It is seen in the fourth or fifth decade of life.

4. MRI shows leptomeningeal enhancement. Periventricular high signal lesions, intra- or extra-axial masses, optic nerve enhancement and spinal cord intramedullary lesions can be seen. Other features of sarcoidosis, such as hilar and mediastinal nodes, and pulmonary involvement may be seen. In 5–15% of cases, lytic areas and coarseness of trabeculi may be seen in small bones of hands and feet.

5. Sarcoidosis can affect pituitary gland, optic nerve, eye (iridocyclitis, choroiditis) meninges, cerebral parenchyma (infarct, transient ischemic attack) spinal cord, (myelopathy, radicuolopathy), brainstem and cerebellum and peripheral nerves (mononeuropathy, polyneuropathy). The patients are treated with steroids in the acute phase.

Case 6.24: Answers

1. Axial T2-weighted image of MRI shows a high signal area in the centre of the pons. The rest of the brain appears normal.

2. Central pontine myelinolysis.

3. Central pontine myelinosis (osmotic demyelination) is produced by rapid correction or overcorrection of severe hyponatraemia, which results in destruction of myelin sheaths as a result of release of myelinotoxic compounds, with preserved axons and neurons. It is common in people with chronic alcohol problems and in chronic intravenous fluid administration. Another theory proposes that, in regions of compact interdigitation of white and grey matter (such as the pons), cellular oedema resulting from fluctuating osmotic forces causes compression of fibre tracts and induces demyelination. During the period of hyponatraemia, the concentration of intracellularly charged protein moieties is altered; reversal cannot parallel a rapid correction of electrolyte status. Risk factors are serum sodium < 120 mmol/L for > 48 hours, aggressive intravenous therapy with hypertonic saline and development of hypernatraemia during treatment. It is also seen in liver transplant recipients, people with burns and Wilson's disease.

4. The most common location is the centre of the pons. Occasionally myelinolysis occurs in extrapontine locations such as basal ganglia, cerebellum, thalamus, caudate nucleus, subcortical white matter, corona radiata and lateral geniculate body. Clinical features are quadriparesis, changing levels of consciousness, locked-in syndrome, pseudobulbar palsy, coma and death.

5. CT shows central hypodensity. MRI shows low signal intensity in T1 and high signal in T2. Differential diagnoses are infarcts, glioma, hypoxia, demyelination, radiation, toxins, Leigh's disease and Wilson's disease. Diagnosis is established by clinical correlation.

Case 6.25: Answers

1. MRI shows a well-defined, broad-based, isointense lesion in the right parietal region, which is enhancing intensely on the contrast scans, with minimal perilesional oedema.

2. Meningioma.

3. Meningioma is the most common benign tumour in brain. It is derived from arachnoid cap cells, which are meningothelial cells that penetrate the dura. The most common locations are the convexity, parasagittal region, sphenoidal ridge and olfactory groove. It can be seen in the ventricles and other sites in the brain. Ectopic meningiomas can be seen outside the brain. Meningomas are seen in middle- and old-aged people, more common in women. It is associated with neurofibromatosis type 2, where meningiomas can be multiple. There is an association with basal cell naevus syndrome.

4. The histological types are fibroblastic, transitional, meningothelial and angioblastic. The last two are aggressive. It is multicentric in 2–10%. Meningiomas can be discrete globular masses or seen as en plaque, which is associated with just hyperostosis. Other variants are cystic meningiomas or lipoblastic meningiomas. On plain skull films, calcification, hyperostosis and prominent vascular grooves are seen. A CT scan shows a well-defined extra-axial mass, which is located outside the brain parenchyma. Meningiomas have a broad base, displace the grey–white matter interface inside and have a cleft between the mass and brain (CSF vascular cleft). The mass is hyper- or isodense, with calcifications and hyperostosis of adjacent bone. After contrast, there is intense enhancement of the mass, with a dural tail of enhancement. There is minimal oedema. MRI shows similar appearance with low signal in T1. The signal in T2 is lower in fibrous types and higher in more aggressive types, and there is intense contrast enhancement with the dural tail. As an extra-axial mass, the meningioma is supplied by branches of the external carotid artery. The most common supply is from middle meningeal artery. In angiography, the tumour fills early with contrast and there is a persistent blush. These may exhibit spoke-wheel configuration.

5. Differential diagnoses of meningioma are glioma (intra-axial), metastasis, lymphoma and haemangiopericytoma, Asymptomatic small meningiomas are followed up. Large meningiomas are surgically resected.

Case 6.26: Answers

1. This is contrast-enhanced MRI of the brain obtained in the sagittal plane. MRI of the brain shows multiple enhancing masses in the inferior cerebellum and upper cervical spine.

2. Haemangioblastoma.

3. Von Hippel–Lindau syndrome.

4. The CT scan of the abdomen shows multiple, hypodense cysts in the pancreas. There is also a small solid tumour in the right kidney, which is a renal cell carcinomas.

5. Haemangioblastoma is a benign tumour of vascular origin. It is commonly seen in the cerebellar hemispheres. It can also be seen in the spinal cord, cerebral hemispheres or brain stem. The lesion can be solid, cystic with a mural nodule or cystic. The CT scan shows a well-defined cyst or a cyst with an enhancing nodule or a solid enhancing lesion. MRI shows a cyst with low signal in T1 and a high signal in T2, with a solid nodule within, which shows intense enhancement. Flow voids are seen in the solid component. Haemorrhage gives high signal in both. Oedema is seen around the tumour. Angiography shows a vascular nidus in the cyst. Draining veins are seen. It is associated with von Hippel–Lindau disease, which is characterised by cerebellar and spinal cord haemangioblastomas, cysts of the pancreas and kidneys, endolymphatic sac tumour, rhabdomyoma of the heart, renal carcinoma, phaeochromocytoma, cystadenoma of the epididymis, islet cell tumour, liver adenoma and paraganglioma. Renal cell carcinomas in von Hippel–Lindau syndrome occur at a younger age, and are frequently multiple and bilateral compared with renal carcinomas in those without the syndrome.

6. Differential diagnoses: **pilocytic astrocytoma** (cerebellar hemisphere, large cyst > 5 cm, thick wall, mural nodule not as vascular; **medulloblastoma** (solid, vermis); **arachnoid cyst** (no mural nodule); **metastasis** (more oedema)

Case 6.27: Answers

1. Non contrast CT scan shows a hyperdense lesion in the right middle cranial fossa, adjacent to the midline, which shows very intense enhancement after contrast. There is some mass effect with some distortion of the right lateral ventricle, but no perilesional oedema is noted.

2. Cerebral aneurysm.

3. Most of the aneurysms are congenital berry aneurysms. Others are atherosclerotic or mycotic, traumatic, neoplastic, or caused by collagen vascular disease and fibromuscular disease. Risk factors are family history, age > 50, female, Marfan syndrome, Ehler–Danlos syndrome, pseudoxanthoma elasticum, neurofibromatosis type 1, polycystic kidney disease and AVM. Multiple aneurysms are seen in fibromuscular hyperplasia, coarctation, Ehlers–Danlos syndrome, AVM, SLE, polycystic kidney disease and coarctation. The most common location of a cerebral aneurysm is the circle of Willis, especially at the bifurcations. The most common location is the anterior communicating artery, posterior communicating artery and (MCA) bifurcation.

4. Aneurysms present with subarachnoid haemorrhage, which is seen as bright blood in the sulci, cisterns and fissures. An aneurysm can be calcified or non-calcified. In the non-contrast scan, it is hyperdense (especially if there is thrombus) or hypodense. Contrast enhancement is homogeneous when there is no thrombus and circumferential if there is central thrombosis. The MRI signal depends on thrombus and flow. There might be signal void if there is fast flow and mixed signal if there is mixed thrombosis. CT angiography and MRA will demonstrate an aneurysm in a non-invasive way replacing the conventional angiogram as a routine diagnositc tool. When an aneurysm ruptures intracerebal haematoma occurs. The underlying aneurysm can be diagnosed based on the location of the haematoma:

   Interhemispheric fissure – anterior communicating artery (AcoA)

   Sylvian fissure: MCA

   Prepontine cistern: basilar artery

   Foramen magnum: posterior inferior cerebellar artery (PICA)

   Corpus callosum: pericallosal artery.

5. Previously all suspected aneurysms were diagnosed with a cerebral angiography. Currently, all patients with suspected aneurysm, based on the presence of subarachnoid haemorrhage, undergo CT angiography or MRA, which gives information about the location, number, size, neck and sac of aneurysm. Surgical clamping of aneurysms is done only when coil occlusion cannot be done. Ten per cent die within 24 hours as a result of haemorrhage, herniation, infarcts and brain-stem haemorrhage. Complete recovery is seen in 5%. Rebleeding is seen 10–20% in 2 weeks, 10–20% in 1 month and 50% in 6 months. Risk of death from surgery is 50% for ruptured and 1–3% for unruptured aneurysms. Endovascular techniques have been developed in recent years whereby these aneurysms can be treated by packing them with platinum coils under radiographic control, thus minimising risks from surgery.

Case 6.28: Answers

1. The CT scan shows a large area of low density in the entire right cerebral hemisphere. There is minimal compression of the right lateral ventricle, but there is no midline shift to the left side.

2. Large non-haemorrhagic infarct in the right cerebral hemisphere in the right MCA territory.

3. Infarct is caused by a thrombotic or embolic occlusion of a large artery, or small vessel occlusion, coagulopathies, cardiac causes, vasculitis and non-arteriosclerotic causes. Cerebral hemispheres are the most common location, with the MCA territory the most commonly affected.

4. Routine CT is not positive until 12–24 hours. MRI is positive within a few minutes of onset of the stroke. Early diagnosis is useful if intra-arterial thrombolysis is contemplated. MRI protocol consists of T1- and T2-weighted images, susceptibility imaging (for haemorrhage), diffusion and perfusion imaging. Earliest signs in CT are dense MCA sign (bright MCA as a result of hyperdense thrombus), insular ribbon sign (hypodense external capsule not distinguishable from insular cortex), loss of differentiation between grey and white matter, low-density basal ganglia and subtle sulcal effacement. CT shows obvious changes from 24 hours. A hypodense wedge-shaped lesion is seen as a result of cytotoxic oedema. Mass effect is seen in the acute stage, with sulcal effacement and herniation. Enhancement of the cerebral gyri may be seen between 7 and 30 days. MRI shows low signal in T1, high signal in T2, with blurring of the grey–white matter junction, meningeal enhancement, enhancement of cortical arteries and gyriform enhancement. Haemorrhagic conversion occurs after 2–4 days because of leakage of blood from ischaemically damaged capillaries after reperfusion. Eventually the infarct liquefies and leaves an area of encephalomalacia and brain atrophy with gliosis. Calcification can be seen in children.

5. Presence of haemorrhage and a massive infarct involving more than 2/3rds of cerebral hemisphere detected on CT scan, history of stroke or serious head injury within 3 months, presence of aneurysm/AVM in brain, history of seizure at onset of strokeand anticoagulated patients with INR > 1.5 are contraindications for thrombolysis.

Case 6.29: Answers

1. CT shows a well-defined hypodensity in the lentiform nucleus of basal ganglia on the left side.

2. Lacunar infarct.

3. Lacunar infarcts are small infarcts < 15 mm, caused by fibrinoid degeneration and occlusion of small perforating vessels, which are the lenticulostriate, thalamoperforating, pontine perforating and recurrent artery of Heubner. It is seen in people with diabetes and hypertension. The upper two-thirds of the putamen, caudate nucleus, thalamus, pons and internal capsule are the common locations.

4. Pure motor syndrome, pure sensory syndrome, ataxia, dysarthria clumsy hand syndrome and abnormal movements are the various types of lacunar infarct syndromes.

5. CT shows well-defined hypodense lesions, < 15 mm in the basal ganglia and thalamus. The lesions show higher signal than CSF due to gliosis. MRI shows low signal in T1 and high signal in T2, Differential diagnosis of T2 bright lesions in MRI are – multiple sclerosis, ischaemic changes, vaculitis, infection (tuberculosis, cysticercosis), haematoma, etc.

Case 6.30: Answers

1. This is high-resolution MRI of the brain. The coronal image through the temporal lobe shows a normal appearance of the left temporal lobe, including the hippocampus. There is slight atrophy of the right hippocampus, with dilatation of the temporal horn. There is also a high signal in the right hippocampus (compare with the left side, which has a signal similar to the normal brain parenchyma)

2. Mesial temporal sclerosis.

3. Epilepsy is a common neurological disorder characterised by recurrent, unprovoked seizures. Causes are mesial temporal sclerosis, developmental venous anomaly, tuberous sclerosis, heterotopias/cortical dysplasias, perinatal hypoxia, infections, traumatic scarring, tumours and vascular malformations.

4. Temporal lobe epilepsy manifests with complex partial seizures. The most common cause of complex partial seizures is mesial temporal sclerosis (35–65%), in which the hippocampus is small. It is usually unilateral, but can be bilateral in 10–15% of cases. The epileptogenic focus involves structures in the mesial temporal lobe such as the hippocampus, amygdala and parahippocampal gyrus. Mesial temporal sclerosis is seen in 65% of temporal lobectomy specimens obtained in temporal lobe epilepsy. Interictal EEGs demonstrate epileptiform discharges over the region of the affected temporal lobe. Whether mesial temporal sclerosis is the cause or the result of temporal lobe epilepsy is debatable. Patients present with complex partial seizures that can become generalised. Interictal EEG demonstrates epileptiform discharges over the region of affected temporal lobe.

5. MRI is the best imaging modality to detect and delineate brain lesions in partial seizures, especially temporal lobe lesions. Thin-section, high-resolution coronal MR images are the most useful for detecting these lesions. In T1-weighted images, the affected side is small as a result of hippocampal atrophy, with associated dilatation of the temporal horn of the lateral ventricle. In T2-weighted images, a high signal is seen in the affected hippocampus, as a result of gliosis and increased free water content. The FLAIR sequence suppresses the fluid in the surrounding temporal horn of the lateral ventricle and makes the high signal in the

hippocampus conspicuous. Quantitative three-dimensional volume measurements can be used. MRI is also useful in diagnosing other causes of epilepsy. MR spectroscopy shows reduced *N*-acetylaspartate. Tumours produce mass effect and show contrast enhancement. Cortical dysplasias are similar to tumours, without enhancement, and have a signal similar to the grey matter of the brain. Cavernous angiomas are the most common vascular malformations associated with seizures. Post-traumatic scarring produces a high signal.

7
MUSCULOSKELETAL
RADIOLOGY
QUESTIONS

Case 7.1

A 37-year-old woman presents with right knee pain and swelling. Clinical examination showed a tender right knee with limited flexion and extension. There is no history of trauma and medical history is unremarkable.

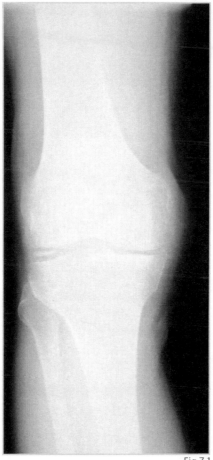

Fig 7.1

1. What are the findings on the X-ray of the knee?
2. What is the diagnosis?
3. What is the differential diagnosis for this appearance?
4. What is the most common cause of this appearance in the lateral compartment of the knee?
5. What are the pathological and radiological features?.

Answers *on pages 427–453*

Case 7.2

A 56-year-old patient with a chronic disease presents with pain in the right foot.

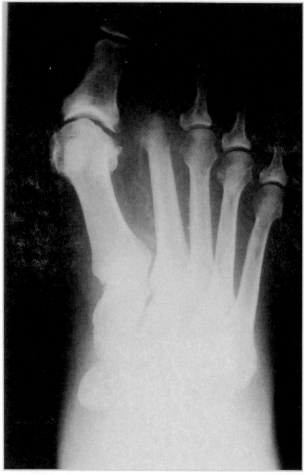

Fig 7.2

1. What are the findings on the X-ray?
2. What is the diagnosis?
3. What is the pathophysiology of this disease process?
4. What are the radiological features?
5. What are the complications?
6. What is the role of imaging in this disease? What is the most important diagnostic dilemma in this condition?

Answers *on pages 427–453*

Case 7.3

A 45-year-old man presents with pain around the wrist and ankle joints. On examination, there is digital clubbing, with swelling, redness and tenderness in the wrists and ankles.

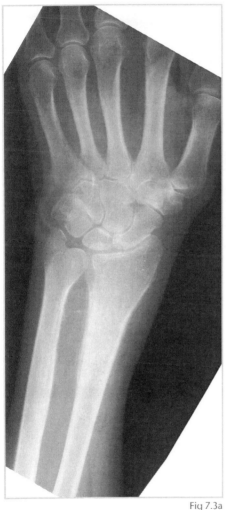

Fig 7.3a

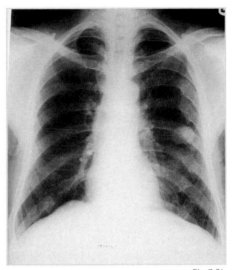

Fig 7.3b

1. What do you see on the X-ray of the wrist?

2. What do you find on the second X-ray?

3. What is the diagnosis and what is the cause?

4. What are the other causes of this condition?

5. What are the pathophysiology and the radiological features?

6. What is the radiological differential diagnosis?

Answers *on pages 427–453*

A 13-year-old boy presented with severe low back pain and fever for 3 days. On examination acute tenderness was noted in the lower lumbar spine. No neurological deficit was detected.

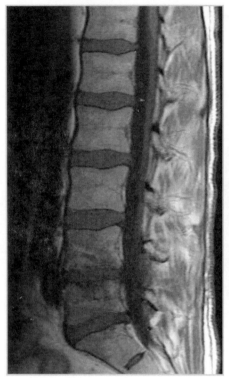

Fig 7.4a

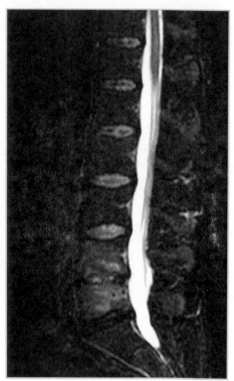

Fig 7.4b

1. What are the observations on MRI?

2. What is the diagnosis?

3. What are the clinical features and what further investigations are required?

4. What are the radiological features?

5. What is the management of this condition?

Answers on pages 427–453

Case 7.5

A 41-year-old woman presents with pain, swelling and stiffness of the hands and feet. She had severe pain and tenderness in the cervical spine.

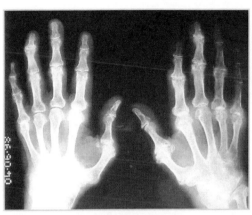
Fig 7.5a

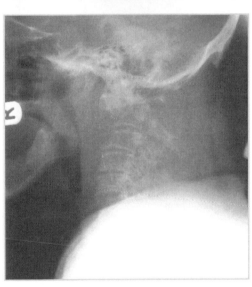
Fig 7.5b

1. What are the findings on the X-rays of the hand and spine?
2. What is the diagnosis?
3. What are the diagnostic criteria?
4. What are the characteristic locations?
5. What are the typical radiological features and complications?
6. What is the differential diagnosis?

Answers *on pages 427–453*

A 45-year-old man presents with pain and swelling in his left foot. On clinical examination, his right great toe is very tender and red.

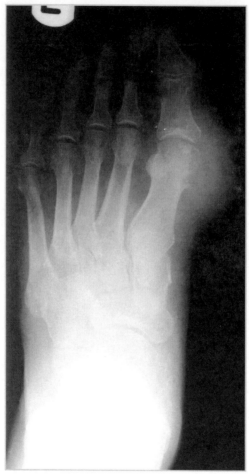

Fig 7.6

1. What are the findings on the X-ray of the foot?
2. What is the diagnosis?
3. What are the pathology and location of this disease?
4. What are the radiological features?
5. What is the differential diagnosis?

Answers on pages 427–453

Case 7.7

A 67-year-old woman presents with severe pain in her right foot. She is known to have diabetes, maintained on insulin. On examination, her foot is warm, red and tender. Lab analysis shows an elevated WBC.

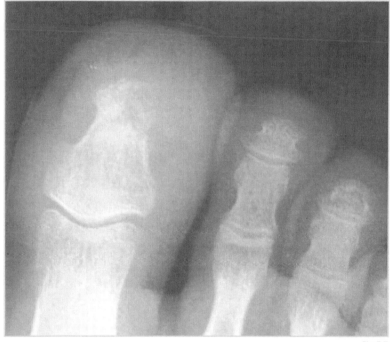

Fig 7.7

1. What do you see on the X-ray of the foot?
2. What is the diagnosis?
3. What are the causes of the disease?
4. What are the clinical features and complications?
5. What are the radiological features and treatment?

Case 7.8

A 69-year-old man presents with severe pain in the left knee. Clinical examination showed a tender right knee, with restriction of joint movements.

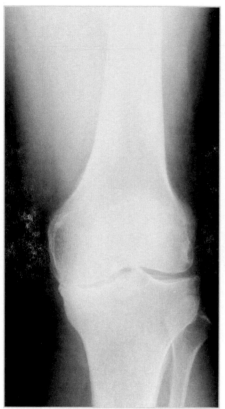

Fig 7.8a

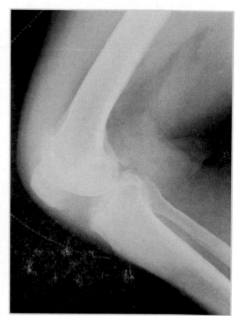

Fig 7.8b

1. What are the findings on the X-ray of the knee?
2. What is the diagnosis?
3. What are the predisposing factors and pathological features?
4. What are the common locations?
5. What are the radiological features and differential diagnosis?

Answers on pages 427–453

Case 7.9

A 45-year-old woman presents with deformities in her fingers and digital swelling.

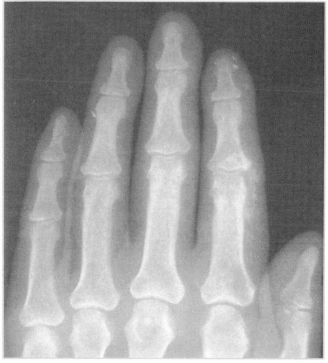

Fig 7.9

1.   What are the findings on the X-ray of the hand?
2.   What is the diagnosis?
3.   What are the radiological features?
4.   What are the common sites of this disease?
5.   What is the differential diagnosis?

Answers on pages 427–453

A 16-year-old girl presents with back pain, fever, night sweats and weight loss.

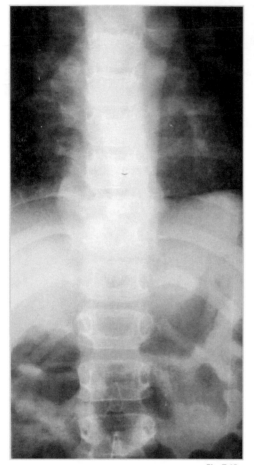

Fig 7.10a

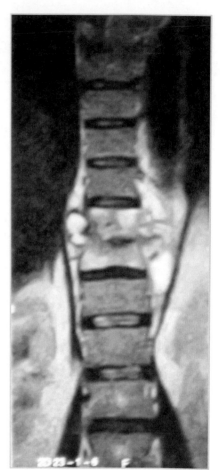

Fig 7.10b

1. What do you see on the X-ray of the spine and MRI?

2. What is the diagnosis?

3. What are the pathophysiology and mode of spread?

4. What are the clinical and radiological features?

5. What is the differential diagnosis?

Answers on pages 427–453

Case 7.11

An 11-year-old boy presents with dull pain in his left leg, which is worse in the night. On examination, there is a red, tender swelling in the medial aspect of the left tibia.

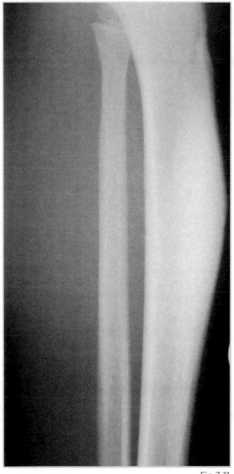

Fig 7.11

1. What are the findings on the X-ray?
2. What is the diagnosis?
3. What are the clinical features and pathology?
4. What are the radiological features?
5. What is the differential diagnosis and the treatment?

Answers *on pages 427–453*

A 14-year-old boy presents with failure to thrive, generalised bone pain and vomiting.

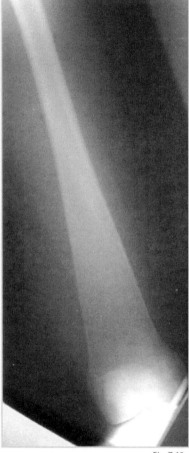

Fig 7.12a

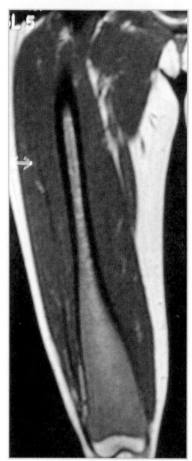

Fig 7.12b

1. What do you note on the X-ray and MRI?
2. What is the diagnosis?
3. What is the aetiopathology?
4. What is the differential diagnosis?
5. What are the clinical and radiological features of this disorder?

Answers on pages 427–453

Case 7.13

A 37-year-old woman presents with pain, tenderness and restricted movements of the right shoulder joint.

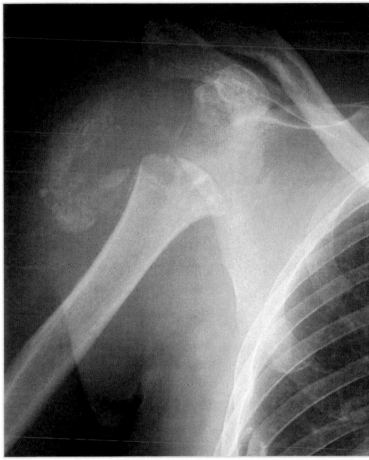

Fig 7.13

1. What are the findings on the X-ray?
2. What is the diagnosis?
3. What is the pathology of this disease?
4. What are the causes and types of this disorder?
5. What are the radiological features and differential diagnosis?

Answers *on pages 427–453*

A 74-year-old woman presents with backache. On examination, there is tenderness in the lower dorsal and upper lumbar vertebrae with restriction of movements.

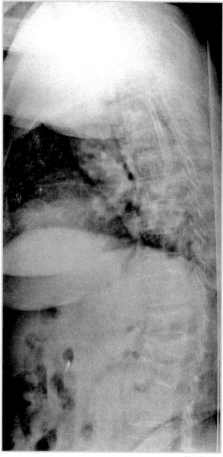
Fig 7.14a

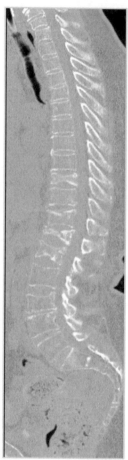
Fig 7.14b

1. What are the findings on the X-ray and CT scan?
2. What is the diagnosis?
3. What are the causes?
4. What are the radiological features? What are the other investigations that might be required in this patient?
5. What are the complications and what is the role of radiology in treatment?

Answers on pages 427–453

Case 7.15

A 61 year old presents with diffuse bone pain. On examination, there is tenderness in the pelvis and spine. Serum calcium and phosphorus are normal, but the serum alkaline phosphatase is elevated. The prostate-specific antigen (PSA) is normal.

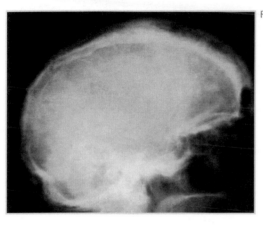
Fig 7.15a

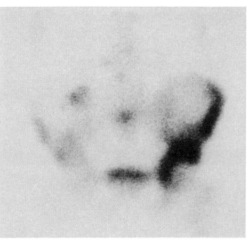
Fig 7.15b

1. What do you see on the X-ray of the skull and the bone scan of the pelvis?
2. What is the diagnosis?
3. What are the aetiology and progression of this disease?
4. What are the clinical and radiological features?
5. What are the complications and differential diagnosis of this disease? What is the treatment?

Answers on pages 427–453

Case 7.16

A 27-year-old woman presents with a skin condition and arthralgias in the hands and feet. On examination, the distal joints in the hands and feet are swollen, red and tender, with restriction of movements.

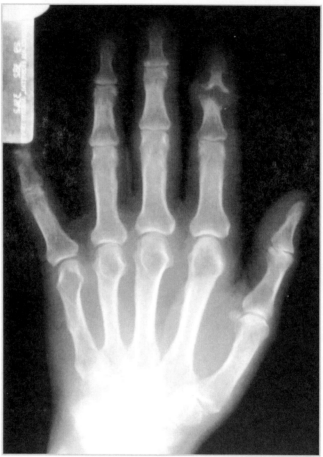

Fig 7.16

1. What are the findings on the X-ray of the hand?
2. What is the diagnosis?
3. What are the pathology and location of this disease?
4. What are the radiological features?
5. What is the differential diagnosis?

Answers on pages 427–453

A 14-year-old boy presents with fever, pain and stiffness of multiple joints, especially the elbow and knee joints. On examination, there is tenderness and restricted movements of multiple joints.

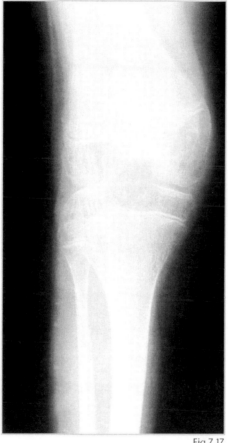

Fig 7.17

1. What do you see on the plain X-ray of the right knee?
2. What is the diagnosis?
3. What are the clinical features?
4. What are the radiological features?
5. What is the differential diagnosis?

Answers *on pages 427–453*

Case 7.18

A 37-year-old woman presents with malaise and body pain. X-rays of the chest and abdomen were done as part of her work-up.

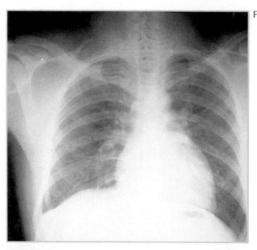

Fig 7.18a

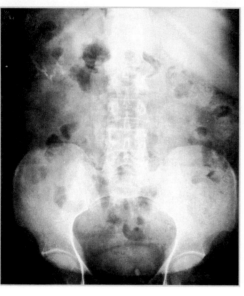

Fig 7.18b

1. What do you observe on the X-rays?
2. What is the diagnosis?
3. What is the aetiopathology of this disease?
4. What is the differential diagnosis?
5. What are the other causes of tthis radiological appearance?

Answers on pages 427–453

Case 7.19

A 13-year-old boy presents with skin rashes, muscular weakness and pain.

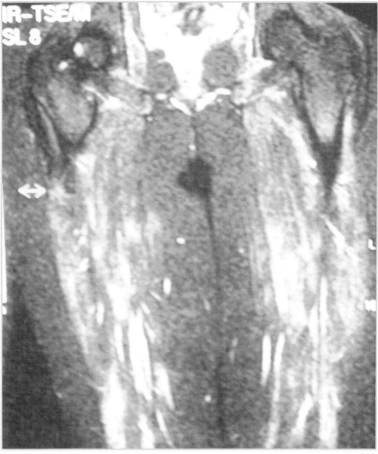

Fig 7.19

1. What do you see on the contrast enhanced MRI of the thigh?
2. What is the diagnosis?
3. What other investigations are needed?
4. What are the clinical features?
5. What are the radiological features and the treatment?

Answers *on pages 427–453*

Case 7.20

A 12-year-old girl presents with pain, tenderness and restricted movements of the right arm. She also has precocious puberty. On examination, she has severe tenderness on the proximal shaft of the right humerus and excessive pigmentation of the skin.

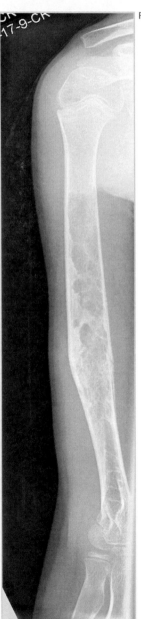

Fig 7.20

1. What are the findings on the X-ray?
2. What is the diagnosis?
3. What are the pathology and clinical features?
4. What are the radiological features and differential diagnosis?
5. What are the complications?

Answers on pages 427–453

Case 7.21

A 75-year-old woman presents with diffuse bone pain, especially in the hip and spine. On clinical examination, there is diffuse bony tenderness and limitation of joint movements.

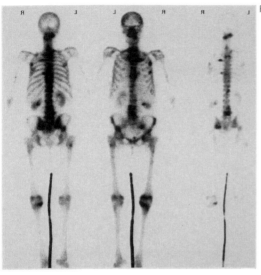

Fig 7.21a

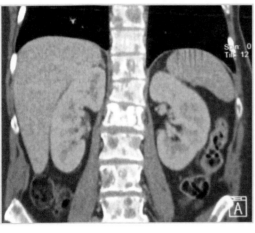

Fig 7.21b

1. What are the findings on the bone scan and the CT scan?
2. What is the diagnosis?
3. What are the causes of this disease?
4. What are the different radiographic appearances of this lesion?
5. What is the differential diagnosis?

Answers *on pages 427–453*

A 4-year-old boy presents with failure to thrive, irritability and bowed legs. On examination there are bilateral knock-knees and an abnormal skull.

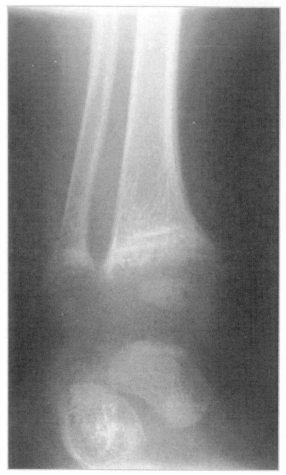

Fig 7.22

1. What are the findings on the X-ray of the ankle?
2. What is the diagnosis?
3. What is the pathophysiology of this disease?
4. What are the causative factors?
5. What are the radiological features and differential diagnosis?

Answers on pages 427–453

Case 7.23

A 5-year-old boy with severe growth retardation and deformities had a skeletal survey.

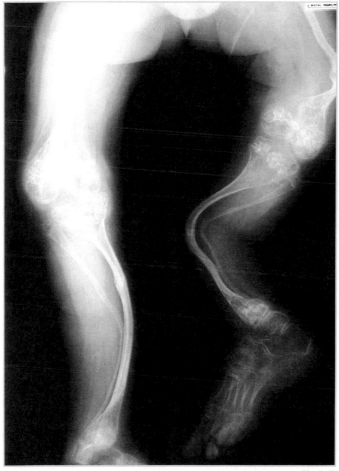

Fig 7.23

1. What are the findings on the X-ray?
2. What is the diagnosis?
3. What are the types of this disease?
4. What are the radiological features?
5. What is the differential diagnosis?

Answers *on pages 427–453*

A 35-year-old man presents with low backache. On examination, there is tenderness in the lower lumbar spine and restriction of flexion and extension.

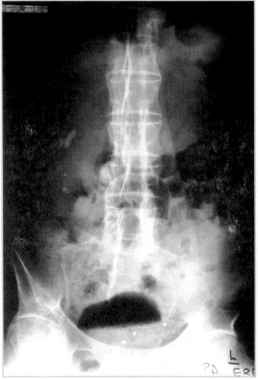

Fig 7.24a

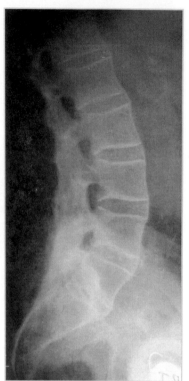

Fig 7.24b

1. What do you find on the AP and lateral view of the lumbar spine?
2. What is the diagnosis?
3. What are the associations and pathology of this disease?
4. What are the radiological features?
5. What are the differential diagnosis and the systemic complications?

Answers on pages 427–453

A 47-year-old man presents with fatigue, malaise, and pain in his shoulders and hips.

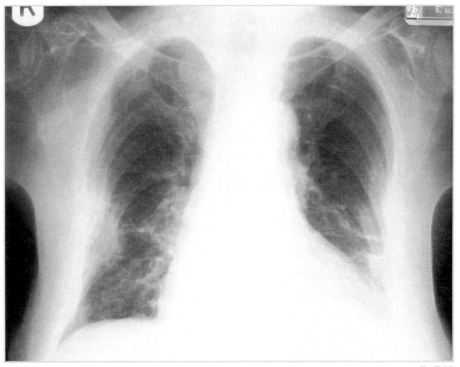

Fig 7.25

1. What do you observe on the chest X-ray?
2. What is the diagnosis?
3. What are the causes and pathology of this disease?
4. What are the clinical and radiological features?
5. What is the differential diagnosis?

Answers *on pages 427–453*

Case 7.1: Answers

1. X-ray of the knee, shows calcification in the lateral compartment of the knee joint, involving the lateral meniscus. There is some narrowing of the medial joint space.

2. Chondrocalcinosis of the lateral meniscus.

3. Chondrocalcinosis is calcification of the cartilage and can be caused by ageing, pseudogout (CPPD), gout, ochronosis, arthritis (rheumatoid, degenerative, traumatic, infections), acromegaly, haemochromatosis, Wilson's disease, haemophilia, hypothyroidism, hyperparathyroidism, hypophosphatasia, familial hypomagnesaemia and diabetes mellitus.

4. CPPD (calcium pyrophosphate deposition disease) – also called pseudogout.

5. CPPD is an arthritis variant, in which calcium pyrophosphate crystals are deposited in hyaline cartilage, synovial tissue, capsule, meniscus, labrum, ligamentum flavum, soft tissues of the hand and fibrocartilage of the temporomandibular joint. The exact physiological dysfunction is not clear. Some noxious event initiates a cascade that causes hypertrophy and degeneration of chondrocytes. Intracellular material extends to the surrounding matrix and alters the calcium-binding effect of matrix proteoglycans. Calcium pyrophosphate crystals grow adjacent to these hypertrophic chondrocytes. There are four clinical presentations of this disease: **pseudogout, tophaceous pseudogout, familial calcium pyrophosphate dihydrate deposition** and **osteoarthritis**. Pseudogout has the same features as gout, but pseudogout crystals are rod or rhomboid shaped and have no or weak positive birefringence. The knee is most commonly affected. The shoulder, elbow, ankle and first metatarsophalangeal (MTP) joint are also affected. The onset is sudden and spontaneous resolution occurs.

Case 7.2: Answers

1. X-ray shows vascular calcification of small arteries in the foot and destruction of the head of the 2nd metatarsal bone. The phalanges of the 2nd toe are missing, suggestive of surgical amputation. There is some degenerative change in the first metatarsophalangeal joint and hallux valgus deformity.

2. Diabetic foot.

3. 25% of diabetics develop foot problem. Diabetic foot is a combination of peripheral arterial disease, neuropathy and infection. Neuropathy affects sensory, motor and autonomic systems (sensory – loss of pain and protective reflexes, autonomic – decreased sweat, thick skin, increased vascularity due to sympathetic imbalance, Motor altered weight distribution causes ulcers at pressure points). Gas in the soft tissue, ulcer, sinus tracts, fractures, cellulitis, abscess, osteomyelitis, septic arthritis and gangrene are the pathological changes resulting from infection. Neuropathic changes are seen in mid foot..

4. X-ray: vascular calcification is seen. Ulcer is seen as a soft-tissue defect. Gas may be seen in soft tissue. There is an increased risk of fractures caused by stress and altered biomechanics. Fracture may be in an advanced state by the time of diagnosis. MRI shows soft-tissue and bone marrow oedema, with a low signal in T1 and a high signal in T2, with no contrast enhancement. In chronic neuropathic joint, the toes, midfoot and ankle are affected. Midtarsal joints are the most common sites. Changes can be hypertrophic or atrophic. In the hypertrophic type, there is bone destruction, fragmentation, loose bodies, disorganisation, debris and effusion. High uptake is seen on a bone scan. No enhancement is seen on MRI or CT, which differentiates it from infection. Deformities and antibiotic-impregnated pellets and postsurgical changes can also be seen.

5. Infection: osteomyelitis is the result of contiguous spread. The first and fifth metatarsal heads are most commonly affected. A plain X-ray is positive after 10–21 days. Increased uptake is seen on a bone scan, gallium scan and of ᵐIn-labelled leukocytes. MRI shows a low signal in T1 and a high signal in T2, with enhancement. Cortical erosion and soft-tissue oedema are also seen. Chronic osteomyelitis shows a mixture of bone destruction and remodelling. Septic arthritis is common in MTP and interphalangeal (IP) joints. Joint effusion, osteopenia, marginal sclerosis, bone erosion and joint space narrowing are seen. Abscess is seen as a focal collection. MRI shows rim enhancement.

6. Imaging is tailored according to the individual patients symptoms. Clinical assessment and high quality plain films play important role in diagnosis. Plain film is useful for detection of ostseomyelitis, soft tissue gas, ulcers, neuropathic joints, antibiotic pellets, deformities. The most important diagnostic dilemma is to determine whether there is active infection superimposed on neuropathic change. Conventional scintigraphic bone scan is non specific and shows increased uptake both in infection and neuropathic joints. However infection seeking scintigraphic agents such as 111-In-labelled WBC scan or ^{99m}Tc-leukoscan, along with conventional bone scan will be able to demonstrate active infection. MRI can also be used to detect features of active infection within bone marrow.

Case 7.3: Answers

1. The X-ray of the right wrist shows a smooth, homogeneous periosteal reaction in the distal radius and ulna. This is more prominent in the medial aspect of the radius.

2. The X-ray of the chest in the same patient shows a rounded mass in the periphery of the left mid-zone.

3. Hypertrophic (pulmonary) osteoarthropathy resulting from lung cancer.

4. Other causes of hypertrophic osteoarthopathy are: tumours (mesothelioma, lymphoma, vascular metastasis, pleural fibroma, thymoma, oesophageal leiomyoma, pulmonary haemangioma), chronic infection (abscess, bronchiectasis, TB, blastomycosis, cystic fibrosis, interstitial fibrosis), gastrointestinal tract (ulcerative colitis, TB, Whipple's disease, Crohn's disease, bowel lymphoma), hepatic (cirrhosis, chronic active hepatitis, liver abscess, bile duct carcinoma), undifferentiated nasopharyngeal carcinoma and pancreatic carcinoma.

5. Hypertrophic osteoarthropathy is caused by release of vasodilators that are not metabolised by the lung, increased flow through AV shunts, reflex peripheral vasodilatation or hormones (oestrogen, growth hormone, prostaglandin). Radiological features are cortical thickening and lamellar periosteal proliferation of new bone. It is initially smooth, later rough, and seen in the diaphysis and metaphysis of long bones. Common sites are the tibia, fibula, radius, ulna, proximal phalanges and femur. It is most conspicuous

in the concavity of long bones on the dorsal and medial aspects. A bone scan shows increased uptake. Soft-tissue swelling of the phalanges is seen.

6. Differential diagnosis for bilateral periosteal reaction is – venous stasis, pachydermoperiostosis, thyroid acropachy, fluorosis, juvenile rheumatoid, psoariasis, Reiter syndrome, congenital syphilis, acute leukemia, scurvy, vitamin A intoxication, metastatic neuroblastoma, healing rickets, tuberous sclerosis and Caffey's disease.

Case 7.4: Answers

1. Pre-contrast T1-weighted MRI shows reduction of the disc space at the L4–5 level, with irregular endplates. There is an abnormally low signal in the L4 and L5 vertebrae. T2-weighted images show a high signal in the corresponding vertebrae. A high signal is seen in the disc.

2. Discitis.

3. Discitis is infection of the intervertebral disc. *Staphylococcus aureus* is the most commonly identified organism. In 70% of children, the causative organism is not identified and can be streptococci, enterococci, *E. coli, Salmonella, Pseudomonas* and *Klebsiella* spp., TB, brucellosis, fungi and parasitic diseases. The infection usually spreads haematogenously. L2–3 and L3–4 are the discs commonly involved. Children classically present with fever, back pain, irritability and a refusal to walk. In children, the discs are well vascularised, the vessels becoming obliterated by 13 years. As a result, isolated discitis can occur in childhood, but by adulthood infection starts in the vertebral body and spreads to the disc.

4. A plain X-ray is normal in the acute phase, but after 2–8 weeks shows narrowing of the disc space and erosions of the endplates of adjacent vertebrae. A bone scan shows high uptake in the affected region. MRI is the imaging method of choice with the highest sensitivity. The MR features are disc space narrowing, a high signal in T2-weighted images and marrow oedema in adjacent vertebrae. Disc enhancement and extension into adjacent soft tissue is often seen. The soft-tissue abscess can extend anteriorly or posteriorly into the spinal canal, causing cord compression. In chronic infection, collapse of the vertebral body and deformity are seen. Blood culture is used for deciding on treatment. CT-guided biopsy can be done if complications develop. The causative organism can be identified.

5. Intravenous antibiotics are given. Immediate surgery is performed if there is spinal cord compression. Deformities are treated by fusion of spinal segments.

Case 7.5: Answers

1. X-ray of the hand and show diffuse osteopenia in the subarticular and periarticular regions. There is joint space narrowing and marginal erosions at the metacarpophalangeal joints. There is marked erosion of the distal ulna and carpal bones, resulting in carpal fusion. X-ray of the cervical spine, shows marked osteopenia, narrowing of disc spaces, atlantoaxial subluxation and dislocation.

2. Rheumatoid arthritis.

3. Diagnosis of rheumatoid arthritis is made if at least four of the following are present: morning stiffness > 1 hour, swelling of more than three joints, symmetrical swelling, typical radiological changes, rheumatoid nodules, positive rheumatoid factor.

4. Common locations are in the hands and feet. In the hand common locations are the metacarpophalangeal (MCP) joints, proximal interphalangeal (PIP) joints, IP joint of the thumb. Earliest changes are seen in the second and third MCP and the third PIP joints. In the feet, the common locations are the medial aspect of metatarsal heads of second and third digits, the medial and lateral aspect of the fifth metatarsal, and IP joints.

5. The radiological changes are periarticular osteoporosis, soft-tissue swelling, symmetrical joint space reduction, marginal erosions and deformities. Deformities in the hand include boutonnière , swan-neck deformity and mallet finger. Other features are odontoid erosion, anterior atlantoaxial subluxation, erosion of posterosuperior margins of ribs, narrow glenohumeral joint space, widened acromioclavicular joint caused by clavicular erosion and protrusio acetabuli. Tenosynovitis, synovial cysts and osteoporosis are also seen. Ultrasonography with Doppler ultrasonography or MRI with contrast is used to detect synovial thickening and proliferation in the earliest stages, so that treatment can be initiated.

6. Differential diagnosis – Osteoarthritis (DIP joints, sclerosis, no marginal erosions), psoriasis (asymmetric, proliferation adjacent to erosions, terminal phalanx involvement), gout (asymmetrical joint involvement, eccentric soft tissue, absent or mild osteoporosis, joint space loss may be absent, erosions with overhanging edges), septic arthritis (joint space loss, cortical destruction, bony ankylosis), chronic inflammatory arthritis (absence of bone erosion, serology negative) and erosive arthritis (proximal and distal IP joints, no osteoporosis, serology negative).

Case 7.6: Answers

1. The X-ray of the right foot shows a large eccentric soft-tissue swelling adjacent to the MTP joint of the first toe. There is also joint space reduction and erosions with overhanging edges. No osteoporosis noted.

2. Gout.

3. Gout is caused by deranged purine metabolism resulting in hyperuricaemia. This can be primary as a result of overproduction of uric acid or a defect in renal urate excretion. Secondary causes result from myeloproliferative disorders, haemolysis, glycogen storage disorders, Lesch–Nyhan syndrome, acquired defect in renal urate excretion (chronic renal failure, drugs, myxoedema, hypo-/hyperparathyroidism, MI and hypertension). The stages of the disease are **asymptomatic hyperuricaemia, acute gouty arthritis, chronic tophaceous gout, gouty nephropathy** and **nephrolithiasis.** The common locations are in the joints of the hands and feet, the first MTP joint being the most commonly affected. Bones, tendons, bursa and the external ear are also affected. Radiological features are not seen 6–12 years after the initial attack and seen in only 45% of patients.

4. An X-ray shows eccentric, juxta-articular, lobulated, soft-tissue swelling, which may show peripheral calcifications, joint effusion, preservation of joint space till late stage, absence of periarticular osteoporosis, erosions with scalloped margins, chondrocalcinosis and punched-out lytic lesions with overhanging margins (elevated osseus spicule separating tophi from adjacent erosion). Renal uric acid stones may be seen.

5. Differential diagnoses: CPPD (degenerative joint disease, with narrowing of joint, cartilage calcification), psoriasis (joint space destruction, involvement of sacroiliac joint), rheumatoid arthritis (marginal erosions, osteopenia, soft-tissue swelling, symmetrical), joint infection (rapid destruction, loss of articular cortex), amyloidosis (bilateral symmetrical, osteopenia), xanthomatosis, osteoarthritis (symmetrical, in elderly people, osteophytes are present).

Case 7.7: Answers

1. The X-ray of the foot shows a focal area of lucent destruction in the right great toe. There is no periosteal reaction. Mild soft-tissue swelling is seen.

2. Acute osteomyelitis of the terminal phalanx of the right big toe.

3. Acute osteomyelitis is infection of bone by an infecting organism, usually *Staphylococcus aureus*. Other organisms are coagulase-negative staphylococci, streptococci, *Bartonella* spp. and *Brucella* spp. Infection can be acquired via the haematogenous or exogenous route. It is common in long bones, starting in metaphyseal sinusoidal veins and resulting in focal oedema, which leads to local tissue necrosis, breakdown of the trabecular bone structure, and removal of bone matrix and calcium. Infection spreads along the haversian canals, through the marrow cavity and beneath the periosteal layer of the bone. Subsequent vascular damage causes ischaemic death of osteocytes, leading to the formation of a sequestrum. Periosteal new bone formation on top of the sequestrum is known as involucrum.

4. Clinically there is bone pain, fever, malaise, irritability, restricted limb movement, swelling, tenderness, warmth and regional lymphadenopathy. Complications include chronic osteomyelitis, metastatic infection, septic arthritis resulting from the transphyseal spread of the infection (children under 2 years of age), angular deformity of bones caused by arrest of bone growth, pathological fractures, bacteraemia and septicaemia, soft-tissue infection and persistent sinuses, and premature epiphyseal fusion.

Musculoskeletal Answers

5. X-rays are normal in the earlier stages. Subtle soft-tissue swelling and displacement of fat planes can be noted. In 10–14 days, a longitudinal lucent destructive lesion with areas of sclerosis and periosteal reaction is seen. A three-phase ^{99m}Tc-labelled bisphosphonate bone scan (perfusion, blood pool, static) is very sensitive and positive in 24 hours, and shows a well-defined focus of tracer uptake in all the phases. It is useful for looking at multifocal sites of osteomyelitis. The uptake on three-phase bone scans is related to blood flow and osteoblastic activity. ^{111}In- or ^{99m}Tc-labelled leukocytes are very specific in localising infections. Ultrasonography can show a hypoechoic collection close to the bone, earlier than radiological detection. MRI is also a very sensitive tool. Osteomyelitis is seen as low signal in T1 and a high signal in T2. MRI is useful in assessing the extent of osteomyelitis and subperisoteal abscess. The inflammatory component enhances on contrast whereas necrotic pus does not. CT can also detect osteomyelitis earlier than an X-ray, but is typically used in chronic osteomyelitis. Primary treatment is a combination of a penicillinase-resistant synthetic penicillin and a third-generation cephalosporin. There are many alternative regimens.

Case 7.8: Answers

1. AP view of the right knee shows joint space reduction of the medial tibiofemoral compartment and marginal osteophyte formation. Lateral view shows joint space reduction in the patellofemoral compartment.

2. Osteoarthritis.

3. Osteoarthritis is degenerative joint disease caused by abnormal forces acting on a normal joint or a normal forces acting on abnormal joints due to cartilage abnormality or subchondral bone abnormality. Aging causes decreased chondroitin sulfate, unsupported collagen fibrils and irreversible hyaline cartilage degeneration. In the early stages, there is cartilage swelling and softening, followed by increased cartilage thickness due to chondrocyte proliferation, followed by cartilage loss caused by proteolytic enzymes being produced and released from chondrocytes themselves. These potent enzymes cause fibrillation, erosion and cracking of articular cartilage.

4. Knee: medial femorotibial > lateral femorotibial > patellofemoral

    Hand: first MCP joint, trapezioscaphoid, distal IP (DIP) > PIP, Bouchard's nodes – osteophytes at PIP joint; Heberden's nodes at DIP joint

    Feet: first MTP

    Hip: femoral and acetabular osteophytes

    Spine: discal disease, apophyseal joints

    Sacroiliac joints.

5. An X-ray shows joint space narrowing, subchondal sclerosis, subchondral cyst formation (geode), effusion and osteophytes at the articular margin. MRI shows increased signal intensity of abnormal cartilage on T2-weighted image. MRI and CT arthrogram are better at detecting loose bodies.

Case 7.9: Answers

1. The X-ray of the hand shows resorption of the tips of the phalanges, with soft-tissue calcification in the soft tissue of the fingers.

2. Scleroderma.

3. The radiological features of scleroderma are: punctate calcifications in the soft tissue of fingertips, axilla, ischial tuberosity, forearm, elbow, lower leg, face, tendons and bursae; soft-tissue swelling of digits (sausage digits); tapered digits resulting from acro-osteolysis (resorption of terminal phalanges); and contractures seen in joints. Central/marginal erosions and joint space narrowing are seen without osteoporosis.

4. Common locations of scleroderma arthritis are the first CMC joint, and MCP, DIP and PIP joints.

5. The combination of soft-tissue calcification and terminal phalangeal bone resorption and diagnostic features of scleroderma. Soft-tissue calcification can be seen in lot of conditions such as hyperparathyroidism, sarcoidosis, hypervitaminosis D, milk alkali syndrome, infestation. Acro-osteolysis is caused by psoriasis, dermatomyositis, thermal injuries, polyvinyl chloride

exposure, epidermolysis bullosa, rheumatoid conditions, Reiter's disease, sarcoidosis, leprosy, pyknodysostosis, progeria, asymbolia, syringomyelia and hyperparathyroidism.

Case 7.10: Answers

1. X-ray of the spine shows narrowing of the disc space at T9–T10 level, with irregular end plates. There is paravertebral soft tissue swelling on both sides. MRI shows narrowing destruction of the disc with narrowing of disc space, irregular end plates and increased signal intensity in T9 and T10 bodies. There are bilateral, lobulated, paravertebral soft tissue masses.

2. Tuberculous spondylitis.

3. Tuberculous spondylitis is caused by *Mycobacterium tuberculosis*. The infection reaches the vertebrae usually by haematogenous spread via Batson's plexus. Infection spreads to adjacent vertebrae in the subligamentous space beneath the anterior and posterior longitudinal ligaments. Contiguous spread occurs through the subchondral plate into the disc space.

4. Spinal TB is common in the lower thoracic and upper lumbar vertebrae, with L1 being the most common site. In the vertebra, it starts in the anterior aspect of the body adjacent to the superior or inferior endplate, from where it spreads to the other parts. Clinically, TB of the spine presents with backache, stiffness and tenderness. No chest lesion is seen in 50% of individuals. The characteristic features of tuberculous spondylitis are narrowing of the disc space and irregular endplates. Collapse of a vertebral body leads to gibbus, kyphotic deformity and vertebra plana. Paravertebral extension causes widening of the paravertebral soft-tissue opacity. Calcification can be seen. Bone density is decreased in chronic cases. An ivory vertebra is seen during the healing phase. A CT scan shows a destructive, stippled bone pattern in the vertebra, with calcified paravertebral soft tissue. MRI is very sensitive and accurate in characterising and evaluating the disease extent. The lesion is centred on the subchondral region, with endplate irregularity. The lesion is a low signal in T1 and a high signal in T2. An abscess can be seen in the epidural or paravertebral space, which shows rim enhancement and calcification.

5. Differential diagnoses are **pyogenic spondylitis** (rapid destruction, no calcification of abscess rim, posterior elements not involved, little new bone formation), **tumour** (multiple lesions, non-contiguous, no disc destruction, no soft-tissue abscess), **brucellosis** (minimal paraspinal mass, lower lumbar spine, gas within disc) and **sarcoidosis**.

Case 7.11: Answers

1. The X-ray of the left leg shows extensive sclerosis, cortical thickening on the anterior aspect of the upper tibial shaft due to periosteal new bone formation. There is no soft-tissue swelling or fracture.

2. Osteoid osteoma.

3. Osteoid osteoma is a benign tumour of osteoid and woven bone, measuring < 1.5 cm (> 1. 5 cm – osteoblastoma). It is common in the second and third decades. Clinically, osteoid osteomas present with pain, which his worse at night and relieved by salicylates.

4. Osteoid osteoma is seen in the metaphysis or diaphysis of long bones or the posterior elements of the spine or flat bones. In the bones, the usual location is in the cortex. Occasionally it is seen in cancellous bone or subperiosteally. The characteristic lesion is a round or oval radiolucent nidus (< 1.5 cm), with a surrounding rim of sclerosis and central calcification. In the spine, there is a painful scoliosis concave to the lesion. When the lesion is intra-articular, effusion, cartilage loss and degenerative changes are seen. Disuse osteoporosis can be present. A CT scan shows low density nidus surrounded by sclerosis and a variable amount of mineralisation. MRI shows nidus isointense in T1 and a low signal in T2 with perinidal oedema. An angiogram shows vascular nidus. Bone scintigraphy shows intense activity over the affected site of the bone.

5. Differential diagnoses: **stress fracture, Brodie's abscess, sclerosing osteomyelitis, syphilis, osteoblastoma, bone island, Ewing's sarcoma metastases, lymphoma** and **subperiosteal aneurysmal bone cyst**. The nidus can be removed surgically or by ablation under CT guidance. The tumour can be percutaneously ablated using radio frequency (RF), ethanol, laser or thermocoagulation. In spinal tumours, complete ablation or resection of the tumour is desirable but not always

feasible. Percutaneous RF ablation is performed by using general or spinal anaesthesia. After localisation of the nidus with 1- to 3-mm CT sections, an osseous access is established and ablation performed at 90°C for 4–5 min by using a rigid RF electrode. The procedure is successfully completed when the electrode by heating to the desired temperature within the nidus.

Case 7.12: Answers

1. There is expansion of the distal metaphysis of the femur. There is no cortical thinning or osteopenia. MRI shows similar changes without signal abnormality.

2. Erlenmeyer flask deformity due to Gaucher's disease. Erlenmeyer flask deformity is characterised by expansion of a distal end of the long bones.

3. Gaucher's disease is a metabolic disorder characterised by deposition of abnormal lipid glucocerebroside in the reticuloendothelial cells of the bone marrow, liver and spleen, due to deficiency of the enzyme, beta glucocerebrosidase. It is most prevalent among Ashkenazi Jewish population and inherited as an autosomal recessive trait.

4. Causes of Erlenmeyer flask deformity: Gaucher's disease, Niemann–Pick disease, anaemia, thalassaemia, sickle cell disease, osteopetrosis, rickets, metaphyseal dysplasia, fibrous dysplasia, hypophosphatasia, achondroplasia, Down syndrome, and rheumatoid arthritis.

5. There are several types: adult/chronic neuropathic form, rapidly fatal infantile/acute neuropathic form and juvenile/subacute neuropathic forms. Skeletal changes in Gaucher's disease are seen predominantly in long tubular bones (especially the distal end of the femur), axial skeleton, hip, shoulder and pelvis. Skeletal changes are seen in 75%. The changes are bilateral and symmetrical. The characteristic finding is Erlenmeyer flask deformity. Other features are diffuse osteopenia, lytic lesions, periosteal reaction, avascular necrosis, bone infarction and H-shaped vertebrae. Other radiological findings are hepatosplenomegaly, lymphadenopathy, multiple hypodense lesions in the spleen and reticulonodular infiltrates in the lung base. Complications are pathological fractures, avascular necrosis, osteomyelitis, myelosclerosis and pulmonary infections. Clinically there is hepatosplenomegaly, impaired liver

function, elevated acid phosphatase, pancytopenia caused by hypersplenism, ascites, haemochromatosis and dull bone pain.

Case 7.13: Answers

1. The X-ray of the right shoulder joint shows resorption of the humeral head, leaving a sharp eburnated margin with subluxation of the gelenohumeral joint. There is extensive fragmentation and debris of bone in the right shoulder joint.

2. Charcot's joint (neuropathic joint) of atrophic type (most likely from syringomyelia or cervical spinal cord injury).

3. Neuropathic joint is a traumatic arthritis caused by loss of sensation and proprioception. There are two theories of formation:

   (a) loss of sensation leads to repetitive trauma and joint destruction

   (b) loss of neural stimuli leads to loss of sympathetic tone resulting in vasodilatation and hyperaemia, and causing bone resorption.

4. The following are the causes:

   Congenital: myelomeningocele, congenital insensitivity to pain, Riley–Day syndrome, Charcot–Marie–Tooth disease

   Central neuropathy: brain/cord injury, syringomyelia, syphilis, spinal tumours, infections, cord compression, MS, alcoholism

   Peripheral neuropathy: diabetes mellitus, peripheral nerve injury/tumour, leprosy, polio

   Others: Raynaud syndrome, scleroderma, rheumatoid conditions, psoriasis, amyloid, uraemia, pernicious anaemia, pain-relieving drugs, steroids

   Morphologically there are two types – atrophic and hypertrophic:

   Atrophic type: this is the most common – osseus resorption, non-weight-bearing joints of upper extremity, usually caused by syringomyelia, peripheral nerve lesion.

   Hypertrophic type: joint destruction, fragmentation, sclerosis, osteophytes

   Mixed pattern

Combined.

The causes of neuropathic joint differ based on the location:

Shoulder – syringomyelia, cord injury.

Hands and feet – Leprosy.

Foot and ankle – Diabetes, syphilis.

Spine – Spinal injury, syphilis, diabetes, congenital insensitivity to pain, amyloidosis.

5. The joints are dislocated and deformed, with degeneration and destruction of articular cortex. Dense subchondral bone is seen as a result of sclerosis and debris is seen because of loose bodies. Usually the joints are painless. Joint changes are seen before the neurological deficit manifests. Bone resorption and fractures are seen. Soft-tissue and vascular calcifications are also seen, and deformities such as licked candy-stick phalanx and scoliosis are also noted. Differential diagnoses for atrophic type: septic arthritis, surgical amputation; differential diagnoses for hypertrophic type: degenerative joint disease, synovial osteochondromatosis.

Case 7.14: Answers

1. Lateral view of the spine, shows generalised osteopenia in the vertebrae. There are multiple anterior wedge compression fractures involving T9, T11, T12 and L1 vertebrae. Sagittal view of the entire spine in CT, shows decreased density of the vertebrae. There are also moderate wedge compression fractures of T9, T11, T12 and L1.

2. Osteoporosis with wedge compression spinal fractures.

3. Types of osteoporosis: **type I** – postmenopausal, **type II** – senile, idiopathic. **Secondary** types are:

Endocrine: steroids, Cushing's disease, hyperthyroidism, hypogonadism, acromegaly

Nutrition: malabsorption, scurvy, alcoholism

Drugs: heparin, steroids

Hereditary: osteogenesis imperfecta, Marfan syndrome, Ehler–Danlos syndrome, homocystinuria, hypophosphatasia, Wilson's disease, alkaptonuria, Menkes syndrome.

4. In the spine, the bones are diffusely osteopenic, with resorption of the horizontal trabeculae but coarse, thickened, vertical trabeculae. **Empty box vertebra/picture framing** is increased due to density of endplates as a result of resorption of spongy bone. Vertebral body compression fractures are very common. They can be wedge, biconcave or true compression fractures. MRI is useful for diagnosing osteoporotic fracture in the setting of backache. The most important use is to differentiate a benign osteoporotic fracture from an acute traumatic fracture and more importantly a malignant fracture. Features of metastatic compression fractures have convex posterior border of vertebral body, abnormal signal intensity of pedicle or posterior element, an epidural mass, encasing epidural mass, focal paraspinal mass and other metastasis. In osteoporotic compression fracture there is a low signal intensity band in T1 and T2, with normal signal in the body, retropulsion of posterior bone fragment and multiple other fractures. In patients with osteoporosis, bone density is measured to predict the risk of developing fractures and getting appropriate treatment. This can be done with single photon absorption or dual photon absorption with radionuclide or dual energy X-ray bone densitometry. This can also be done with CT and ultrasonography (calcaneum).

5. Fractures and pain are complications of osteoporosis. In severe osteoporotic compression fracture with pain, percutaneous vertebroplasty may be undertaken under fluoroscopic or CT guidance. Vertebroplasty is a procedure aimed at preventing vertebral body collapse by injecting polymethymethacrylate cement into the vertebral body. Indications are painful compression fractures refractory to conservative therapy. Ideal candidates are those who present within 4 months of fracture, with midline non-radiating back pain that increases with weight bearing, and exacerbated by palpation of the spine.

Case 7.15: Answers

1. X-ray of the skull shows a cotton wool appearance of the skull vault as a result of extensive sclerosis and thickening of the tables of the skull with expansion of the diploic space. Bone scan of the pelvis shows extensive uptake in the left iliac bone, which appears expanded. Few foci of increased uptake are also seen in the rest of the pelvic bones.

2. Paget's disease.

3. Paget's disease is a multifocal disease of exaggerated bone remodelling. The exact aetiology is not known. Infection by paramyxovirus is one of the proposed aetiologies. There are three stages:

Osteolytic phase: with intense osteoclastic activity and resorption of bone

Mixed phase: osteoclastic and osteoblastic activity – lytic and sclerotic lesions are seen

Late quiescent phase: decreased osteoblastic activity with decreased bone turnover – sclerosis.

4. Paget's disease may be asymptomatic. Fatigue, neuropathy, enlarging head, brainstem compression, pain, hearing loss, blindness, facial palsy and hyperthermia are the common clinical features. The serum calcium and phosphorus are normal, but serum alkaline phosphatase is increased and hydroxyproline is increased in urine he common locations are pelvis, spine, proximal femur, skull, scapula, distal femur, proximal tibia and proximal humerus. Mostly they are polyostotic. Peak incidence is in sixth decade and is more common in men.

Skull – Early stage is osteoporosis circumscriptia – a geographical lytic area in the anterior frontal bone, followed by cotton wool appearance of mixed lysis and sclerosis. There is widening of diploic space, basilar impression and sclerosis of skull base.

Long bones –There is expansion of bones with coarsened trabecula, cortical thickening and cyst like areas. The appearance is like a candle flame or blade of grass, with a V shaped defect starting in the subarticular part of epiphysis and advancing into the diaphysis. Deformities are anterior or lateral curvature, such as shepherd's crook deformity of femur. Multiple marginal or incremental fractures along the bones is so common that they may be regarded as features of the disease than complications.

Pelvis – protrusio acetabuli

Spine – Picture frame type – expansion of body with sclerosis at margins/**ivory vertebra** – completely scerlotic with ossification of ligaments/ expansion of bone with coarse trabeculae,

Bone scan shows intense uptake the active phase and normal in burned out cases. MRI shows reduction of marrow cavity size, low signal in T1, high signal in T2 in active stages and low signal in burnt out cases.

5. Differential diagnoses are metastasis, lymphoma, vertebral haemangioma and fibrous dysplasia. In metastasis there is no cortical expansion and no coarsening of trabeculae. Complications are: **neoplasia** (1–20% risk) (chondrosarcoma, osteosarcoma, fibrosarcoma and malignant fibrous histiocytoma). Radiologically osteolysis develops in previous Paget's disease, increasing soft-tissue mass and pain; **fractures** (vertebral compression fractures, banana fractures on convex surfaces of long bones); **deformity** (shepherd's crook, lentosis ossia, ivory vertebra); **brain-stem compression** by basilar invagination and hydrocephalus; **spinal stenosis; osteoarthritis; narrowing of neural foramina**; and high-output **cardiac failure**.

Treatment is with calcitonin, bisphosphonates or mithramycin.

Case 7.16: Answers

1. The X-ray of the hands shows erosion of the articular margins of middle and distal phalanges at the DIP joint of the right second digit with marginal erosions and proliferative periosteal new bone. The is soft tissue swelling and widening of DIP joint space.

2. Psoriatic arthropathy.

3. Psoriatic arthropathy is a seronegative spondyloarthropathy seen in 20% of patients with psoriasis. Pathologically, there is synovial inflammation, fibrosis and bony proliferation at joint margins, tendon insertions and subperiosteum. The arthritis can be a true psoriatic arthritis or psoriatic arthritis resembling rheumatoid or concomitant psoriasis and RA. Usually, it affects the lower and upper extremities in an asymmetrical fashion. Terminal IP joints are the most commonly affected. Sacroiliac joints and lumbar spine are often affected.

4. The typical radiological changes are asymmetrical joint space reduction with no osteoporosis, periosteal reaction and osseus excrescences. In the hand and foot, DIP, PIP and MCP joints are involved. There is soft-tissue swelling of digits, destruction of DIP joints, pencil-in-cup deformity, erosions with ill-defined margins and proliferation of periosteal new bone. Similar changes are seen in the DIP joint of the first toe. Ivory phalanx and acro-osteolysis are also seen. Bilateral symmetrical sacroiliitis, floating osteophytes in vertebrae, atlantoaxial subluxation and apophyseal joint narrowing and sclerosis are also seen.

Musculoskeletal Answers

5. Differential diagnoses: ankylosing spondylitis (bilateral symmetrical sacroiliitis, less common peripheral skeletal involvement), Reiter syndrome and RA (osteoporosis, symmetrical erosions.)

Case 7.17: Answers

1. The X-ray of the right knee joint shows a widened epiphysis and metaphysis and prominent intercondylar notch but no evidence of bone erosion. The bones are diffusely osteopenic.

2. Juvenile rheumatoid arthritis.

3. Juvenile rheumatoid arthritis is seen in children aged under 16 years and is common in girls. There are many clinical types:

Juvenile onset, adult type: 8–10 years; RA factor positive; poor prognosis; erosive changes and extensive periosteal reaction, protrusio acetabuli

Polyarthritis of ankylosing spondylitis type: boys, 9–11 years; peripheral arthritis; fused bones, common in greater trochanter, heel spur; iridocyclitis.

Still's disease: systemic (fever, rash, lymphadenopathy, hepatosplenomegaly, pericarditis)/polyarticular/pauciarticular; common in carpometacarpal joints; girls aged 2–4, 8–11 years; periosteal reaction in phalanges, broad bones, early maturation and fusion.

4. Juvenile arthritis involves large joints such as the hips, knees, ankles, wrists and elbows. Periarticular soft-tissue swelling, late onset of bony changes, thinned cartilage, ballooned-out widened epiphysis and metaphysis, juxta-articular osteoporosis, erosions, cyst-like lesions away from the joint line and ankylosis are the radiological features. In the cervical spine, there is a decreased size of bodies, atlantoaxial subluxation and fractures, and ankylosis of sacroiliac joint. On the chest X-ray pleural and pericardial effusion, and lung nodules may be seen. The distinctive radiological features are the location of the disease, periosteal new bone formation, late onset of bone erosion and generalised growth disturbance.

5. Differential diagnoses: **haemophilia** – expansion of joint space, wide epiphysis; **septic arthritis** – joint destruction, joint space narrowing.

Case 7.18: Answers

1. The chest X-ray is essentially normal. On close observation, there is a linear, serpiginous calcification in the right side of neck. The second X-ray of the abdomen shows similar calcification in the right upper quadrant of the abdomen.

2. Worm calcification, caused by guinea-worm infection (*Dracunculus medinensis*).

3. Guinea-worm infection is acquired by ingesting water that contains larvae. The larvae are inside a tiny crustacean, *Cyclops* spp. The larvae are released in the stomach or duodenum, the acidity of which kills *Cyclops* spp. The larvae penetrate the mucosa, mature and mate in the abdomen or retroperitoneum. After maturation, the female worm migrates to subcutaneous tissue, usually in the lower extremity, where the larvae exit through the skin, into the water supply.

4. Other causes of worm calcification are cysticercosis, loiasis, *Armillifer armillatus*, Bancroft's filariasis and hydatid disease. Cysticercosis produces oval rice grain calcifications, oriented along the muscle bundles. *Armillifer* sp. produces small calcifications in the hands and feet. Filariasis produces calcifications in the lower extremities. Hydatid cysts produce curvilinear calcification of the cyst wall, but the entire cyst can be calcified when the organism (*Echinococcus granulosus*) dies.

5. Other causes of soft-tissue calcification are:

Metastatic calcification (deposition of calcium in normal tissues): hyperparathyroidism, hypoparathyroidism, hypervitaminosis D, milk alkali syndrome, sarcoidosis, idiopathic hypercalcaemia, metastasis, leukaemia

Dystrophic calcification (areas of tissue injury): renal osteodystrophy, gout, pseudogout, ochronosis, pseudohypoparathyroidism, pseudo-pseudohypoparathyroidism, diabetes mellitus, scleroderma, dermatomyositis, SLE, neuropathic, frostbite, myositis ossificans, calcific tendonitis, infestations, atherosclerosis, Monkeberg's sclerosis, venous calcifications, infarction, Ehler–Danlos syndrome, pseudoxanthoma elasticum, Werner syndrome, calcinosis, necrotic tumour and tumoral calcinosis.

Case 7.19: Answers

1. MRI of the thighs shows bilateral diffuse increased signal within the thigh muscles.

2. The clinical features and MRI findings suggest dermatomyositis/pyomyositis.

3. Blood test for muscle enzymes, electromyography (EMG) and muscle biopsy are required for confirmation. As dermatomyositis can be a paraneoplastic syndrome an X-ray of the chest is required for excluding bronchogenic neoplasm. Gastroscopy, colonoscopy and barium studies may also be required.

4. Dermatomyositis is an idiopathic inflammatory myopathy with characteristic cutaneous findings. Diagnostic criteria are progressive proximal symmetrical weakness, elevated muscle enzymes, abnormal findings on EMG and muscle biopsy, and cutaneous disease. The characteristic feature is a heliotrope rash, which is a violaceous or dusky erythematous rash seen symmetrically in the periorbital region, and Gottron's papules, which are violaceous papules usually seen over the dorsum of the hand and extensor surfaces, but also on the feet, elbow or knee. Proximal muscle weakness is a characteristic features. Muscle tenderness can occasionally be seen. Calcinosis, myocarditis, pulmonary fibrosis, arthritis and dysphagia are other features resulting from multisystemic involvement. Creatine kinase is elevated, as are aldolase, lactate dehydrogenase and antimyosin antibodies.

5. MRI is useful for confirming diagnosis and selecting a site for biopsy. On MRI, there is a symmetrical high signal in proximal muscles. T1-weighted and STIR (fat suppression) images are acquired in the axial and coronal planes. High signal in STIR indicates myositis and a biopsy is done in areas showing maximum areas of inflammation. The muscle signal decreases after initiation of steroid therapy. Low signal in T1 and atrophy of muscles are seen in chronic involvement. The first line of treatment is with steroids. Calcium and Vitamin D are given to prevent steroid induced osteoporosis. If there is no improvement, cytotoxic agents, methotrexate and azathioprine are given. Once subcutaneous calcification develops, response to therapy is poor.

1. The X-ray of the right arm shows a well-defined lucent lesion in the metaphysis of the proximal tibia, with a surrounding rim of sclerosis (rind sign). There is also a pathological fracture, but no periosteal reaction or soft-tissue extension.

2. The radiologial findings are consistent with fibrous dysplasia. The clinical diagnosis is McCune–Albright syndrome, which includes polyostotic fibrous dysplasia, precocious puberty and pigmentation.

3. Fibrous dysplasia is a skeletal developmental anomaly of the bone-forming mesenchyme, with a defect in osteoblastic differentiation and maturation. The medullary bone is replaced by fibrous tissue, which has a characteristic ground-glass appearance on a plain X-ray. Clinically there are four forms: **monostotic** (70%), **polyostotic**, **craniofacial** and **cherubism**. It is commonly seen between age 3 and 15 years. The monostotic form is more common in the ribs, femur, tibia or craniofacial bones. The polyostotic form is more common in the femur, tibia, pelvis, ribs and craniofacial bones. Fibrous dysplasia may be associated with endocrinopathies in 2–3% of cases (precocious puberty in girls, hyperthyroidism, hyperparathyroidism, acromegaly, diabetes mellitus and Cushing syndrome). An elevated ALP is seen. Clinical features are pain, tenderness, deformity, scoliosis, endocrine changes and café-au-lait spots.

4. The usual appearance of fibrous dysplasia is a lucent lesion in the diaphysis or metaphysis, with endosteal scalloping, with or without bone expansion, and the absence of periosteal reaction. Usually, the matrix of the lucency is smooth and relatively homogeneous (ground glass). Irregular areas of sclerosis may be present with or without calcification. The lucent lesion has a thick sclerotic border and is called the rind sign. The lesion may extend into the epiphysis only after fusion. The dysplastic bone may undergo calcification and endochondral bone formation. In the skull, the lesion is convex and expands the outer table. The tables are intact but thinned. A CT scan shows a lucent lesion with attenuation values of 70–130 HU. On MRI, the lesion has a low-to-intermediate signal in T1 and a high signal in T2. Fluid–fluid levels are seen. Differential diagnoses of a well-corticated lucent lesion in metaphysis of children include simple bone cyst, enchondroma, fibrous cortical defect/non-ossifying fibroma, giant cell tumour, haemangioma, primary hyperparathyroidism, neurofibromatosis and Paget's disease (older patients).

Musculoskeletal Answers

5. The complications of fibrous dysplasia are fracture, deformities including severe coxa vara (shepherd's crook deformity), premature fusion of ossification centres with dwarfism, leg length discrepancy, hypophosphataemic rickets and osteomalacia. Malignant conversion is seen in 1% (osteosarcoma, fibrosarcoma, chondrosarcoma).

Case 7.21: Answers

1. The bone scan shows multiple hot areas in the spine, ribs and peripheral skeleton. There is markedly decreased uptake in the rest of the body. Coronal views on the CT scan shows multiple destructive, lytic lesions in the spine.

2. Bony metastasis.

3. Common primaries causing bony metastases are breast, prostate, lung, kidney, uterus, stomach, thyroid, kidney, colon, lymphoma, neuroblastoma and Ewing's sarcoma.

4. Metastasis can be:

   Lytic: lung, breast, thyroid, kidney, colon, neuroblastoma

   Blastic: prostate, breast, lymphoma, carcinoid, adenocarcinoma of gastrointestinal, transitional cell carcinoma of bladder, pancreas, neuroblastoma

   Mixed blastic and lytic: breast, prostate, lymphoma

   Expansile lesion: kidney, thyroid

   Permeative: Burkitt's lymphoma

   Sunburst periosteal reaction: prostate, retinoblastoma, neuroblastoma, gastrointestinal tract

   Calcification: breast, osteosarcoma, testes, thyroid, ovary, mucinous adenocarcinoma of gastrointestinal tract

   With soft-tissue mass: thyroid kidney

   Children: neuroblastoma, retinoblastoma, rhabdomyosarcoma, hepatoma, Ewing's tumour.

5. Differential diagnoses of metastasis are: osteopoikilosis, multiple myeloma, primary bone tumours including lymphoma and varied forms bone infection. Bone scan, PET scan and MRI are very sensitive in the diagnosis of bone metastasis.

Case 7.22: Answers

1. The X-ray of the ankle shows an increased distance between the shaft and epiphyseal centre with cupping and fraying of the metaphyseal margin. Distal epiphysis of the tibia has a horizontal margin.

2. Rickets.

3. Rickets is a metabolic abnormality affecting endochondral bone growth, in which the zone of preparatory calcification does not form, with heaping of maturing cartilage cells, and failure of osteoid mineralisation in the shaft with elevated periosteum.

4. Causes of rickets:

Primary vitamin D deficiency

Malabsorption: gastrectomy, enteropathy, enteritis, biliary obstruction, biliary cirrhosis, pancreatitis

Primary hypophosphataemia, vitamin D deficiency rickets

Hypophosphatasia, pseudohypophosphatasia

Fibrogenesis imperfecta osseum

Axial osteomalacia

Hypoparathyroidism, hyperparathyroidism, thyrotoxicosis, Paget's disease, fluorides, neurofibromatosis, osteopetrosis, malignancy, macroglobulinaemia, ureterosigmoidostomy.

5. Radiological features: rickets is commonly seen in the metaphysis of long bones such as the wrists, ankles and knees. The X-ray shows delayed formation of poorly mineralised epiphysis and epiphyseal plates are wide and irregular. Increased distance is seen between the end of the shaft and the epiphysis. Cupping and fraying of metaphysis, metaphyseal spurs, coarse trabeculation, periosteal reaction, deformities such as bowed legs and bowing of diaphysis and frontal bossing are other features. Children present with irritability, bone pain, tenderness, craniotabes, rachitic rosary, bowed legs, delayed dentition, swelling of wrists and ankles. Differential diagnoses: metaphyseal dysplasia, healing scurvy.

Case 7.23: Answers

1. The X-ray shows massively deformed bones in both legs. The bones show gross cortical osteopenia. There are multiple fractures with callus formation.

2. Osteogenesis imperfecta tarda.

3. Osteogenesis imperfecta is a connective tissue disorder that is characterised by micromelic dwarfism, bone fragility, blue sclerae and abnormal dentition. The clinical types are osteogenesis imperfecta congenita (at birth, autosomal dominant [AD], type II, lethal), osteogenesis imperfecta tarda (not at birth, sporadic, types I and IV, non-lethal).

   Sillence classification:

Type	Features	Inheritance
I	Normal stature, minimal deformity, blue sclera, hearing loss, dentition abnormal	AD
II	Perinatal, osteopenic calvaria, beaded ribs, compressed femurs, lone bone deformities, platyspondyly, lethal	AD, mosaic
III	Progressively deforming, sclera lightens with age, hearing loss, abnormal dentition, short stature	AD, AR (autosomal recessive), mosaic,
IV	Mild deformity, variable short stature, hearing loss, abnormal dentition, variable sclera	AD, mosaic
V	Similar to type IV, hypertrophic callus, dense metaphyseal bands, interosseus membrane ossification; unique histology	Unknown
VI	Similar to type IV, unique histological features	Unknown

4. The characteristic radiological features are decreased skull ossification, wormian bones, biconcave vertebral bodies, pelvic deformity due to infolding of the lateral walls, obliteration of root canals in the teeth, short and bowed long bones, progressive deformities of limbs and spine into adulthood, rib fractures, and multiple fractures with exuberant callus formation.

5. Complications are hearing loss and death from intracranial haemorrhage. Differential diagnoses are achondrogenesis, congenital hypophosphatasia and campopelic dysplasia and non-accidental injury (battered baby syndrome).

Case 7.24: Answers

1. The X-rays show bilateral symmetrical sclerosis of the sacroiliac joints. Calcification of the interspinous and supraspinous ligaments, with bamboo spine appearance, is noted. Lateral view shows squaring of the vertebral bodies and calcification of the anterior longitudinal ligament and syndesmophytes.

2. Ankylosing spondylitis.

3. Ankylosing spondylitis is an autoimmune seronegative spondyoarthropathy, that primary affects the axial skeleton (aacroiliac joints, thoracolumbar, lumbosacral junction, sternal joint, pubic symphysis). In peripheral skeleton, hip joint is the most commonly affected. Shoulder joint, insertions of tendons in pelvis and proximal femur are also affected. Osteoblastic reaction causing complete ankylosis may be present. Associations are ulcerative colitis, regional enteritis, iritis, cardiac conduction defects and aortic insufficiency.

4. The earliest changes are seen in the sacroiliac joints. There is bilateral symmetrical sclerosis of the joint margins, mainly on the iliac side. Joint space irregularity, erosions and ankylosis are seen in the late stages. In the spine, the vertebrae are squared with straight or convex anterior margins. Other features are reactive sclerosis of vertebral body corners and ballooning of discs. The hallmark is formation of marginal syndesmophytes, which are dense spicules bridging the vertebral bodies. This gives the appearance of bamboo spine on the AP view as a result

of syndesmophytes and ossification of interspinous and supraspinous ligaments. Complications are fractures, pseudoarthrosis and atlantoaxial subluxation. In the chest, upper lobe bullae, fibrosis and cavitation are seen.

5. Differential diagnosis includes other seronegative spondyoarthropathies, such as Rieter's syndrome (asymmetric SI joint, absent or minor paravertebral ossification), psoriasis (unilateral /asymmetric SIJ, paravertebral ossification rarely seen, small joints involvement), inflammatory bowel disease (clinical features of inflammatory bowel disease),late stage of rheumatoid disease (joint space narrowing, small joints involvement), deposition disease (CPPD, gout, ochronosis) and osteitis condensans illi. Asymmetrical involvement is seen in psoriasis, Reiter syndrome and juvenile rheumatoid arthritis. Unilateral sacroilitis is seen in infection and osteoarthritis.

Case 7.25: Answers

1. In the chest X-ray there is a horizontal area of lucency surrounded by sclerosis in the lateral margin of the right scapula. The heart is enlarged but the lungs are clear.

2. Looser's zones in the right scapula indicate that the patient has osteomalacia.

3. Osteomalacia is incomplete mineralisation of normal osteoid tissue after growth plate closure (rickets – before growth plate closure). Normal bone mineralisation depends on many factors that supply calcium and phosphate to the bones. Vitamin D maintains calcium and phosphate homoeostasis through its action on bone, the gastrointestinal tract, kidneys and parathyroid glands. Vitamin D is acquired through diet or produced by the skin on exposure to ultraviolet light. Sequential hydroxylation in the liver and then the kidneys produces 1,25-dihydroxyvitamin D_3. Dysfunction in any of these metabolic steps results in osteomalacia. Renal osteodystrophy is the most common cause of osteomalacia in adults and results from phosphate loss from renal tubules. Abnormal quantities of osteoid coat the surface of the trabeculae and line the haversian canals in the cortex.

4. Osteomalacia starts insidiously with pain in the spine, legs and arms, with tenderness. The radiological features are osteopenia, coarsening trabecula, Looser's zones and occasionally complete fractures. Looser's zones (milkman pseudofractures) are a type of insufficiency or stress fracture. It is strongly suggestive but not diagnostic of osteomalacia. They are radiolucent areas occurring at right angles to the cortex and extend across a portion of the bone diameter. Characteristic sites are axillary margins of the scapula, ribs, pubic rami, proximal end of femur and ulna. Occasionally, they are bilateral and sclerotic margins can be seen. Other features of renal osteodystrophy such as osseous resorption, soft-tissue calcification, osteopenia and amyloid deposition can also be seen. A CT scan and MRI can be used to diagnose indeterminate fractures.

5. Looser's zones are also seen in chronic renal disease, fibrous dysplasia, hyperthyroidism, Paget's disease, renal osteodystrophy and X-linked hypophosphataemia.

COLOUR IMAGES

Case 1.2

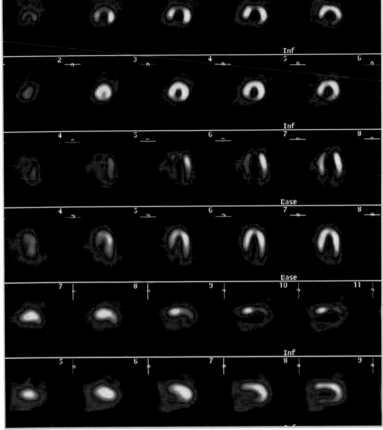

Fig 1.2

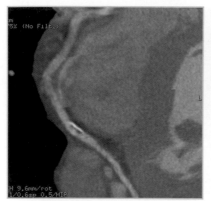

Fig 1.3a

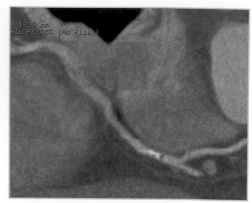

Fig 1.3b

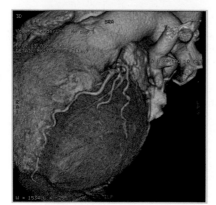

Fig 1.3c

Case 1.20

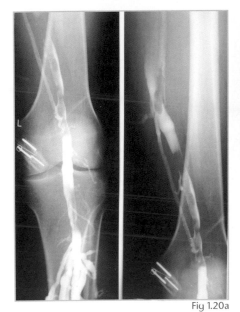

Fig 1.20a

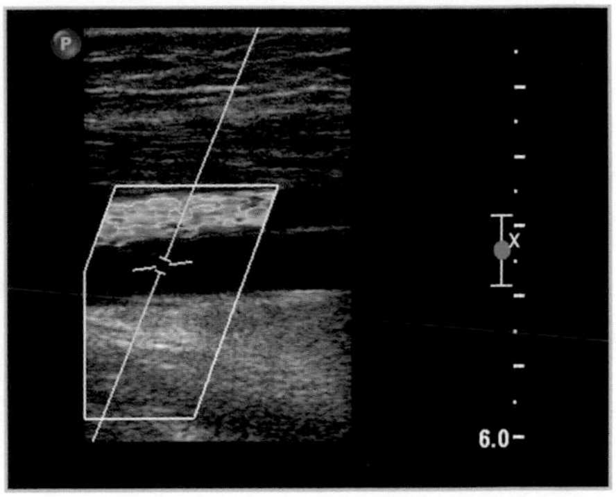

Fig 1.20b

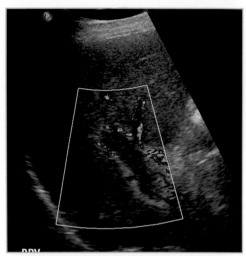

Fig 3.9a

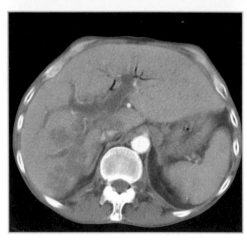

Fig 3.9b

INDEX

abdominal bloating/distension 3.7, 3.9, 3.12, 3.13, 3.17, 3.18, 3.27, 3.31, 3.36, 4.1
  sudden onset 3.30, 4.2
abdominal bruit 4.13
abdominal mass 3.2, 4.2, 4.9
  cystic 3.41
  right upper quadrant 3.16, 3.34
abdominal pain/tenderness 3.2, 3.28, 3.33, 3.35, 3.40–42, 3.44, 4.18, 5.2, 5.6, 5.14, 5.18
  colicky 3.3
  with distension 3.7, 3.9, 3.12, 3.18, 3.27, 4.1
  epigastric 3.1, 3.5, 3.25, 3.41
  intermittent 3.26
  left lower quadrant 3.32
  left side 2.34
  left upper quadrant 5.11
  persistent 5.9
  renal origin 4.8, 4.10, 4.11, 4.17
  right iliac fossa 3.24
  right upper quadrant 3.10, 3.11, 3.16, 3.31, 3.34
  severe 3.20, 3.38
  sudden onset 3.30
achalasia cardia 3.21
acidosis 3.30
acoustic neuroma 6.21
acute respiratory distress syndrome (ARDS) 2.27
adrenal calcification 5.9
adrenal haemorrhage 5.9
air crescent sign 2.3
alcohol problems 2.1, 2.5, 2.30
ALP, elevated 7.15
alveolar proteinosis 2.33
amnesia 6.23
anaemia 3.14, 3.29
anaerobic organisms

cerebral abscesses 6.11
emphysematous cholecystitis 3.16
empyema 2.34
liver abscess 3.11
aneurysm
  aortic 1.5
  cerebral 1.6, 6.27
  coronary artery 1.5
  left ventricle 1.5
  rupture 6.1
aneurysmectomy 1.12
angiomyolipoma 4.14
angiotensin-converting enzyme (ACE), elevated levels 2.17
ankle, pain/swelling/tenderness 7.3
ankylosing spondylitis 7.24
anthracosis 2.22
aorta
  aneurysm 1.5
  coarctation 1.6, 6.1
  dissection 1.1, 1.5
  stenosis 1.1
aortic arch, right-sided 1.7
aortic valve
  bicuspid 1.1, 1.6
  replacement 1.5
apical impulse 1.12, 1.17
arm, pain 2.38, 6.5, 7.20
Arnold–Chiari I malformation 6.2
arteriovenous malformation (AVM) 6.1, 6.16, 6.27
arteritis 1.5, 1.15, 1.18
arthritis, traumatic 7.13
asbestos exposure 2.21, 2.23
ascariasis, small bowel 3.26
ascites 3.27
Asian ethnicity 1.15, 2.45
Aspergillus spp. 2.3, 2.47, 6.11

aspiration pneumonia 2.5, 2.30
astrocytoma 6.3, 6.5
atherosclerosis 1.5
atrial septal defect (ASD) 1.19
autosomal dominant polycystic kidney disease (ADPKD) 4.4
axilla, swelling 5.18

back pain/tenderness 2.43, 5.10, 5.11, 5.16, 7.4, 7.10, 7.14, 7.24
  see also spinal pain/tenderness
balloon angioplasty 1.3, 1.6
barium enema
  after-effects 3.32
  ulcerative colitis 3.40
barium study of the small bowel 3.38
Beck's triad 1.8
bedwetting, persistent 4.5
berry aneurysm 1.6, 6.27
bird of prey sign 3.18
bladder outlet obstruction 4.2
Blalock–Taussig shunt 1.7
bloating 3.36
body
  pain 5.8, 7.18
  swelling 3.10
Boerhaeve syndrome 3.23
bone marrow transplantation 2.47, 3.43, 6.11
bone pain/tenderness 3.36, 5.6, 5.13, 7.12, 7.15, 7.21
bowel
  ischaemia 3.30
  obstruction 6.24
bowel sounds
  absent 3.7
  decreased 3.18, 3.30, 3.36, 3.44

brain
  infarct 6.28, 6.29
  tuberculoma 6.19
breast cancer 2.50
breath sounds, decreased
  2.6, 2.8, 2.9, 2.12, 2.16,
  2.20, 2.21, 2.23, 2.28,
  2.34, 2.39, 2.40, 2.44,
  2.46
breathing, bronchial 2.1,
  2.3, 2.5, 2.10, 2.13, 2.15,
  2.18, 2.22, 2.24, 2.30,
  2.33, 2.37, 2.38, 2.41,
  2.45, 2.47, 2.48
breathing difficulties see
  dyspnoea
bronchial atresia 2.16
bronchiectasis 2.18
bronchiolitis obliterans
  2.37
bronchoalveolar lavage
  (BAL) 2.33
bronchogenic cyst 2.40
Budd–Chiari syndrome
  3.10
bypass surgery 1.3

calcification 1.13, 1.19,
  2.23, 2.29, 6.13, 7.18
calcium channel block-
  ers 6.1
calcium pyrophosphate
  deposition disease
  (CPPD, pseudogout) 7.1
Candida albicans 3.22
Caplan syndrome 2.24
carcinoid tumour of the
  lung 2.19
cardiac failure 1.7, 1.10
cardiac tamponade 1.8
cardiomegaly see heart,
  enlarged
cardiomyopathy, hyper-
  trophic 1.17
Carney's triad 2.36
cephalisation 1.10
cerebellar signs, positive
  6.26
cerebral abscess 6.11
Charcot's joint 7.13
chest pain 1.6, 1.8–13,
  1.17, 2.3, 2.6, 2.10, 2.11,
  2.14, 2.19, 2.21, 2.26,

2.33, 2.36, 2.38, 3.8,
  3.15, 3.21, 5.17
chronic 2.32
on exertion 1.2, 1.19
gradual onset 2.8
in immunosuppressed
  patient 2.41, 3.22
intermittent episodes
  1.3
left-sided 1.3
new onset 2.23
post-endoscopy 3.23
right-sided 1.9, 2.34
severe 1.1, 1.5
sudden onset 1.1, 1.9,
  2.5, 2.9, 2.39, 2.47
trauma-related 2.46
worse on breathing 1.14
chest trauma 2.46
chest wall
  paraesthesia 2.43
  tenderness 2.38
chills 3.16, 4.7
cholangiocarcinoma 3.33
cholangiography 3.35
cholecystitis, emphyse-
  matous 3.16
choledochoduodenal fis-
  tula 3.5
cholelithiasis 3.3
chondrocalcinosis 7.1
chronically ill patient
  2.35, 2.48, 3.44, 5.10,
  5.11, 7.2
Churg–Strauss disease
  2.10
cirrhosis 3.12, 3.34
claw (meniscus) sign 3.39
coalworkers' pneumoco-
  niosis 2.22, 2.42
coarctation 1.1
cocaine 1.1, 1.18
coffee-bean sign 3.18
colon
  angiodysplasia 3.37
  bleeding 3.37
  carcinoma 3.28
  cathartic 3.40
  polyposis 3.29
commissurotomy 1.11
confusion, sudden onset
  6.24
connective tissue disor-

ders 1.18, 2.4, 2.25, 7.23
consciousness
  altered 6.6, 6.10
  loss 1.4, 6.12, 6.17, 6.20
constipation 5.6
cor pulmonale 2.4
cord/dense triangle sign
  6.8
coronary artery
  aneurysm 1.18
  disease 1.2, 1.3
  enlargement 1.18
coronary sinus defect 1.19
costovertebral angle, tenderness 4.6, 4.10
cough 2.1, 2.3, 2.6–8,
  2.14–16, 2.19, 2.22, 2.25,
  2.31, 2.44, 3.6, 3.19
chronic 2.42, 6.23
dry 2.50
intermittent 2.29
non-productive 2.33
postoperative 2.30
productive 2.16, 2.18,
  2.20, 2.45, 2.48
crackles 2.2, 2.7, 2.18,
  2.26, 2.28, 2.29
craniopharyngioma 5.5
crepitations 2.17, 2.25
Crohn's disease 3.24,
  3.40
crows' feet 2.23
crying, incessant 3.39
CT
  coronary angiography
    1.3
  high resolution (HRCT)
    2.18
  non-contrast 5.14, 6.1
  pulmonary angiography
    1.9
cupola sign 3.20
cyanosis 1.7, 1.16, 2.45
cystic fibrosis 2.48
cystitis 4.18

Dawson's fingers 6.7
deafness, sensorineural
  6.21
deep venous thrombosis
  (DVT) 1.20
deja vu 6.30
delta sign, empty 6.8

demyelination, osmotic 6.24
dental caries 5.8
dermatomyositis 7.19
developmental delay 6.3, 6.13
dextrocardia 2.15
diabetes 3.13, 7.7
diabetic foot 7.2
diarrhoea 3.31, 3.39, 3.41, 3.42, 3.43, 3.44
bloody 3.40
digits
clubbing 2.1, 5.7, 7.3
swelling 5.7
see also fingers
discitis 7.4
disorientation 6.17
diverticulitis 3.32
doge's cap sign 3.20
Dor procedure (LV reconstructive surgery) 1.12
Dracunculus medinensis(guinea worm) 7.18
drowsiness 6.17
duodenal ulcer 3.5
dypsnoea 1.10
dyspepsia 3.3
dysphagia 3.6, 3.8, 3.14, 3.15, 3.19, 3.21, 3.22
dyspnoea 1.2, 1.3, 1.7, 1.8, 1.10–13, 1.16, 1.19, 2.5, 2.7, 2.10, 2.11–13, 2.17, 2.19, 2.21, 2.22, 2.25, 2.30–34, 2.36, 2.38, 2.40, 2.42, 2.44–46, 2.49, 3.10, 5.17, 6.23
chronic 2.42
in a chronically ill patient 2.48
on exertion 1.6, 1.17
gradual onset 2.7, 2.8
in immunocompromised patient 2.41
increasing 2.50
long-standing 2.23, 2.37
severe 2.4
sudden onset 1.9, 2.5, 2.9, 2.28, 2.39
trauma-related 2.46
dysuria 4.18

Ebstein's anomaly 1.16
Echinococcus granulosus 2.13, 7.18
Ehler–Danlos syndrome 1.1, 1.5, 1.18, 3.17, 6.1, 6.27
Eisenmenger syndrome 1.19
elbow joint 7.17
emphysema, panacinar 2.4
emphysematous cholecystitis 3.16
empyema 2.1, 2.34
endoscopic retrograde cholangiopancreatography (ERCP) 3.35
eosinophilic granuloma 5.16
epilepsy 6.30
Epstein–Barr virus 6.9
Erlenmeyer flask deformity 7.12
Escherichia coli
emphysematous cholecystitis 3.16
liver abscess 3.11
pneumonia 2.5
pyelonephritis 4.17
eyes
grittiness 5.7
red 2.17

facial swelling 1.4
failure to thrive 1.7, 5.15, 7.12, 7.22
falciform ligament sign 3.20
falls 3.42
familial adenomatous polyposis (FAP) 3.29, 3.40
fatigue 1.12, 1.13, 2.45, 3.28, 3.37, 5.10, 5.17, 7.25
fatty liver (steatosis) 3.13
feet, arthralgias pain/swelling, ROM 7.16
fever 1.18, 2.1, 2.2, 2.5, 2.9, 2.10, 2.13, 2.14–16, 2.18, 2.20, 2.32–34, 2.40, 2.44, 2.45, 3.11,

3.16, 3.24, 3.35, 3.40, 4.4, 4.7, 4.8, 4.17, 6.8, 6.11, 7.10
fibrosis, massive 2.22
fibrous dysplasia 7.20
figure of 3 sign 1.6
fine-needle aspiration (FNA) biopsy 5.1
fingers
clubbing 5.7
Dawson's 6.7
deformities/swelling 7.9
see also digits
flank pain 4.4, 4.7, 4.16
Fleishner's sign 3.31
flushing 2.19, 3.42
foot
diabetic 7.2
pain/swelling/stiffness 7.5–7
football sign 3.20
foreign body 2.20, 3.23
fractures, traumatic 2.27
Fraumeni syndrome 6.22
fullness 3.5, 3.25
fungal infection
cerebral abscesses 6.11
lungs 2.3, 2.47
oesophagitis 3.22

gait disturbance 6.26
gallstones 3.3
Garland's triad 2.17
gastric cancer 3.2
gastric ulcer 3.25
gastro-oesophageal reflux disease 3.19
gastrointestinal bleeding 3.37
Gaucher's disease 7.12
glioblastoma multiforme 6.22
gloved finger sign 2.16
goitre, retrosternal 5.4
Golden S sign 2.6
Goodpasture syndrome 2.28
Gottron's papules 7.19
gout 7.6
graft-versus-host disease (GVHD), acute 3.43
Gram-negative organisms

empyema 2.34
lung abscess 2.1
pneumonia 2.5
Graves' disease 5.7
great toe, tenderness 7.6
groin, swellings 5.18
growth retardation 5.5,
7.23
guinea-worm infection
7.18
gynaecomastia 3.12

haemangioblastoma 6.26
haematemesis 3.2, 3.4
haematoma
extradural 6.17
intraparenchymal 6.12
MRI appearance 6.12
subdural, chronic 6.6
haematopoietic stem cell
transplantation 2.47
haematuria 4.10, 4.14,
4.18
haemochromatosis 5.14
haemophilia 5.12
Haemophilus influenzae 2.1,
2.5
haemoptysis 1.11, 2.2, 2.3,
2.6, 2.10, 2.23, 2.28,
2.31, 2.41, 2.46
haemorrhage
adrenal 5.9
intraventricular 6.20
pulmonary 2.28
subarachnoid 6.1
haemorrhagic stroke 1.14
hand, swelling 5.7
hand pain, intermittent
5.7
hands, pain/swelling/stiff-
ness 7.5, 7.16
head and neck, swelling
2.12
headache 1.4, 1.6, 5.2, 5.3,
5.5, 5.15, 6.6, 6.9, 6.12,
6.14, 6.16, 6.17, 6.19,
6.22, 6.23, 6.25, 6.26
severe 6.1, 6.8, 6.11, 6.27
sudden onset 6.1, 6.3,
6.15
heart
apex displaced 1.17
enlarged 1.8, 1.10, 1.11,

1.16, 1.17, 1.19
located on right side
2.15
heart disease
congenital 1.7, 1.16, 1.17
ischaemic 1.2
heart sounds 1.8, 1.11, 1.13,
1.19, 2.44
heartburn 3.5, 3.8, 3.19
Helicobacter pylori 3.5
hemianopia, bitemporal
5.3, 5.5
hemiparesis
left 6.11
right 6.8, 6.9, 6.22
hepatitis B 3.34
hepatocellular carcinoma
(HCC) 3.34
hepatomegaly 3.13
hiatus hernia 3.8
hip, pain 5.12, 7.21, 7.25
HIV/AIDS 2.41, 6.9, 6.14
hoarseness 2.11, 2.12
hollow viscus, perforation
3.20
Homan's sign 1.20
horseshoe kidney 4.11
HRCT imaging technique
2.18
hydatid cysts 2.13, 7.18
hydrocephalus 6.1, 6.20
hydromyelia 6.18
hydropneumothorax 2.39
hydroureteronephrosis
4.15
hyperparathyroidism 5.6
hypertension 1.1, 1.15, 4.1
medically controlled 1.5
uncontrollable 4.13
unresponsive to medica-
tion 5.2
hypertrophic pulmonary
osteoarthropathy 7.3
hyperuricaemia 7.6
hypogastric area, tender-
ness 4.18
hyponatraemia, overcor-
rection 6.24
hypotension 3.30
hypoxia, sudden onset
2.27

iatrogenic injury 3.23

idiopathic pulmonary
fibrosis 2.7
ileus, adynamic/paralytic
3.7
immotile cilia syndrome
2.15
immunocompromised
patients 2.14, 3.22, 6.11
infections, recurrent 5.15
infectious disease, long-
standing 2.14
infective endocarditis 1.6,
1.11
inferior vena cava (IVC),
filter/stent 1.9, 1.14,
1.20
inflammatory bowel dis-
ease 3.35, 3.40
intercondylar notch, wid-
ening 5.12
intercostal recession 2.45
interstitial pneumonia 2.7
intracanalicular neuroma
6.21
intracranial pressure, high
6.10
intravenous urogram
(IVU) 4.1, 4.2, 4.5
delayed film 4.15
intussusception 3.39
inverted V sign 3.20
iron, excess deposition
5.14
irritability 7.22
itching 3.43

jaundice 3.4, 3.9, 3.10,
3.12, 3.33, 3.34, 3.35,
5.14
jejunal diverticulosis 3.17
joint contractures 2.25
joint disease, chronic
2.24
joint movements, limita-
tion 7.21
joint pain 2.10
juvenile rheumatoid
arthritis 7.17

Kaposi's sarcoma 2.41
Kartagener syndrome
2.15
Kawasaki's disease 1.18

Kerley lines 1.10, 2.41
kidney
  abnormalities 4.11, 4.12
  stones 4.6
Klebsiella spp.
  emphysematous chole-
  cystitis 3.16
  lung abscess 2.1
  pneumonia 2.5
  pyelonephritis 4.17
knee
  calcification 7.1
  haemophilic arthropa-
  thy 5.12
  pain/tenderness 5.12,
  7.1, 7.8, 7.17
knock-knees 7.22
Kussmaul's sign 1.13
Kveim–Slitbach test 2.17

lacunar infarct 6.29
LAD artery, enlargement
  1.18
leather bottle stomach
  3.2
left ventricle (LV) aneu-
  rysm 1.12
leg veins, filling defects
  1.20
Legionella pneumonia 2.5
legs
  bowed 7.22
  pain/swelling 1.14, 1.20,
  5.7
    worse at night
  7.11
leptomeningeal enhance-
  ment 6.23
leukaemia 2.47
ligamentum teres sign
  3.20
limbs, weakness 6.2, 6.5,
  6.7, 6.8
linitis plastica 3.2
liver
  abscess 3.11
  cirrhosis *see* cirrhosis
  enlarged 3.9, 5.14
  hard and nodular 3.4
  tumours 3.34
liver function test, abnormal 3.34
loin pain 4.6, 4.14, 4.15

loin-to-groin pain 4.6
Looser's zones 7.25
Lufsichel's sign 2.6
lumbar region
  mass 4.4, 4.9
  tenderness 4.7
lumps 1.18
lung
  abscess 2.1
  benign tumour 2.36
  cancer 2.6, 2.20, 2.36,
  2.38, 7.3
  carcinoid tumour 2.19
  collapse 2.6, 2.20
  consolidation 2.5
  contusion 2.46
  crackles 1.10, 1.11
  fungal infection 2.3,
  2.47
  honeycomb 2.18, 2.24,
  2.25
  hydatid cyst 2.13
  hyperinflated 2.4
  opacification 2.9
  rheumatoid 2.24
  scleroderma 2.25
  solitary nodule 2.36
  see also pulmonary
lung function tests 2.7,
  2.25, 2.31, 2.37
lymph nodes
  enlarged 1.18
  palpable 2.12
lymphangioleiomyomato-
  sis 2.31
lymphangitis carcinoma-
  tosis 2.50
lymphoma 2.12, 5.18, 6.9

McCune–Albright syn-
  drome 7.20
Macleod syndrome 2.49
malabsorption 3.36, 3.44
malaise 1.15, 2.29, 4.10,
  7.18, 7.25
malignant tumours 1.4,
  2.8
manual work 2.21, 2.22
Marfan syndrome 1.1, 1.5,
  1.18, 6.1, 6.27
mechanical ventilatory
  assistance 2.27
Meckel's diverticulum

3.38
medullary sponge kidney
  4.8
memory loss 6.6
meningioma 6.25
mesothelioma, malignant
  2.21
meta-iodobenzylguanine
  (MIBG) scan 5.2
metacarpal/metatarsal
  bones, short 5.8
metastases
  bony 7.21
  cerebral 6.10
micturition *see* urination
mitral stenosis 1.11
Monad's sign 2.3
Morgagni hernia 2.26
MR angiography (MRA)
  1.6, 4.12, 4.13
MRI
  contrast-enhanced 6.26
  high-resolution 6.30
  T2-weighted 6.4, 6.7
multiple endocrine neo-
  plasia type 1 (MEN-1)
  syndrome 3.42
multiple myeloma 5.13
multiple sclerosis (MS)
  6.7
muscle weakness 2.11,
  6.18, 7.19
myasthenia gravis 2.11
Mycobacterium bovis 3.31
Mycobacterium tuberculosis
  2.2, 3.31, 4.16, 7.10
mycotic infection 1.5, 1.18
myelinolysis, central pontine 6.24
myelofibrosis 5.17
myocardial infarct (MI),
  recent 1.12

nausea 3.3, 3.13, 3.20,
  3.43
nausea and vomiting 4.17,
  6.11
neck
  pain 5.4, 6.5
  stiffness 6.8
  swelling 5.1, 5.7
necrobiotic nodules 2.24
neoplasm *see* malignant

tumour
nephrocalcinosis 4.8
neurocysticercosis 6.15
neurofibroma, spinal 2.43
neurofibromatosis 6.21,
6.22, 6.27
neuropathic joint 7.13
neurosarcoidosis 6.23
neutropenia 2.47
night sweats 2.2, 2.5, 2.9,
7.10
see also sweating
northern exposure sign
3.18
nystagmus 6.2, 6.26

odynophagia 3.22
oedema
face and neck 1.4, 2.12
generalised 1.10, 1.13
legs 1.14, 1.20
oesophageal cancer 3.15
oesophageal perforation
3.23
oesophageal varices 3.4
oesophageal web 3.14
oesophagitis 3.22
Ortner syndrome 1.11
osteoarthritis 7.9
osteogenesis imperfecta
tarda 7.23
osteoid osteoma 7.11
osteomalacia 7.25
osteomyelitis, acute 7.7
osteopenia, diffuse 7.5
osteoporosis 7.14
ostium primum/secun-
dum 1.19

Paget's disease 7.15
pain sensation, loss 6.18
palpitations 1.11, 1.16, 1.17,
5.2
Pancoast's tumour 2.38
pancreatitis 3.1, 3.41
parasitic infections 6.14,
6.15, 7.18
parathyroid adenoma 5.6
parathyroid hormone
(PTH) 5.8
patent ductus arteriosus
(PDA) 1.7
Paterson–Kelly syndrome

3.14
percussion
dullness 2.2, 2.9, 2.21,
2.34
hyperresonance 2.39
peribronchial cuffing 1.10
pericardectomy 1.13
pericardial effusion 1.8
pericardial knock 1.13
pericardiocentesis 1.8
pericarditis, constrictive
1.13
periosteal reaction 5.7,
7.3
pertechnate scan 3.38
phaeochromocytoma 5.2
pharyngeal pouch 3.6
photophobia 6.27
picture framing 7.14, 7.15
pituitary adenoma 5.3
plantar response, brisk
6.28
pleural effusion 1.10, 2.9
pleural plaque 2.23
Plummer–Vinson syn-
drome 3.14, 3.15
pneumatosis coli, ischae-
mic 3.30
pneumoconiosis, coal-
workers' 2.22, 2.42
Pneumocystis jiroveci pneumonia 2.14
pneumomediastinum
2.35
pneumonia 2.5, 2.7, 2.14,
2.29, 2.30
in bone marrow trans-
plant recipients 2.47
pneumoperitoneum 3.19,
3.20
pneumothorax 2.4, 2.24,
2.39
polyarteritis nodosa (PAN)
1.18, 4.10
polyarthritis of ankylosing
spondylitis type 7.17
polychondritis, relaps-
ing 1.1
polycystic kidney disease
1.18, 4.4, 6.1, 6.27
postoperative patient
2.30
pregnancy 1.1

proptosis 5.7
prosthetic valve 1.1
pseudocysts, pancreatic
3.41
pseudohypoparathy-
roidism 5.8
Pseudomonas spp.
pneumonia 2.5
pyelonephritis 4.17
pseudoxanthoma elasti-
cum 6.27
psoriatic arthropathy
7.16
puberty, precocious 7.20
pulmonary embolism (PE)
1.9
pulmonary function tests
see lung function tests
pulmonary haemorrhage
2.28
pulmonary hamartoma
2.36
pulmonary hypoplasia
2.44
pulmonary metastases
2.32
pulmonary plethora 1.19
pulmonary venous drain-
age, anomalous 2.44
pulses, abnormal 1.15
pulsus paradoxus 1.13
pyelonephritis 4.17
pyomyositis 7.19
pyuria 4.16

quadriparesis 6.24

radiation pneumonitis
2.8
rectal bleeding 3.28,
3.29, 3.37, 3.38, 3.39
reflexes, exaggerated 6.2,
6.4, 6.5, 6.7, 6.28, 6.29
reflux 3.19
regurgitation 3.19
renal angiography 4.10
renal angiomyolipoma
4.14
renal angle
mass 4.15
tenderness 4.8, 4.16,
4.17
renal arterial stenosis 4.13

renal calculus 4.6
renal cell carcinoma 4.9
renal disease 2.28
renal ectopia 4.12
renal fossa, tenderness 4.14
renal infections, recurrent 4.12
renal osteodystrophy 5.10
renal papillary necrosis 4.7
respiratory distress see breathing difficulty
respiratory infections frequent 1.16 recurrent 2.49
restriction of movement 5.10, 5.12, 5.16
retroperitoneal fibrosis 4.1
rheumatic fever 1.11
rheumatoid arthritis 2.24, 7.5
rhonchi 2.4, 2.31, 2.35, 2.49
rib fractures 2.46
rib notching 1.6
Rich focus 6.19
rickets 7.22
right bundle-branch block (RBBB) 1.16
right heart failure 1.13 strain 1.9
Rigler's sign 3.20
road traffic accident see trauma
rugger jersey spine 5.10

sarcoidosis 2.17, 6.23
schwannoma 6.21
scimitar syndrome 2.44
scintigraphy, thyroid 5.1
scleroderma 2.25, 3.44, 7.9
sclerosing cholangitis 3.35
sclerosis, mesial temporal 6.30
seizures 6.3, 6.11, 6.14, 6.22, 6.23, 6.25 focal 6.19

intractable 6.60
recurrent 6.13
sudden onset 6.15
serum creatinine level, increased 4.15
sheep farming 2.13
shipbuilding 2.23
shoulder joint 7.13, 7.25
sickle cell anaemia 5.11
sigmoid diverticulosis 3.32
sigmoid volvulus 3.18
silicosis 2.42
sinus tenderness 2.10
sinus venosus 1.19
skeletal survey 7.23
skin excessive pigmentation 7.20 nodules 2.43 rash 3.43, 7.19 symptoms 7.16 vascular naevi 3.12
skull abnormalities 7.22 hair-on-end appearance 5.15 punched-out lesions 5.13
small bowel ascariasis 3.26 Crohn's disease 3.24 obstruction 3.7 TB 3.31
speech disturbance 6.10
spinal cord acute inflammation 6.4 compression 2.43 tumours 6.3, 6.5
spinal fractures, wedge compression 7.14
spinal pain/tenderness 2.43, 5.10, 5.13, 7.4, 7.15, 7.21, 7.24
spleen enlarged 3.9, 5.17, 5.18 infarcts 5.11
sprue 3.36
sputum, purulent 2.16
ST-segment elevation 1.12
staphylococci cerebral abscesses 6.11 pneumonia 2.5

Staphylococcus aureus discitis 7.4 empyema 2.34 liver abscess 3.11 lung abscess 2.1 osteomyelitis 7.8 pneumonia 2.5
steatorrhoea 3.36
Steirlin's sign 3.31
Still's disease 7.17
stomach, intrathoracic 3.8
stools, loose/bloody 3.24
streptococci aerobic liver abscess 3.11 cerebral abscesses 6.11 lung abscess 2.1 pneumonia 2.5
stroke 6.28
Sturge–Weber syndrome 6.13, 6.16
superior mesenteric artery, angiography 3.37
superior sagittal sinus, thrombosis 6.8
superior vena cava (SVC) syndrome 1.4
suprasellar mass 5.5
swallowing difficulty 5.1
sweating 1.3, 5.4, 5.7 see also night sweats
Swyer–James syndrome 2.37, 2.49
syncope episodes 6.2 frequent 1.17
syphilis 1.5, 1.18, 3.2, 3.26, 6.5, 7.13
syringohydromyelia 6.2
syringomyelia 6.18
systemic lupus erythematosus (SLE) 1.1
systolic murmur 1.1, 1.6, 1.17, 1.18

tachycardia 1.15, 2.39, 3.1
tachypnoea 2.10, 2.22, 2.26, 2.37, 2.40, 2.44
tapeworm (Taenia solium) 6.15
TB

miliary 2.45
pulmonary 2.2
renal 4.16
small bowel 3.31
spinal 7.10
see also tuber-
⁹⁹ᵐTc-labelled bisphosphonate bone scan 7.8
⁹⁹ᵐTc-labelled dimercap-
tosuccinic acid (DMSA)
scan 4.3
⁹⁹ᵐTc-labelled red blood
cell (RBC) scan 3.37
⁹⁹ᵐTc-Sestamibi 5.6
technetium–thallium sub-
traction imaging 5.6
Tell's triangle sign 3.20
temperature sensation,
loss 6.18
tetany 5.8
tetralogy of Fallot 1.7
thalassaemia 5.15
thallium stress test 1.2
thrill, palpable 1.11
thymoma 2.11
thyroid acropachy 5.7
thyroid gland, enlarge-
ment 5.4
thyroid nodule 5.1
tinnitus 6.21
toxoplasmosis, cerebral
6.14
transverse myelitis 6.4
trauma 1.1, 1.5, 1.18, 6.12,
6.17
road traffic accident
2.27, 2.46, 6.12, 6.20
unremembered 6.6
tuberz-, *see also* TB
tuberculoma 6.19
tuberculous autonephrec-
tomy 4.16
tuberculous spondylitis
7.10
tuberous sclerosis 2.31,
6.3

Turcot syndrome 6.22
Turner syndrome 1.1

ulcerative colitis 3.40
ulcers
duodenal 3.5
gastric 3.25
in Zollinger–Ellison syn-
drome 3.42
Urachus sign 3.20
ureter, congential abnor-
malities 4.5
ureteric colic 4.6
urinary tract infections,
recurrent 4.3, 4.5, 4.11
urination
frequency 4.18
painful/difficult 4.2,
4.8, 4.15, 4.17
urine collecting system,
obstruction 4.15

valve replacement 1.11
varicella pneumonia 2.29
venogram 1.20
venous pulsations, promi-
nent 1.13
venous thrombosis
cerebral 6.8
deep (DVT) 1.20
portal 3.9
ventilation–perfusion
scan (V/Q) scan 1.9
vertebra plana 5.16
vertebrae
empty box 7.14
H-shaped 5.11
L3 point tenderness
5.16
vertebral bodies, dense
5.17
vesicoureteric reflux 4.3
videofluoroscopic barium
swallow 3.19
viral infections 6.4
visual disturbances 5.3,

5.5, 6.7
voiding cystourethrogram
(VCUG) 4.3
vomiting 3.3, 3.6, 3.7, 3.8,
3.18, 3.20, 3.25, 3.42,
3.43, 6.8, 6.12, 7.12
Von Hippel–Lindau syn-
drome 6.26

weakness
bilateral 6.4, 6.23
left-sided 6.6, 6.10, 6.12
limbs 6.2, 6.5, 6.7, 6.8
right-sided 6.16, 6.29
sudden onset 6.4, 6.28
Wegner's granulomatosis
2.10
Weigert–Meyer rule 4.5
weight gain 5.3
weight loss 1.15, 2.2, 2.13,
2.14, 3.2, 3.14, 3.15, 3.17,
3.24, 3.26, 3.31, 3.33,
3.40, 3.41, 5.4, 5.17, 5.18,
7.10
Wells' clinical prediction
guide 1.20
wheezing 2.4, 2.37
whirl sign 3.18
white blood cell (WBC)
count, raised 2.1, 7.7
Wolff–Parkinson–White
syndrome 1.16
Wolman's disease 5.9
worm calcification 7.18
wrist joint 7.3
Wunderlich syndrome
4.14
Wyburn–Mason syndrome
6.16

Zencker's diverticulum
3.6
Zollinger–Ellison syn-
drome 3.5, 3.42